Janneke van Kalkeren

CW01649034

Techniques in the Behavioral and Neural Sciences

Volume 4

Series Editor

JOSEPH P. HUSTON

Düsseldorf

ELSEVIER

AMSTERDAM · NEW YORK · OXFORD

Manual of Microsurgery on the Laboratory Rat

PART I

General Information and Experimental Techniques

Editors

J.J. VAN DONGEN, R. REMIE, J.W. RENSEMA and G.H.J. VAN WUNNIK

Maastricht and Weesp, The Netherlands

ELSEVIER

AMSTERDAM · NEW YORK · OXFORD

© 1990 Elsevier Science Publishers B.V. (Biomedical Division)

All rights reserved. No part of this publication may be reproduced, stored in a retrieval system or transmitted in any form or by any means, electronic, mechanical, photocopying, recording or otherwise without the prior written permission of the Publisher, Elsevier Science Publishers B.V. (Biomedical Division), P.O. Box 1527, 1000 BM Amsterdam, The Netherlands.

No responsibility is assumed by the Publisher for any injury and/or damage to persons or property as a matter of products liability, negligence or otherwise, or from any use or operation of any methods, products, instructions or ideas contained in the material herein. Because of the rapid advances in the medical sciences, the Publisher recommends that independent verification of diagnoses and drug dosages should be made.

Special regulations for readers in the U.S.A.:
This publication has been registered with the Copyright Clearance Center Inc. (CCC), Salem, Massachusetts. Information can be obtained from the CCC about conditions under which the photocopying of parts of this publication may be made in the U.S.A. All other copyright questions, including photocopying outside the U.S.A., should be referred to the publisher.

ISBN Volume:0-444-81138-9 (Hardback)
0-444-81139-7 (Paperback)
ISSN Series: 0921-0709

1st edition 1990
2nd printing 1991

Published by:
Elsevier Science Publishers B.V.
(Biomedical Division)
P.O. Box 211
1000 AE Amsterdam
The Netherlands

Sole distributors for the U.S.A. and Canada:
Elsevier Science Publishing Co., Inc.
655 Avenue of the Americas,
New York, NY 10010
U.S.A.

This book is printed on acid-free paper.

Library of Congress Cataloging in Publication Data

Manual of microsurgery on the laboratory rat / editors, J.J. van Dongen ... [et al.].
p. cm. -- (Techniques in the behavioral and neural sciences ; v. 4-)
Includes bibliographical references and index.
Contents: Pt. 1. General information and experimental techniques.
ISBN 0-444-81138-9
1. Experimental microsurgery. 2. Rats--Surgery. I. Dongen, J. J. van (Johan J.) 11. Series.
RD33.6.M265 1990
617′.05--dc20 90-14041
CIP

PRINTED IN THE NETHERLANDS

Foreword

The use of animals for research purposes can be justified only under a set of strict conditions. Amongst these is the condition that persons who are involved in animal experiments are competent. During the last decade animal experimentation has come more and more under the control of legislative regulations.

The 1986 EC Council Directive regarding the protection of animals used for experiments and other scientific purposes, states that experiments shall be performed solely by competent authorized persons (art. 7).

In the USA, requirements for training are regulated in the Animal Welfare Act (1986). Research institutions must provide training on humane care and use of animals, and on methods to minimize pain and limit the numbers of animals. In several countries courses are being organized in order to meet these demands. Most of these courses are at a basic level and do not deal with surgical techniques. This is understandable since only a limited number of persons are involved in research projects which include surgical procedures. For this latter group there is, however, evident need for more advanced training.

This book can be seen as an important teaching tool for this group of persons. The comprehensive text and clear illustrations with many essential details were prepared in order to support practical training.

Pain and discomfort are not always avoidable in experiments that involve surgical procedures. Although the book does not deal with the moral aspects of animal experimentation, an ethical judgement prior to the performance of the experiments is considered by the authors as a matter of extreme importance. Also, it is seen as a *conditio sine qua non* that persons involved in experiments are adequately trained. I know that

I am in line with the objectives of the authors when I say that this book aims to improve competency in order to contribute to a more responsible use of animals in research.

L.F.M. van Zutphen, Ph.D.
Professor and Head of the Department of
Laboratory Animal Science
Veterinary Faculty, University of Utrecht
The Netherlands

Preface

Microsurgery is defined as: "intricate surgery performed on tissues, etc., using a specially designed operating microscope and miniature precision instruments". By definition, it therefore is an auxiliary technique, applicable in various biomedical disciplines. It started its development in ENT- surgery but it was followed by a vast array of other disciplines, which developed and used microsurgical techniques in their specific fields of interest. Numerous techniques and their applications have been described eversince; however, these publications could seldom be used as educational tools to master a certain technique.

Whilst giving courses on microsurgical techniques on the laboratory rat, it became apparent that an up-to-date didactically justified manual was needed, for the training of workers in the biomedical sciences.

To meet with the afore mentioned objectives we have chosen a special set–up, which shows the reader step by step, using accurate drawings and descriptive text, how to perform the operations. To complete the manual, and make the techniques even more accessible, video tapes have been made.

Section I of this manual contains general information about the rat, its anatomy, anaesthesia and the operation microscope. For easy reference, a number of steps which are frequently used in the operations, are described in the section about general techniques.

Section II describes experimental techniques, related to freely moving animals, which offer far more realistic and refined models (absence of anaesthetic side effects, stress, etc.). This also has the effect of reducing the number of experimental animals needed. Besides refinement and reduction of animal experiments, replacement is, whenever possible, amongst our main objectives. We therefore hope, that this manual will be of use to students, animal technicians, and researchers in the fields of behavioural science, neuroscience, pharmacology, toxicology and physiology who all need to study and use animal experiments.

We realize that the techniques described in this manual are not the ultimate, and we would appreciate any commentary, which would lead to improvement. We do not want to pass over in silence the fact that the production of the manual together with the video tapes, would not have been possible without the moral support of our wives and children. We therefore thank: Ada van Dongen, Ilse and Robert, Liesbeth Remie and Theo, Edith Rensema, Serge, Martijn, Petra and Judith, Vivianne van Wunnik, Ivo and Bart.

Johan van Dongen
René Remie
Hans Rensema
Ger van Wunnik

Address for correspondence:
Microsurgical Developments (MD)
P.O. Box 2045
6201 CC Maastricht
The Netherlands

Acknowledgements

During the realization of this manual, we have not only enjoyed substantial help but also a lot of moral support. We experienced that both expert opinions as well as friendship from many people are of vital importance. Therefore it is with great pleasure that we take this opportunity to thank all those who have contributed in some way to the realization and completion of this manual.

We would like to express our gratitude to:

Mrs. M. Eversden for her linguistic advice. Mr. H.L. Bartels for his microsurgical expertise, his enthusiasm and his cooperation. Prof. Dr. C. Greep for his support in the initial phase. Mr. K. Crul for the discussions and management advice. Mr. H. van Dijk, photographer, for some excellent pictures.

Our advisory board, in alphabetical order:

Prof. Dr. P.J.C. van Breda-Vriesman, for his ideas and expertise in the field of experimental microsurgery.

Prof. Dr. J. Drukker, for his support during the final phase in the completion of the manuscript.

Dr. W. J. Pereboom, for his advice, his continuous support, and the fruitful discussions about our mutual philosophy concerning animal experiments.

Prof. Dr. P.H. Robinson, for his enthusiasm and his interest in experimental microsurgery.

Prof. Dr. J. Zaagsma, for his interest in the in vivo experimental pharmacology and his support to this project from the beginning.

Prof. Dr. L.F.M. van Zutphen, for his support, his enthusiasm and the discussions about laboratory animal science, which convinced us of the fact that the manual could actually help in an adequate training of people who are going to perform animal experiments.

The support of Duphar B.V., Weesp, the Netherlands and Zeiss Nederland B.V., Weesp, the Netherlands is gratefully acknowledged.

Introduction

During the past decades, research in life sciences has been growing exponentially. The experimental animal most frequently used in this area, particularly in the physiological and pharmacological and related disciplines, undoubtedly is the rat. Although a great number of general and specialized textbooks, monographs, symposium proceedings and journals dealing with the results from animal experiments are available, information on basic as well as specialized techniques used in this research is far less accessible.

This book, being the first Part of the Manual of Microsurgery on the Laboratory Rat, clearly fills a gap. It is comprised of two sections, dealing with general aspects and with more specialized experimental techniques, respectively. Section I, consisting of seven chapters, describes in a concise way numerous details of basic principles and techniques, most relevant not only for the microsurgeon but also for all workers preparing and using rats for in vivo experiments. In section II permanent cannulation of four major blood vessels, the thoracic duct and the bile duct (double fistula), portacaval shunting, perfusion of the isolated gut in situ as well as intra-uterine operations are discussed. All procedures are described step-by-step and in great detail including the instruments and materials; most importantly, they are clarified by magnificent illustrations of an astonishing realistic quality which show all relevant details.

The application of such 'permanent' techniques enables the study of numerous physiological and pharmacological questions in the unanaesthetized freely moving rat under stress-free conditions. For several reasons this is a major advantage. Firstly, the interfering effects of anaesthetics on the homeostasis of organ functions regulated by endogenous neuronal and humoral factors, and on the effects of exogenously applied drugs, can be avoided. Secondly, several techniques, alone or in combination, allow the investigation of local processes under optimal physiological conditions. An example of which is the study of the local regulation of the evoked noradrenaline overflow from the portal vein sympathetic varicosities by different presynaptic receptors by Remie et al. (quoted in Chapter 11). Thirdly, because the animals can be kept alive for a prolonged period of time, the adaptive effects of experimental interventions of all kinds, including pathophysiological conditions and the chronic effects of drugs, can be studied. Finally, and most importantly, such techniques reduce the number of animals considerably, because the same animal can be used repeatedly, thus contributing to animal welfare.

I hope and expect that this book will be recognized by researchers of different disciplines to be a most useful and instructive manual for preparing and performing animal experiments.

J. Zaagsma, Ph.D.
Professor and Chairman of the
Department of Pharmacology and
Therapeutics
University of Groningen
The Netherlands

List of contributors

A.P.M.G. Bertens, Veterinary anaesthesiologist
Department of Laboratory Animal Science
University of Utrecht
Utrecht, the Netherlands

J.J. van Dongen, Experimental microsurgeon
University of Limburg
Maastricht, the Netherlands

M. Eversden, Linguistic adviser
Microsurgical Developments (MD)
Maastricht, the Netherlands

F.A. de Haas
Zeiss Nederland B.V.
Weesp, the Netherlands

R. Remie, Pharmacologist, Experimental microsurgeon
Department of Pharmacology
Duphar B.V. Weesp, the Netherlands

J.W. Rensema, Medical artist
Department of Anatomy and Embryology
University of Limburg
Maastricht, the Netherlands

J.C. van der Wal, Anatomist
Department of Anatomy and Embryology
University of Limburg
Maastricht, the Netherlands

G.H.J. van Wunnik, Video director
Department of Medical Sociology
Laboratory of Behavioural Sciences
University of Limburg
Maastricht, the Netherlands

Contents

I. GENERAL INFORMATION

Manual of Microsurgery on the Laboratory Rat, Part I
Van Dongen, Remie, Rensema and Van Wunnik (eds)
© 1990 Elsevier Science Publishers B.V. (Biomedical Division)

CHAPTER 1

The rat as an experimental animal

Including the 1985 NIH Principles for the utilization and care of vertebrate animals used in testing, research, and training

R. REMIE, J.J. VAN DONGEN, J.W. RENSEMA and G.H.J. VAN WUNNIK

1.1. Introduction

Of all laboratory animals the rat (*Rattus norvegicus*) is one of the most commonly used in biological and medical research and is probably the most investigated animal on earth. Numerous models of diseases in man have been developed in the rat. Rats are an obvious choice as they are strong, inexpensive, easy to handle, they require minimal space and are low on maintenance costs. Furthermore, if selected carefully, they have narrow genetic variations and thus demonstrate little biological variation in response to stimuli. The early history of the rat is rather unclear. The spread of the animal (*Rattus rattus* and *Rattus norvegicus*) probably began with the opening of trade routes with countries in the Far East. Southeast Asia is thought to be the main centre of origin of these rodents. The *R. rattus* has been more successful in warmer regions, while the *R. norvegicus* clearly liked a colder climate.

Table I shows the taxonomic classification of the laboratory rat (adapted from Robinson 1979).

The introduction of the rat into the laboratory probably started at the end of the 19th century. At that time breeding colonies were established. Nowadays a great number of strains are available, and within one strain the animals are almost identical and well defined. The exact ancestry of most stocks of the laboratory rat is unknown. Many of the modern strains of rats, however, take their origin from the stocks of the Wistar Institute of Anatomy and Biology in Philadelphia, which made a major contribution to both breeding and husbandry of the laboratory rat. In 1906 the Wistar Institute started a random bred (heterogeneous) colony, which was com-

TABLE I

Class: Mammalia
Subclass: Theria
Infraclass: Eutheria
Order: Rodentia
Suborder: Myomorpha
Superfamily: Muroidea
Family: Muridae
Subfamily: Murinae
Genus: Rattus
Species: norvegicus

mercially available, and an inbred colony which was maintained by strict brother × sister matings resulting in the "King Albino" (PA). Nowadays over 130 strains are listed and at least 50 are known to have descended wholly or partially from the commercial Wistars. Other outbred strains contributing to this development are the Sprague-Dawley and the Long-Evans strain, both originating from the USA (Lindsey, 1979).

Particular aberrations of the normal genetic code have provided mutants which can be of special interest as models of disease, such as hypertension, anaemia, muscular dystrophy, obesity, jaundice, metabolic disorders as well as rats that are sensitive or resistant to tumours (see Robinson, 1979 and Festing, 1979, for an overview).

Besides all the above mentioned advantages, one of the disadvantages of the rat seems to be its small body size and the difficulty of operating. This, however, is not the case if one uses the appropriate instruments, adequate suture materials, and good surgical technique. If one possesses average manual dexterity, it is possible to carry out most of the operations described in this manual, which are usually carried out on much larger animals.

1.2. Principles

Principles for the utilization and care of vertebrate animals used in testing, research and training, cited from: Governmental activities relating to the use of animals in research (1985).*

The development of knowledge necessary for the improvement of the health and well-being of humans as well as other animals requires *in vivo* experimentation with a wide variety of animal species. Whenever U.S. Government agencies develop requirements for testing, research, or training procedures involving the use of vertebrate animals, the following principles shall be considered; and whenever these agencies

*For guidance throughout these Principles the reader is referred to the *Guide for the Care and Use of Laboratory Animals* prepared by the Institute of Laboratory Animal Resources, National Research Council.

actually perform or sponsor such procedures, the responsible institutional official shall ensure that these principles are adhered to:

I. The transportation, care and use of animals should be in accordance with the Animal Welfare Act (7 U.S.C. 2131 et seq.) and other applicable Federal laws, guidelines, and policies.

II. Procedures involving animals should be designed and performed with due consideration of their relevance to human or animal health, the advancement of knowledge, or the good of society.

III. The animals selected for a procedure should be of an appropriate species and quality and the minimum number required to obtain valid results. Methods such as mathematical models, computer simulation, and *in vitro* biological systems should be considered.

IV. Proper use of animals, including the avoidance or minimization of discomfort, distress, and pain when consistant with sound scientific practices, is imperative. Unless the contrary is established, investigators should consider that procedures that cause pain or distress in human beings may cause pain and distress in other animals.

V. Procedures with animals that may cause more than momentary or slight pain or distress should be performed with appropriate sedation, analgesia, or anesthesia. Surgical or other painful procedures should not be performed on unanesthetized animals paralyzed by chemical agents.

VI. Animals that would otherwise suffer severe or chronic pain or distress that cannot be relieved should be painlessly killed at the end of the procedure or, if appropriate, during the procedure.

VII. The living conditions of animals should be appropriate for their species and contribute to their health and comfort. Normally the housing, feeding, and care of all animals used for biomedical purposes must be directed by a veterinarian or other scientist trained and experienced in proper care, handling and use of the species being maintained or studied. In any case, veterinary care shall be provided as indicated.

VIII. Investigators and other personnel shall be appropriately qualified and experienced for conducting procedures on living animals. Adequate arrangements shall be made for their in-service training, including the proper and humane care and use of laboratory animals.

IX. Where exceptions are required in relation to the provisions of these Principles, the decisions should not rest with the investigators directly concerned but should be made, with due regard to Principle II, by an appropriate review group such as an institutional animal research committee. Such exceptions should not be made solely for the purpose of teaching or demonstration.

6

References

Festing, M.F.W. (1979) Inbred strains in biomedical research, Macmillan, London and Basingstoke.

Governmental activities relating the use of animals in research (1985) Laboratory animal welfare: U.S. government principles for the utilization and care of vertebrate animals used in testing, research and training. Ilar News, volume XXVIII, 4: 7–14.

Lindsey, J.R. (1979) In: The Laboratory Rat, vol. I, by Baker, Lindsey and Weisbroth, pp. 2–33. Academic Press, New York.

Robinson, R. (1979) In: The Laboratory Rat, vol. I, by Baker, Lindsey and Weisbroth, pp. 37–50. Academic Press, New York.

Manual of Microsurgery on the Laboratory Rat, Part I
Van Dongen, Remie, Rensema and Van Wunnik (eds)
© 1990 Elsevier Science Publishers B.V. (Biomedical Division)

CHAPTER 2

The use of different strains

R. REMIE, J.J. VAN DONGEN and J.W. RENSEMA

Inbred strains of laboratory rats have made a substantial contribution to biomedical research. Much of the progress made in immunology and transplantation research would not have been possible without the availability of inbred strains. A strain is regarded as inbred when it has been mated brother × sister for 20 or more consecutive generations. Festing (1979) discussed in detail the properties of these strains and formulated seven criteria, which are:

1. Long-term genetic stability. This is of extreme importance since background data on the characteristics of the strain can be used for a long period of time.
2. Isogenicity. The strain consists of genetically identical individuals.
3. Homozygosity.
4. International distribution. Enabling an international comparison of research results.
5. Identifiability. Many inbred strains can be identified by their immunological and biochemical characteristics.
6. Uniformity. Compared with outbred animals, inbred strains are more uniform.
7. Individuality. Because each inbred strain represents a unique genotype, this often leads to a phenotype which has special characteristics like high blood pressure, behaviour, response to infections, or spontaneous diseases. This makes them of great interest when elucidating the pathogenesis of these diseases.

A fine example of such an inbred strain is the spontaneously hypertensive rat (SHR), discovered by Kozo Okamoto. He and his co-workers succeeded in breeding a rat having a genetic disorder producing hypertension, by selective inbreeding of Wistar rats from the Animal Centre Laboratory, Kyoto University Faculty of Medicine (Wistar-Kyoto or WKY). In 1963 the strain had reached its sixth generation and in

October 1969 the twenty-first generation was obtained by continued brother × sister matings (Okamoto, 1972).

Though the inbred strains are well defined, most countries or even laboratories have their own sublines, which may have become genetically contaminated. It therefore goes without saying that one has to be careful in comparing rats originating from different sublines, and it is good practice always to state the exact source from whence the animals were obtained.

It is of utmost importance to control the quality of the animals at all stages of their production and maintenance, in order to minimize disease, to maximize genetic purity, and to standardize environmental and nutritional variables (see control of rat breeding). Uniformity in an inbred strain can easily be tested by means of a skin transplantation. In the case where the donor and recipient display some genetic difference, the transplant will rapidly be rejected.

Besides the inbred strains, random-bred strains are available. In these strains the mating is at random, and in large populations the amount of inbreeding will be low. It is, however, difficult to maintain a genetically stable outbred strain because of the lost genetic information by unavoidable inbreeding. This could eventually lead to small changes in the population causing different responses in animals to stimuli, compared with reactions of their ancestors. The main advantage of an outbred strain is that they breed prolifically and are therefore cheap. The major disadvantage is, however, that only a few outbred strains are available internationally, meaning that experiments carried out on those animals are localized.

Besides inbred and outbred strains, there are congenic lines of inbred strains which are often used in transplantation immunology. A congenic line can be developed in several ways (Festing, 1979). One of the simplest systems is the so-called "cross-intercross-backcross" method, resulting in animals which are almost identical to the inbred strain, with the exception of the gene one wanted to introduce (Figure 2.1.).

Control of rat breeding

After World War II the need for improving the standards and logistics of laboratory animals was realized, and the Institute of Laboratory Animal Resources (ILAR) was established in the year 1952. One of the Institute's first achievements was the publication of the "Handbook of Laboratory Animals", which presented the "state of the art" with regard to genetic standards, nutrition, diseases, and uses of laboratory animals. It also gave the names of about 25 commercial producers of rats, only a few of which are still in business today. Another step forward in the control of rat breeding started in the 1940s at the National Institute of Health (NIH) in Bethesda, Maryland. Nowadays the "NIH Rodent Repository" represents a collection of strains and stocks of rodents, and lagomorphs of known genetic characteristics, maintained to provide a defined source of breeders. The Repository supplies breeding stocks for scientific purposes to universities and commercial breeders both nationally and internationally. In the United Kingdom the Laboratory Animals Centre (LAC) was founded in 1947. Its primary aim was to improve the quality and the availability of laboratory animals in the United Kingdom. However, it also covers areas such as: information, supply of animals, training and research. The information is published in the LAC News, LAC Manuals and several News Letters one of which is the Rat News Letter.

Specified pathogen-free

Since latent diseases can influence a great number of functional parameters, animals used in research must of course be healthy and every investigator would unreservedly agree that the most stringent precautions should be taken to prevent diseases from being introduced into an animal colony. For this reason there has been an increased tendency to use animals of a known health status, the so-called "specified" or "specific pathogen-free" (SPF) rats. These are rats freed of certain specific pathogens by the use of "gnotobiotic" technology (from the Greek gnosis, knowledge and bios, life). The pathogens known to be absent must be indicated. Figure 2.2. schematically shows the standardization of the micro flora in rats.

Although the gnotobiology provides easy methods for eliminating pathogens from rodent stocks, it has proven virtually impossible to maintain them free of pathogens for extended periods of time. Many factors play a role in the development of latent infections or disease. Routine monitoring of the animals and their environment is essential, and a good husbandry practice is a prerequisite for optimal results (Baker, 1979).

References

Baker, D.E.J. (1979) Reproduction and breeding In: The Laboratory Rat, vol. I, by Baker, Lindsey and Weisbroth, pp. 154–166. Academic Press, New York.

Festing, M.F.W. (1979) Inbred strains in biomedical research. Macmillan, New York.

Okamoto, K., Yamori, Y., Ooshima, A., Park, C., Haebara, H., Matsumoto, M., Tanaka, T., Okuda, T., Hazama, F. and Kyogoku, M. (1972) Establishment of the inbred strain of the spontaneously hypertensive rat and genetic factors involved in hypertension. In: Spontaneous hypertension; its pathogenesis and complications. Ed. Kozo Okamoto, Igaku Shoin Ltd. Tokyo. Springer-Verlag, Berlin, Heidelberg, New York.

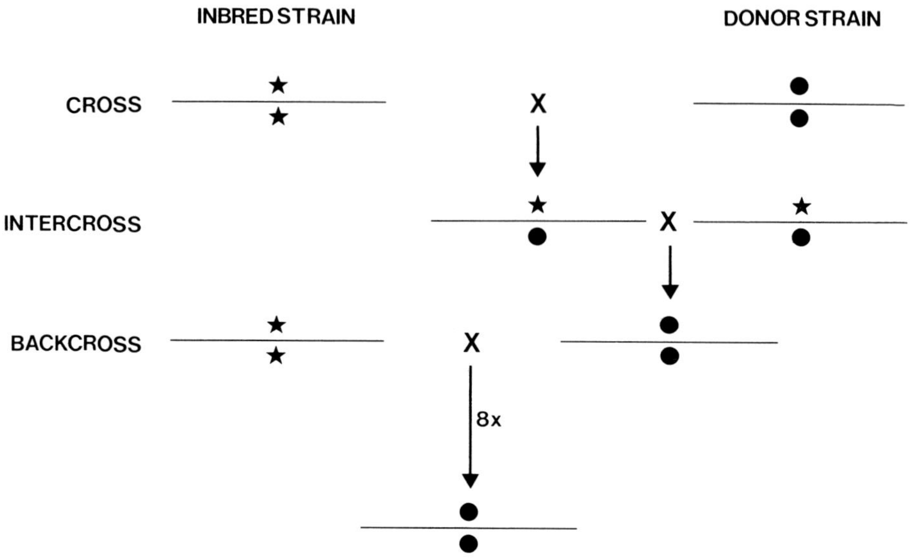

Figure 2.1. The congenic line.
The cross-intercross method for backcrossing a recessive gene on to an inbred strain. The result being a congenic line of the inbred strain.

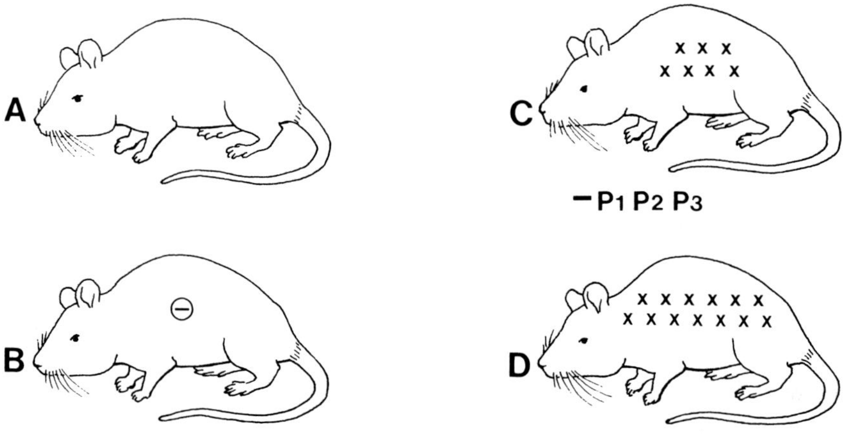

Figure 2.2. Standardization of the micro flora in the rat.
A. The gnotobiotic rat (germ-fee or axenic rat).
B. The gnotobiotic rat inoculated with one known microorganism.
C. The specified or specific pathogen-free rat, which is free from the pathogens P1, P2 and P3.
D. The conventional rat with an unknown microflora.

Manual of Microsurgery on the Laboratory Rat, Part I
Van Dongen, Remie, Rensema and Van Wunnik (eds)
© *1990 Elsevier Science Publishers B.V. (Biomedical Division)*

CHAPTER 3

General principles of microsurgery

R. REMIE, J.W. RENSEMA, G.H.J. VAN WUNNIK and
J.J. VAN DONGEN

3.1. The microsurgeon

Initially the study of microsurgical techniques makes many mental and physical demands. You have to develop an ability to concentrate on the visual image, as seen through the microscope, and become familiar with the magnified objects. You must also develop an awareness of the fact that even simple movements in a significantly smaller world are more complex than they are "life-size". Under the operating microscope not only are the objects enlarged, but at the same time your movements are magnified between 8 and 40 times. Also the physical ability required to coordinate ones movements, decreases in proportion to the magnification.

Individual preparation
Listed below are some suggestions to improve your performance.
– Try to avoid any mental stress. Make sure that you have no appointments, and that you cannot be disturbed by telephone calls etc. You need to be able to devote all your time to the exercise. It is unrealistic to expect to perform well when your attention is divided or you act hastily.
– Try to sleep well and avoid heavy physical exertion during the 24 hours preceding the surgical exercise, as this will interfere with your fine muscular control and will increase your tremor.
– Do not change any habits relating to your intake of coffee, as radical increase or decrease will increase your tremor.
– Do not despair or become discouraged when something has gone wrong. If you encounter a difficulty, evaluate it and try to do something about it before you continue.

– Do not work for too long at a stretch. If possible take a 10 minute break every hour, otherwise you will lose concentration and your coordination and learning ability will be reduced.

3.2. Anatomy

A thorough knowledge of the rat's anatomy is essential as it will reassure you whilst performing an operation. Do not start an operation until you are familiar with all the structures in the area of interest. Animals killed after being used in an experiment make ideal learning material. Use the operation microscope to look in detail at all kinds of tissue and learn how to handle the tissues with your instruments. For example, try dissecting some blood vessels to see how much tension they can withhold. As you will see, the majority of functions during microdissection are performed by slight pronation and supination movements of the fingers and forearm. Small spreading movements parallel to the blood vessel (or other structures), will prevent tearing of branches (Figure 3.2.1.). Even while dissecting dead animals try to use atraumatic techniques, i.e. do not grab the whole thickness of the blood vessel between the jaws of your forceps. Pick it up only by its outer layer, the adventitia. The least damage you cause to the blood vessels and the surrounding tissues the better. In addition to the work on the anatomy that you will find in this manual, it would be useful to study Greene's work (1963) and the more recent work of Hebel and Stromberg (1986).

3.3. Planning

Both planning and preparation of an operation are important, and commonly underestimated. You should commence an operation preferably in the morning, in order to provide optimal post-operative care. The same applies to surgery at the end of the week, unless proper attention can be provided over the weekend period.

Always be sure before commencing an operation, that you have everything you need at your disposal. Almost every operation requires special equipment such as cannulae, syringes, hypodermic needles, specialized instruments and sometimes specialized drugs or solutions. It is most frustrating when you have to leave the operating theatre to search for things you urgently require, not to mention the break it causes in the aseptic technique.

When you want to master a new technique or must do an operation you have not carried out for a long time, it is important to (re)study the anatomy of the area of surgery and surgical techniques to ensure the optimum result. A detailed knowledge of both the anatomy and the required techniques will prevent unnecessary manipulation of tissues, thereby reducing tissue damage, haemorrhagic risk and infection. The result being healthy and well prepared animals, which are likely to give the best response in the subsequent experimental study.

3.4. Asepsis

Although the rat has a remarkable resistance to the development of wound infection it is, however, frivolous to neglect aseptic technique for the surgical procedures. Surgery in the laboratory rat must be governed by the same basic principles as those for surgery on human beings. Asepsis (the method of achieving a germfree condition) is very important in (micro)surgery and, unfortunately, the opinion amongst researchers that rodents are especially resistant to surgical infections is still widespread. Most surgeons operate on rats without taking any precautions to minimize the initial contamination of the surgical area. This neglect can lead to infection or even to the untimely death of the rat. Another outcome of bad aseptic technique is the reduction of long term patency rates of inserted cannulae (Popp and Brennan, 1981). In our hands permanent jugular vein cannulae can remain patent for up to six months when both cannulae and surgical instruments are sterilized before use, in addition to the standard precautions (see below). When using unsterile cannulae and instruments, the patency is drastically reduced to between one or two weeks. But not only patency is affected, also the recovery of the animal is delayed and the time needed to return to the pre-operative weight is extended.

A high level of aseptic technique can be achieved using the following procedures:

- Sterilization (generally achieved by autoclaving) of surgical instruments and all materials that are permanently implanted in the animal.
- The use of sterile suture materials, hypodermic needles and syringes.
- The use of sterile solutions (saline and heparin).
- A clean operating area, including a silicon rubber plate (30 × 25 × 1 cm) which can easily be sterilized or disinfected using 0.5% of an aqueous chlorhexidine solution or 70% ethanol.
- The use of proper scrub when washing hands such as Betadine–scrub (a polyvinylpyrrolidone-iodine solution), Hibi-scrub (chlorhexidine solution), or disinfection with Sterillium (isopropanol, n-propanol and ethylhexadecyl-dimethylammonium-ethylsulphate).

In addition to the above mentioned precautions, when possible all animals should be administered an antibiotic, for example a single dosage of 150 mg/kg amoxycillin subcutaneously (s.c.) or ampicillin (150 mg/kg s.c.) given 10 min prior to the operation will give adequate protection against infections.

3.5. Surgical instruments

In order to proceed with microsurgery it is essential to own your own set of instruments (Figure 3.5.1.). These should be of a good quality and must be well maintained. Do not begin with old, worn out or obsolete equipment. Once you have acquired your set, do not lend it out. Your set should consist of:

Microsurgical instruments:

- Jewellers forceps (No.5, Dumont)
- Jewellers forceps 45°-angled (Dumont)
- Vessel stretcher or vessel dilator
- Needle holder (Barraquer-type), without a lock
- A pair of ring handled dissecting scissors with gently curved blades
- A pair of fine 45°-angled iridectomy scissors (Wecker-type)
- Vessel clamps:
  - One 10 mm double approximator (Acland)
  - Two 12 mm single clamps (Acland, Biemer or Heifetz)

Non-microsurgical instruments:

- Anatomical or dissecting forceps (straight)
- Anatomical or dissecting forceps (90°-angled)
- A pair of fine toothed forceps.
- A pair of ring handled scissors (straight, sharp/sharp or sharp/blunt)
- A needle holder (Matthieu or Castroviejo)
- An artery forceps, baby-Mosquito or micro-Halsted clamp
- Towel clips (Backhaus)
- Baby Dieffenbach Serrefines (bulldog haemostatic clamps)
- Bulldog clamp, modified to resemble a Satinsky vascular clamp
- An instrument case

Microsurgical instruments should preferably be 11–12 cm in length, as longer instruments are difficult to handle. Dumont's jewellers forceps come highly recommended because they are of extremely high quality. Dumont's angled jewellers forceps can also be used as a needle holder. An advantage of the Barraquer needle holder is that the round grips allow easy rotating movements, made with the fingers only and not with the total wrist. The clamps can be divided into venous and arterial types, the latter having a higher shutting strength. One must be careful with clips that have a very high shutting strength, as they can cause damage to the vascular wall. We use either Acland-Clips or Biemer-Clips, which are available for both arteries and veins, or the intracranial aneurysm clips made by Weck (Heifetz).

Microsurgical instruments are very delicate and require careful handling and cleaning. Always clean your instruments immediately after surgery, using a haemolytic enzyme solution like Hemosol. Then rinse the instruments in tap water. Before the instruments are stored they must be dried and oiled using standard instrument oil.

Should you drop one of your instruments, repair may be possible with the aid of a fine oilstone, or some jewellers emery paper. This work must of course be carried out under the microscope.

The instruments should be held in a pencil grip. The pencil grip is the most delicate and accurate method for microdissection and microsuturing. The relative positions of the hands to the instruments are shown in detail in the drawings. Take a good look at them and copy the positions as shown. Remember that only your fingertips move while the rest of your hand should rest on a stable object like the operating table. If you neglect these basic rules you will soon find out that you make unwanted movements inhibiting your work. Start by holding your instruments in a writing (pencil) position as depicted in Figure 3.2.1., this position guarantees optimal stability in your struggle against unwanted movements.

For further information about the handling of the non-microsurgical instruments, the reader is referred to the works of Anderson and Romfh (1980), Kirk (1978) and Wind and Rich (1987).

3.6. Standby equipment

The bipolar coagulator

The bipolar coagulator is an indispensable surgical instrument that contributes to high grade haemostasis and increases speed, leading to a higher efficiency of operation. Learn to use the coagulator properly with an appropriate pair of clean oiled bipolar forceps as this will reduce sticking of the forceps to the tissue.

The electrical clipper

Rats have very thin hairs and not all electrical clippers can be used to shave them. An efficient and reliable clipper is the one from Aesculap (Figure 3.6.1.), the Favorita II (GT 104). This clipper has a large range of cutterheads, of which the most suitable for rats is the one with 1/20 mm clipping height. The use of the clipper is illustrated in Chapter 7 (General techniques).

The light source

Some of the operations described in this manual can be carried out without the use of an operation microscope. A portable cold-illumination lighting system from which the intensity can be regulated will then be very effective. Moreover, the flexible fibre-optic arms can be equiped with small focussing lenses in order to obtain diffuse or pinpoint lighting. Other halogen lamps can also be used, although these mainly do not have heat filters which necessitates more frequent moistening of the operating area. Proper lighting is of enormous help for surgery, so do not commence an operation with inadequate lighting. Always have some spare halogen lamps available, as the average lifetime for these kind of lamps is only about 50 hours.

The operating table

In your struggle to avoid unwanted movements, the operating table is of major importance. It is very important that the table is placed on an extremely stable frame, to minimize vibrations (Figure 3.6.2.). As shown in Figure 3.6.3. the table consists of a main part in which two half circles are cut away in order to give maximum support to the arms of the surgeon(s), and two small panels used for small standby equipment. The material of which the table is made must be smooth and easy to clean (e.g. PVC).

The rat board

The rat board should be approximately 35 cm long and 25 cm wide. It is best made of 7–10 mm thick silicon rubber, as this is easily cleaned, sterilized if necessary, and it readily accepts needles to secure the instruments and clamps.

References

Anderson, R.M. and Romfh, R.F. (1980) Technique in the use of surgical tools. Appleton-Century-Crofts, New York.

Greene, E.C. (1963) Anatomy of the rat. Hafner Publishing Company, New York and London.

Hebel, R. and Stromberg, M.W. (1986) Anatomy and embryology of the laboratory rat. BioMed Verlag, Birgit Hebel D-8031 Wörthsee, FRG.

Kirk, R.M. (1978) Basic surgical techniques. Churchill Livingstone, Edinburgh, London and New York.

Popp, M.B., Brennan, M.F. (1981) Long-term vascular access in the rat: importance of asepsis. Am. J. Physiol. 241 (Heart Circ. Physiol. 10):H606-H612.

Wind, G.G. and Rich, N.M. (1987) Principles of surgical technique. Urban & Schwarzenberg, Baltimore-Munich.

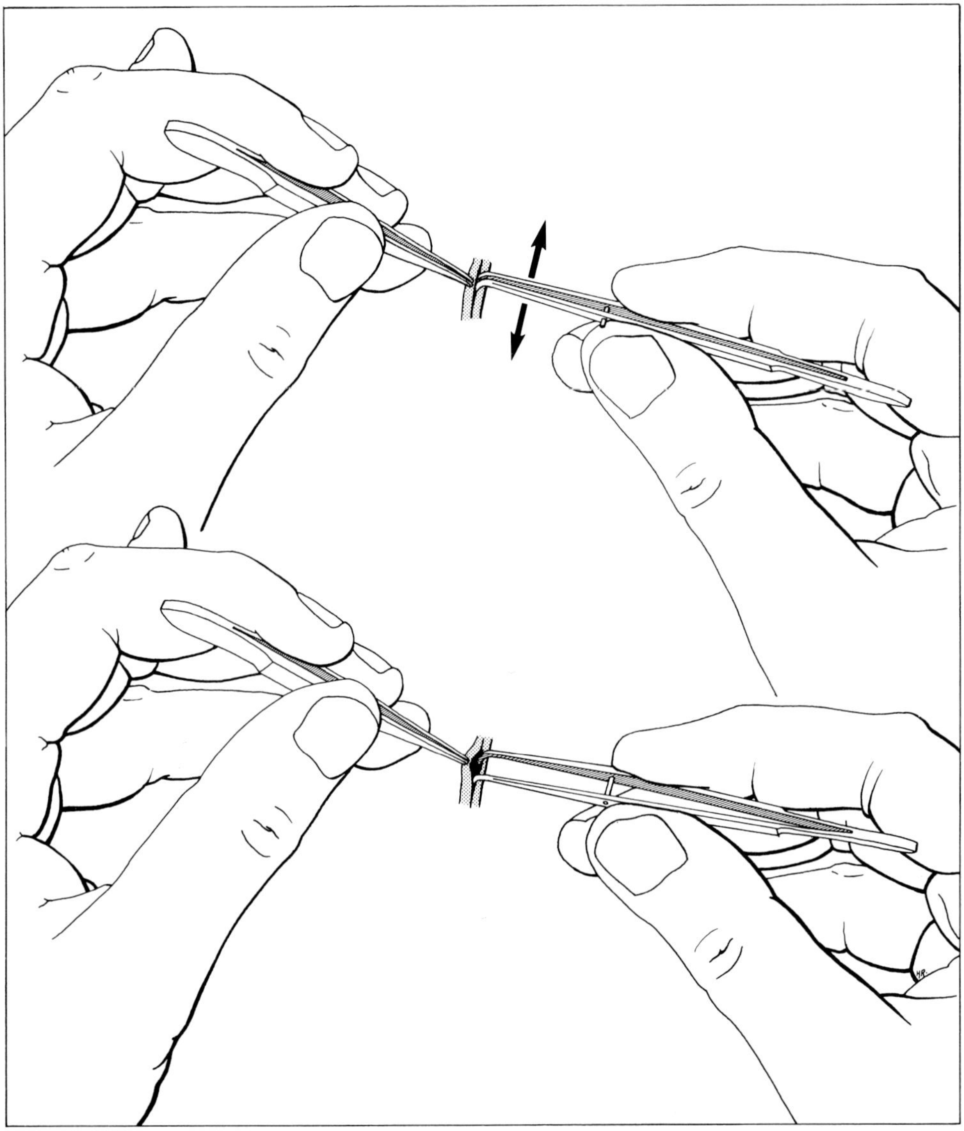

Figure 3.2.1. Blunt dissection.
Dissection of tissues is best achieved by repeatedly spreading the tips of the forceps. The left hand instrument supports the adventitia.

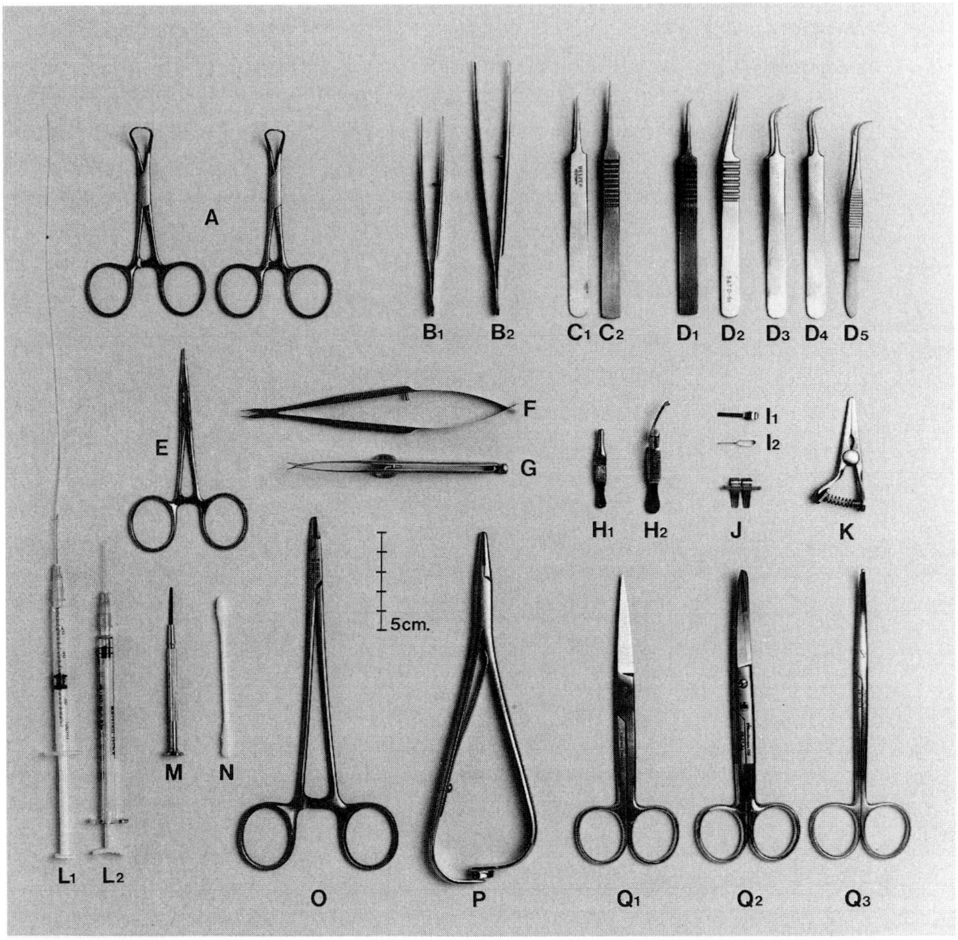

Figure 3.5.1. The surgical instruments.

A	towel clips (Backhaus)
B_1	small straight anatomical forceps
B_2	large straight surgical forceps
C_1/C_2	straight jewellers forceps
D_1	angled jewellers forceps
D_2	vessel stretcher
D_3/D_4	curved jewellers forceps
D_5	curved anatomical forceps
E	artery forceps (baby-Mosquito)
F	needle holder (Barraquer-type), without a lock
G	45°-angled iridectomy scissors (Wecker-type)
H_1	baby Dieffenbach serrefine (bulldog haemostatic clamps)
H_2	large bulldog clamp modified to resemble a Satinsky vascular clamp
I_1	vessel clamp (Heifetz)

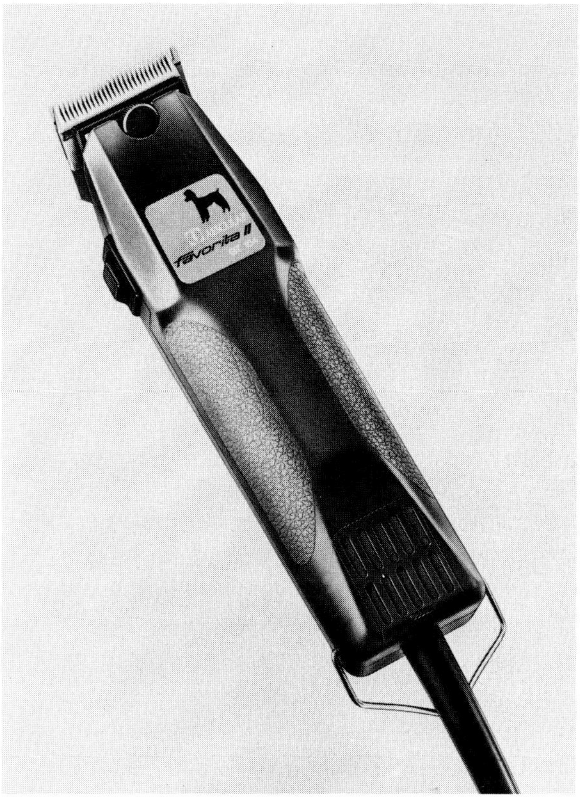

Figure 3.6.1. The electrical clipper.

←

I_2 vessel clamp (Biemer)
J 10 mm double approximator (Acland)
K bulldog clamp (Pilling)
L_1/L_2 1 ml syringes
M screw driver
N cotton wool stick
O straight slender needle holder
P needle holder (Matthieu)
Q_1 ring handled preparation scissors straight, sharp/sharp
Q_2 ring handled preparation scissors curved, blunt/sharp
Q_3 ring handled preparation scissors curved, blunt/blunt
(photo: H. van Dijk, Maastricht, the Netherlands)

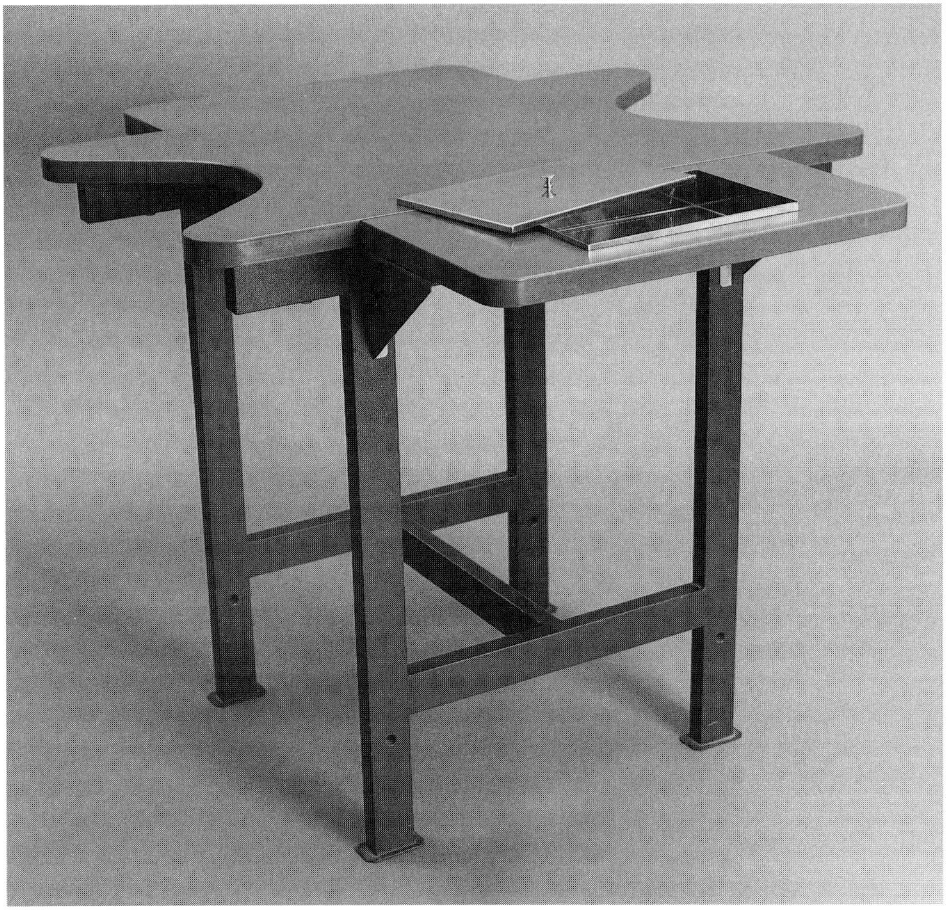

Figure 3.6.2. The operating table (I).
Picture showing the operating table and the stable frame (photo: H. van Dijk, Maastricht, the Netherlands).

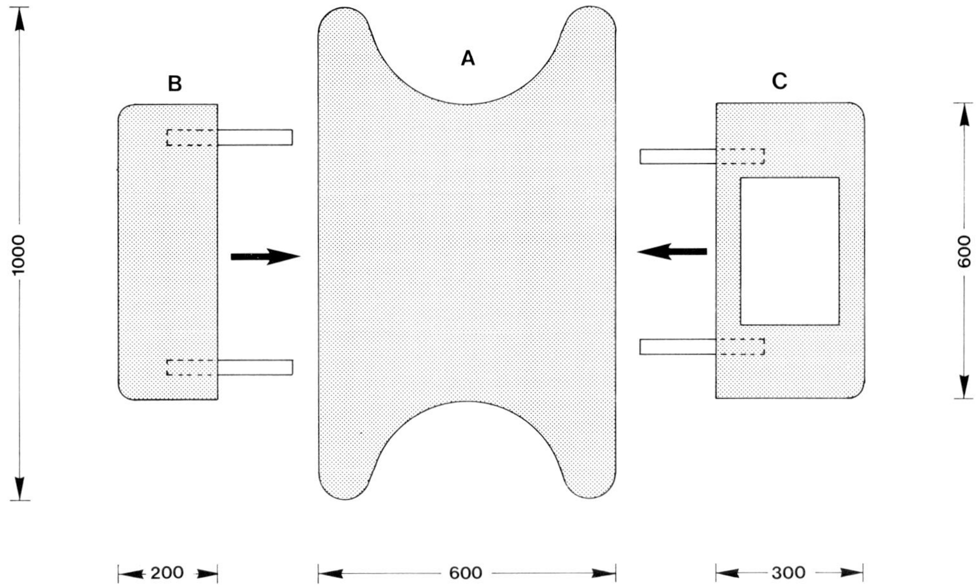

Figure 3.6.3. The operating table (II).
Dimensions of the operating table consisting of a central table top (A) and two tables on the side (B and C). The dimensions of the cut-away section in part C depend on the size of your instrument case. The table top should be at least 30 mm thick (all dimensions in millimetres).

Manual of Microsurgery on the Laboratory Rat, Part I
Van Dongen, Remie, Rensema and Van Wunnik (eds)
© *1990 Elsevier Science Publishers B.V. (Biomedical Division)*

CHAPTER 4

The operation microscope

F.A. DE HAAS, R. REMIE, J.J. VAN DONGEN, J.W. RENSEMA and M.EVERSDEN

4.1. Introduction

This chapter is about the development of the operation microscope. Today – 1990 – there are many types of operation microscopes available, together with a number of instruments which have directly derived from the operation microscope. All these instruments share the same basic design, but vary in peripheral details. For simplicities sake the whole group falls under the term, "the operation microscope".

The first successful attempts at microsurgery were carried out at the beginning of this century by Axel Carrel. Despite the absence of suitable instrumentation for observation of the operation area, and with only the crude surgical instruments of that time at his disposal, he successfully carried out some organ transplants in animals. In 1920 Carl Zeiss created the well known surgery-spectacles, a pair of 2 × magnifiers in an adjustable spectacle frame, which were the first real optical aid. The original Zeiss surgical loupes, as they are called, are still in use today, sixty years after their introduction (Figure 4.1.1.).

In the late thirties, surgery of the inner ear was still difficult to perform, because of the lack of suitable instrumentation, the only optical aid in existance being the above mentioned surgery-spectacles.

Just before World War II, leading eye- and ENT-surgeons asked Carl Zeiss to develop a mobile and versatile instrument to observe the operation field, with a high power magnification, to discern details that previously could not be seen. The instrument needed to have a large working distance combined with very strong illumination, casting no shadows. Furthermore, the instrument needed to be freely movable in any direction. It would have to project a natural (not mirror) stereoscopic image, with a large depth of focus. In 1938 these wishes were considered to be pure science fiction.

The Carl Zeiss scientists took up the challenge. To an optical specialist it was clear that they had to use another famous Zeiss instrument as a basis, the binocular telescope, invented by professor Ernst Abbe in 1887. It would have to be adapted for focussing on objects at a very short distance. The light path inside was parallel, so they could fit a magnification changer in, without having to use correctional optics, thus avoiding loss of light.

It took several years of hard work and research, until Carl Zeiss in 1952 could present the operation microscope to leading ENT-surgeons like professor Wullstein in Germany, and professor Jongkees in the Netherlands. The miraculous operation microscope (Opmi 1, as it later became known) fulfilled every single wish, and on its introduction it was simply science fiction which had become a reality (Figure 4.1.2.).

The instrument was equipped with a strong coaxial light source, for which the tungsten bulb had to be specially modified. The illumination cast no shadow because it was coaxial with the optical observation system. The rays run parallel through the system and create an image at infinity, both paths of the binocular (stereo) microscope going jointly through one objective, using a five step changer to alter the magnification factor. The magnification factor of the microscope body multiplied by the focal length-factor of the binocular tube, multiplied by the magnification of the eyepieces, provides a total range of $0.4\times$ to $40\times$. The focal distance of the main objective determines the working distance. Main objectives with focal distances from 50 mm, 125 mm, and up to 200 mm were available from the beginning. The longer the working distance, the lower the magnification factor.

The Opmi 1 gives an upright unreversed stereoscopic image, which is so very important for manipulating under the microscope, because one observes a natural image, not a mirror image.

Even today, very few users know that the binocular tube with eyepieces of their operation microscope is a perfect high quality binocular telescope.

The instrument presented in 1952 made it possible to look and manipulate inside narrow tube-shaped structures. This combined with the long working distance and the hitherto unknown depth of focus, made it ideally suited to the purposes of ENT-surgery, and for many other disciplines as was proved in later years. The microscope was presented on a rollable stand with a whole range of couplings which could be used as required in selecting the preferred approach to the operating field. At the same time Zeiss offered alternative stands for the operation microscope, enabling it to be used for different purposes such as table stands for the preparation of and operating on small animals.

4.2. Microsurgery

Due to the fact that ENT was the first discipline to use the operation microscope as a routine, it were experiences within this discipline which led to the development of more refined surgical techniques. This resulted in the famous microsurgical seminars given by professor van den Broek in Nijmegen (The Netherlands).

As microsurgical operations tend to last for many hours, and are very strenuous for both surgeons and their assistants, it is important to make any improvements which can help to relax tension in the operating theatre. Instrumentation is one of the first factors to be considered.

From its initiation the operation microscope has been an instrument that projects an image at infinity, which means that the user(s) can operate with it for long periods as there is no visual stress. This is the huge advantage of the Zeiss operation microscope, compared to those constructed to the Greenough principle which require constant re-focussing on the image.

However, still more demands for adaptation were made within the field of microsurgery. The construction of highly refined instrumentation has greatly benefitted from the tremendous progress in all fields of technology which have been made in the second half of the twentieth century. Not least because of the very special demands made by the spacecraft industry. A whole catalogue of new inventions are incorporated within the series of operating microscopes today, but the original optical system has remained principally unaltered.

As microsurgery requires great manual dexterity, often two surgeons have to work together. Therefore many attempts have been made to couple two operation microscopes together. None of the attempts proved very practical, until in the early seventies the Opmi 7 was constructed, at the instigation of U.S. neurosurgeons. The Opmi 7 was an instrument with motorized zoom magnification change. The body had no focussing system, vertical focussing being performed via the motorized stand. Two or more surgeons, positioned on either side of the operation area, could look comfortably into one instrument and observe a natural view, thus being able to assist one another (Figure 4.2.1.). Opmi 7 served its purpose, but with the evolution of medical and instrumental technology its function has been mainly taken over by the Opmi 6 variation (Figure 4.2.2.).

For acquiring preparational skills using operation microscopes on laboratory rats, the study of the work of Lang and Muchel (1981) is highly recommended.

4.3. Short description and manual

An operating microscope equipment in general consists of the following units:
- The stand
- The couplings
- The illumination
- The optical part

The stand

This is an important, though often neglected part of the microscope equipment. The stand is designed for precise and stable positioning of the microscope over the operation area. It must equalize and minimize vibrations. It must hold the microscope over the operation area, but in no way inconvenience surgeons and assistants, nor may it contaminate them or the sterile area.

The stand contains the power supply for the illumination of the microscope and, if desired, for the motorized zoom-focussing and xy-movements, as well as for other electrical and electronical functions.

For many disciplines, specially adapted stands are available (Figures 4.3.1. and 4.3.2.). For example, ceiling mounts for eye- and neurosurgery and drivable mounts for ENT and for plastic surgery, and chair mounts for gynaecology. Table mounts are often used in experimental surgery and quality control.

The couplings

The Opmi can be mounted directly onto the stand. The movability in this case is less extensive. If it is necessary to make topple, turn or tilt movements, a wide choice of couplings are available for every discipline. One of the most widely used couplings is the xy-coupling, which moves the microscope slowly to and fro. This is activated by a foot switch.

The illumination

Practically all microscopes are now equipped with a fibre illumination (cold light). The tungsten halogen bulb – 12 Volt/100 Watt – is housed in the stand and by way of glass fibre, its light is projected into the microscope body.

A specially designed optical system brightly illuminates the operation field, and most importantly it does it homogeneously. With the latest microscopes, the operator himself determines the area to be illuminated.

The optical part

– The objective

This is a big loupe with a certain focal distance, e.g. f=200 mm. The focal distance more or less equals the working distance of the system.

– The microscope body

This contains the primary part of the observation system (which can be completed by a tube with eyepieces as needed) and the optics for the coaxial illumination. The coaxial illumination and the observation system share the same main objective. By this vehiculum the famous shadowless illumination is achieved. As a rule, in the observation system in the microscope body, either a Galilei-changer or a zoom-changer are placed to set the desired magnification.

The factor (γ) of the chosen magnification is shown on the changer. In the Galilei-changer these factors are: 0.4 – 0.63 – 1.6 – 2.5.

The motorized instruments are activated by all types of switches; footswitches, handswitches, switches which are operated by head movements of the surgeon, even voice operated switches are available.

The hand operated Opmi's have a button for fine focussing by means of a rack and pinion, and a knob for setting the desired magnification.

– The tube

There is a tube for each position of the microscope. When the microscope is used in vertical position, looking down, the inclined tube is used, and when it is used in horizontal position, looking straight forward, a straight tube is applied.

For special applications tubes that can be tilted at 60° and 180° angles are available, so that the operator can always perform comfortably in the sitting position.

The focal distance of the optics of the tube is inscripted on it, e.g. f = 125 mm. The tube projects a real image of the object inside the eyepiece.

– The eyepiece

The eyepieces are available in the fixed magnifications of either 8 ×, 10 ×, or 12.5 ×. An eyepiece acts as a magnifying glass, enlarging the intermediate image projected by the microscope system. The eyelens is adjustable with a range plus or minus 5 dioptre (dpt). This is to allow for the eyepieces to be adapted to any visual inadequacies of users who operate with or without spectacles. For this reason the exit pupils of the operation microscope eyepieces, have been positioned further outside the eyelens. Eyepieces are equiped with flexible eyecups.

For the user without glasses, the eyecups act as a guide by having the exit pupil of the eyepieces coinciding with the user's pupils. The flexible eyecups can be turned inside out, to act as protective rings for spectacle wearers. The above mentioned coincidence is important to ensure a full view on the extremely large field of modern wide angle eyepieces.

– The optical splitters

As light rays are parallel up to the entrance optics of the tube, projecting an infinite image, all sorts of adapters may be placed between the microscope body and tube without influencing the quality of the image. These adaptors split part of the image projecting rays, either permitting two or more surgeons or assistants to observe exactly the same operation area in natural orientation, or (if desired, or as in some cases is necessary) in the orientation that is required (Figure 4.2.1.). Other beam splitters can be used at the same time for photography and video. Using a stereo beam splitter, two surgeons can operate together with four hands, working opposite each other across the operation area.

– The magnification
Vt = total magnification
fob = focal distance 1/2 objective
foc = focal distance 1/2 eyepiece
Voc = the magnification of the eyepiece
γ = the factor of the changer- or zoom-system
Vt = f tube/f objective $\times \gamma \times$ Voc
Example: Vt = 125/200 $\times$ 1 $\times$ 10 = 6.25 $\times$.

4.4. Settings of the microscope (do this before sterilization)

– Switch on microscope and illumination.
– Check the functions, focus, zoom etc.
– Set the microscope at its lowest magnification; adjust tube to correct pupil distance and set the focussing eyepieces to 0-dpt; place the instrument directing at a distance approximately equal to the focal length of the main objective. Now you should see an image; try to improve contour sharpness by repeating the focussing at the highest magnification.

Reference

Lang, W.H. and Muchel, F. (1981) Zeiss microscopes for microsurgery. Springer-Verlag. Berlin, Heidelberg, New York.

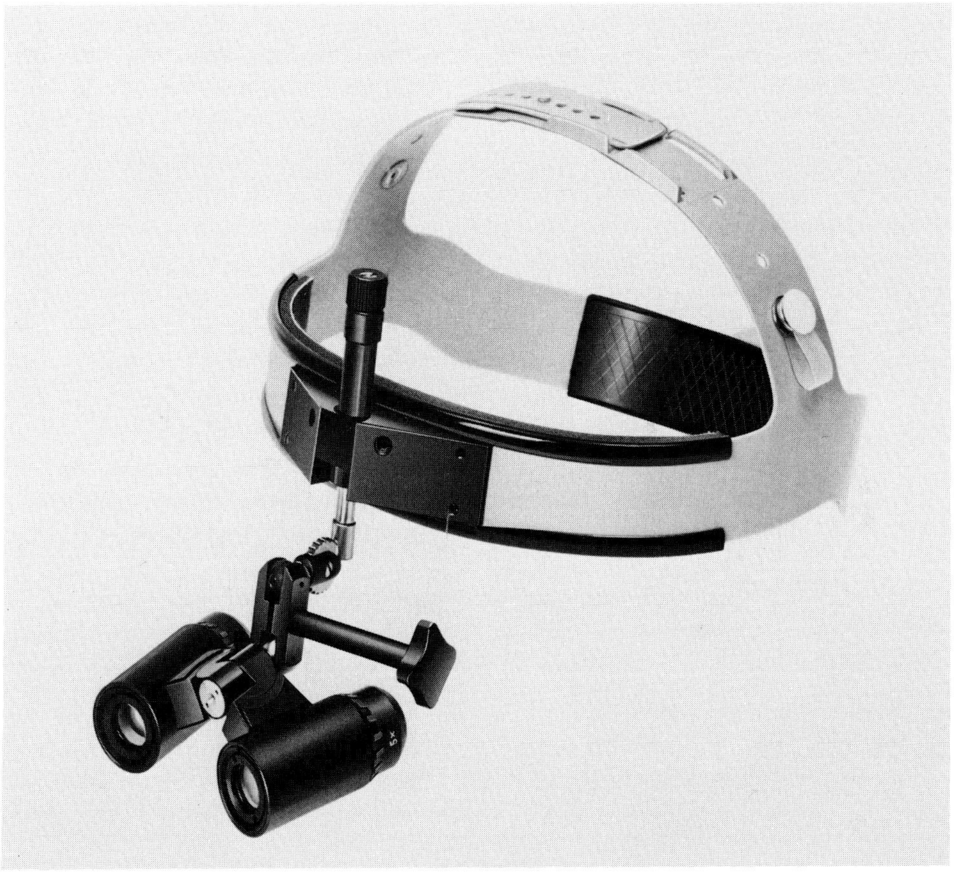

Figure 4.1.1. The prism magnifying headband.

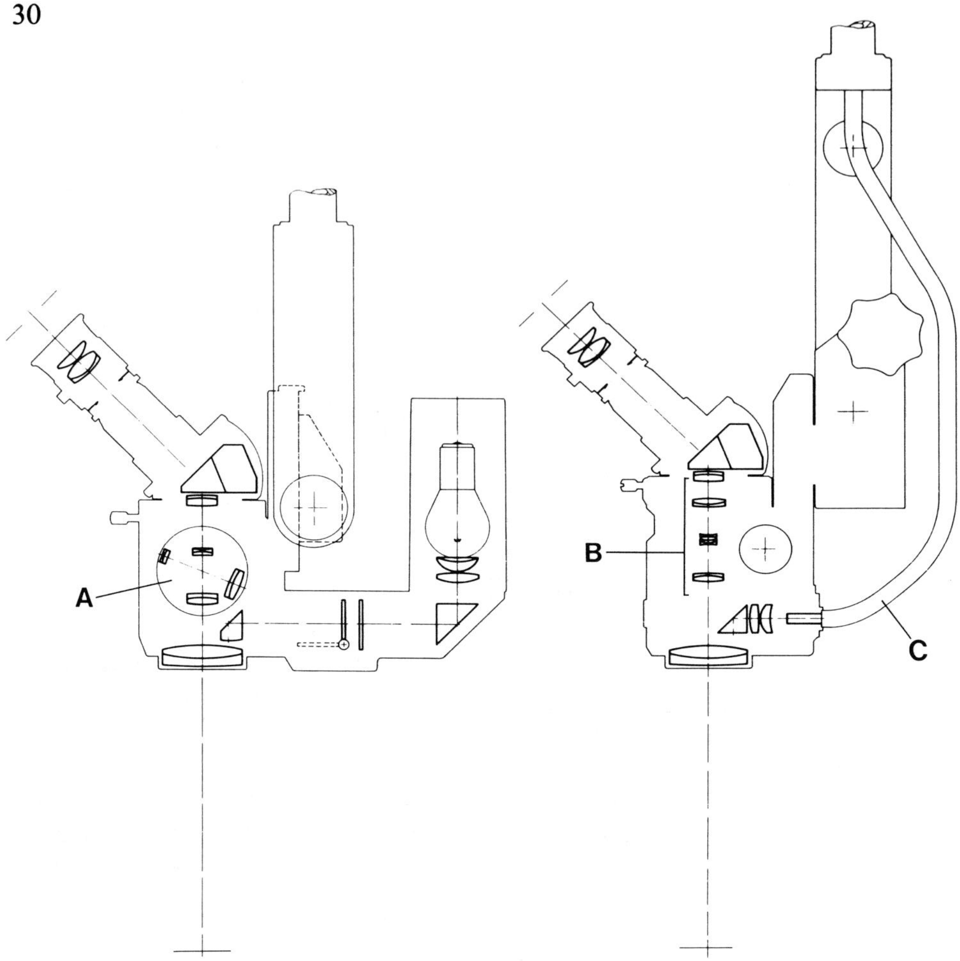

Figure 4.1.2. The Opmi 1.
Design principle of the Opmi 1 with 5-stage magnification changer (A) (left), and with a zoom system (B), and integral fibre-optics illumination (C) (right).

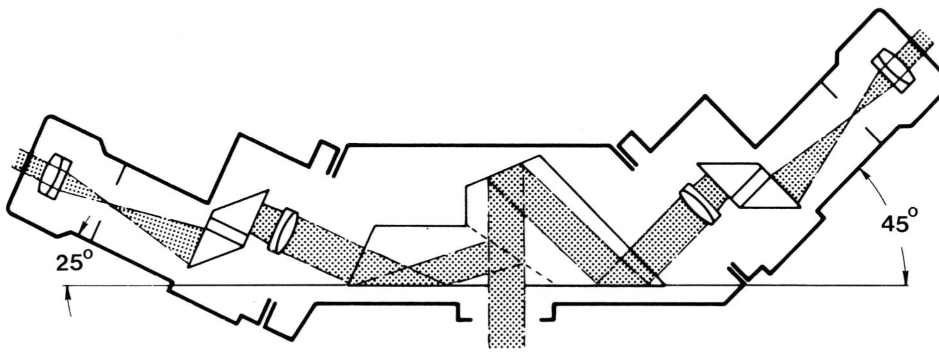

Figure 4.2.1. Beam path of the stereo beam splitter.

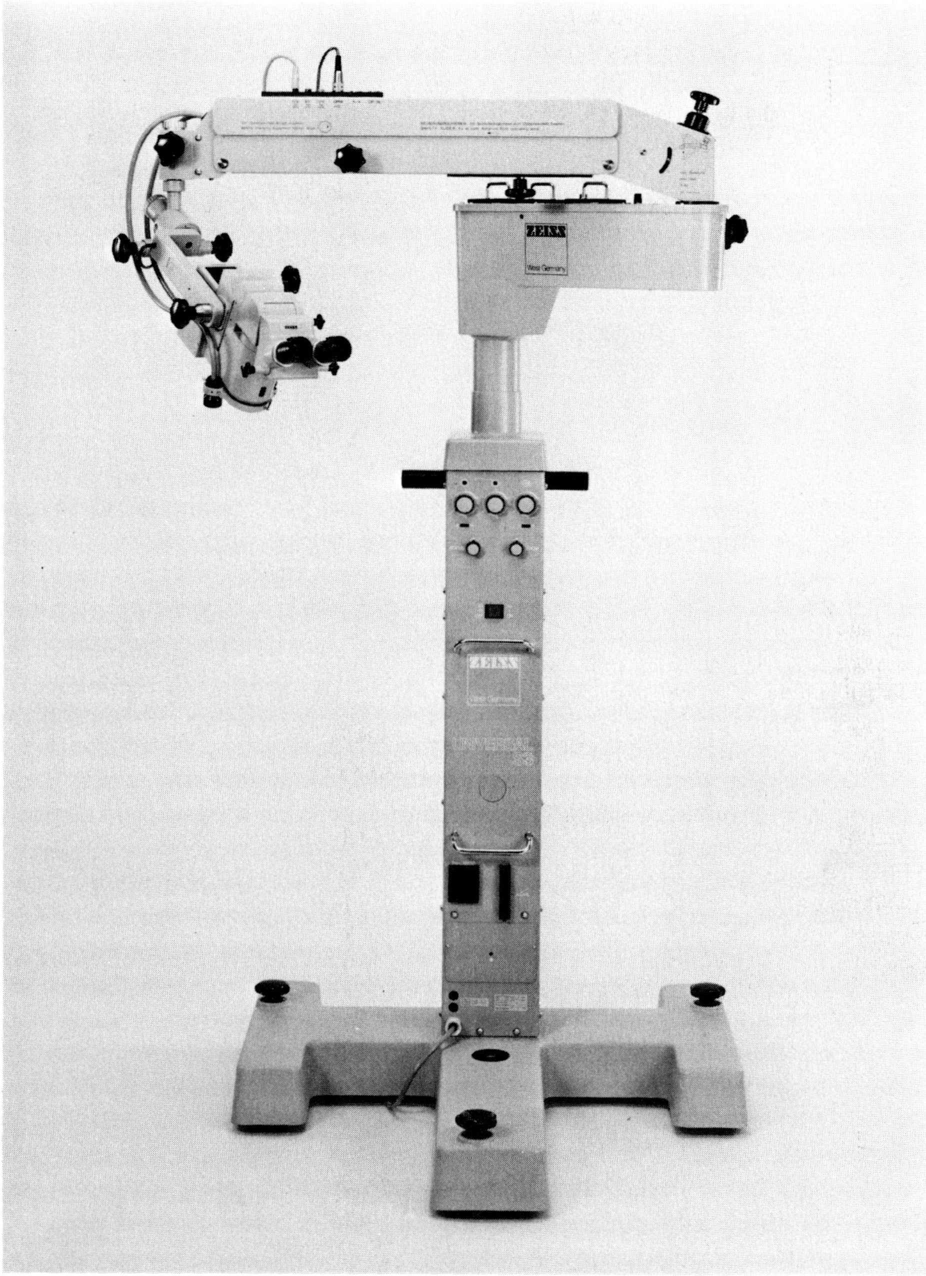

Figure 4.2.2. The Opmi 6 with S 3 motor stand.

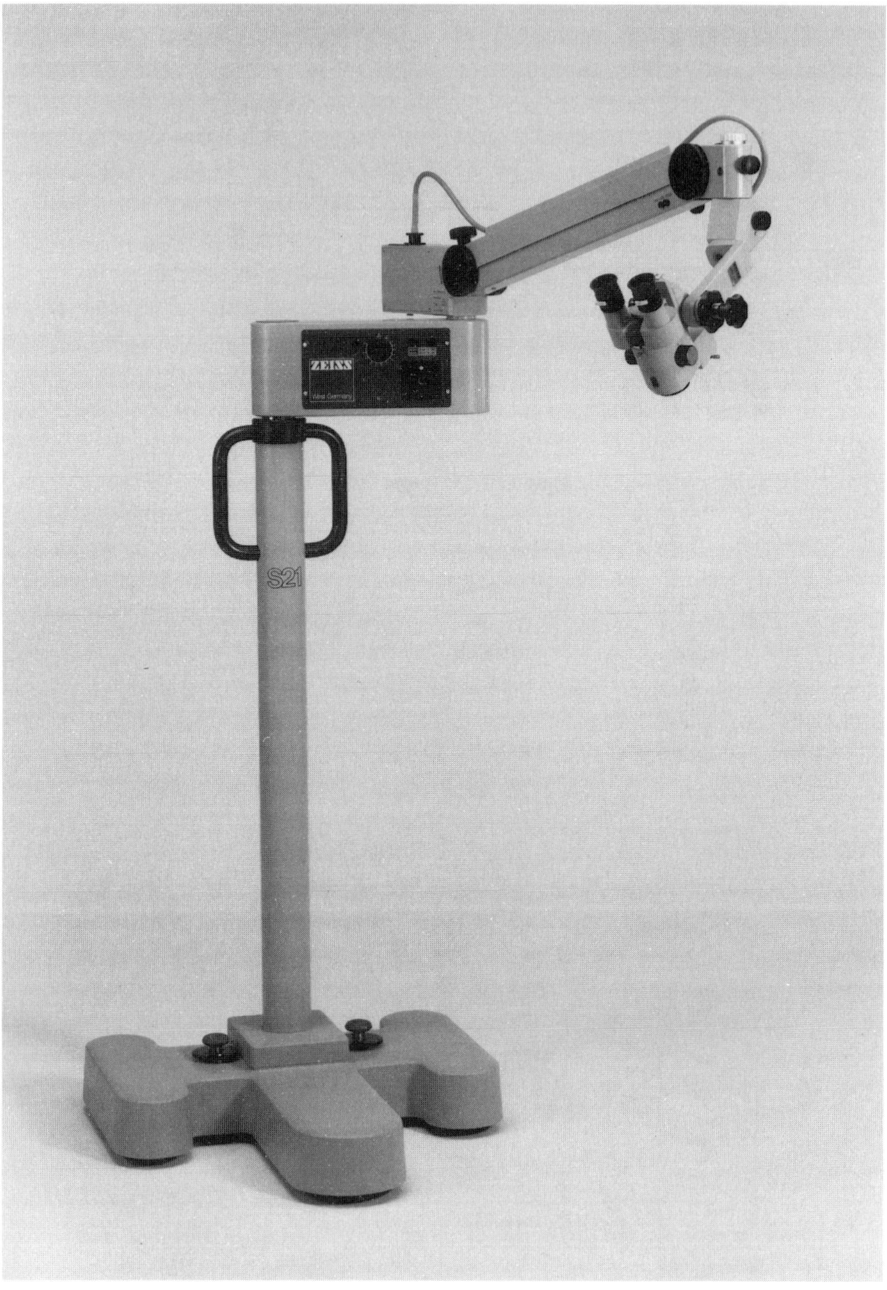

Figure 4.3.1. The Opmi 9 with S 21 stand.

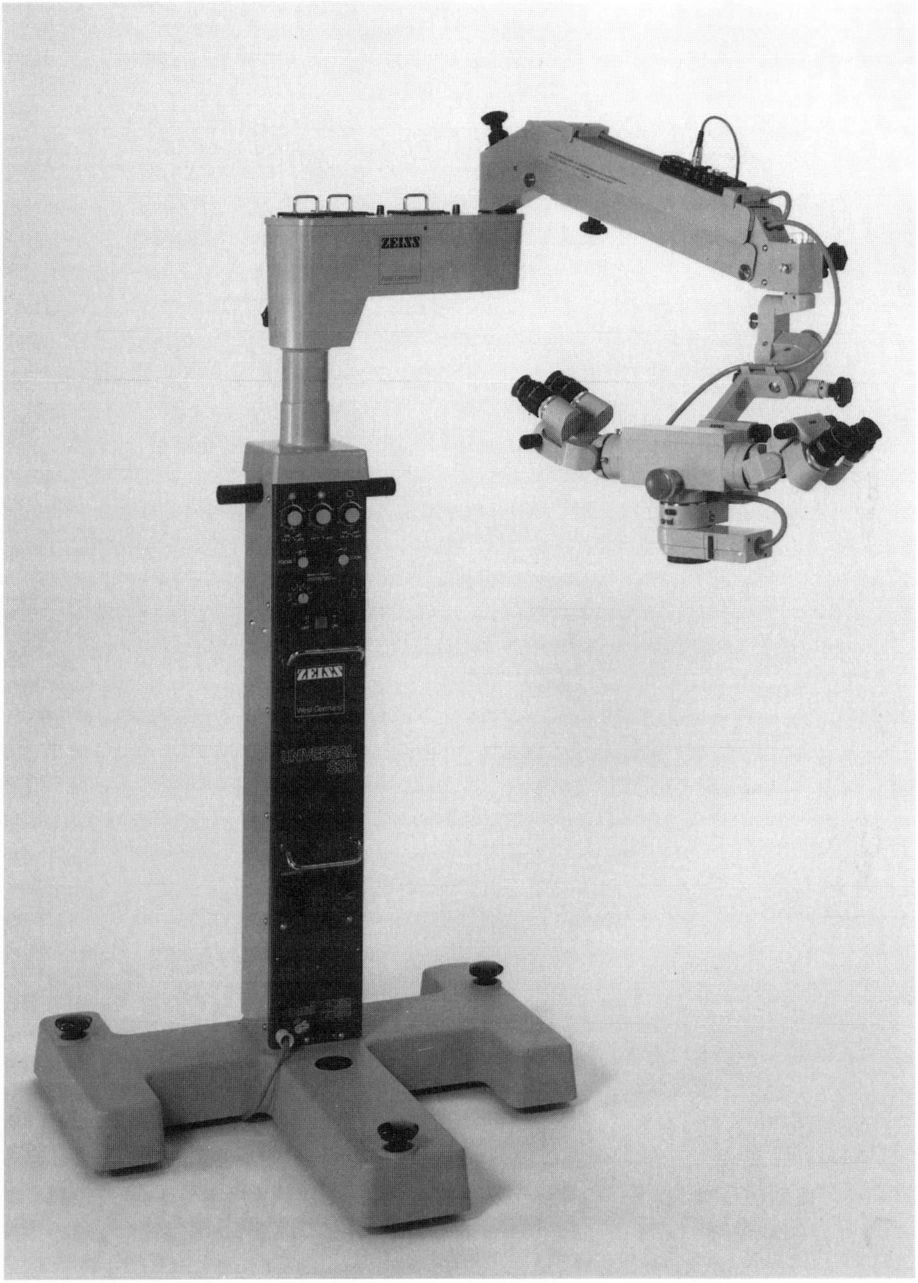

Figure 4.3.2. The Opmi MD with S 3 motor stand.

Manual of Microsurgery on the Laboratory Rat, Part I
Van Dongen, Remie, Rensema and Van Wunnik (eds)
© 1990 Elsevier Science Publishers B.V. (Biomedical Division)

CHAPTER 5

Brief anatomy of the rat

J.J. VAN DONGEN, J.C. VAN DER WAL, J.W. RENSEMA, M. EVERSDEN and R. REMIE

5.1. Introduction

Within this chapter the circulatory system as well as the anatomy of the main thoracic and abdominal viscera are described using the Nomina Anatomica Veterinaria (NAV, 1983). Only the Latin names appearing in the Nomina are given. There are many anatomical variations or irregularities which can occur caused, for example, by inbred degeneration or alterations in tissue structures during growth. The origin of blood vessels can vary, and organs can be positioned differently from those described by others (Greene, 1963; Lambert, 1965; Rowett, 1965; Castaing et al., 1980; Hebel and Stromberg, 1986: Boekelaar, 1985).

The Latin terms for artery and vein are abbreviated to A. and V. respectively in the singular, and Aa. and Vv. in the plural. An English schematic survey of the circulatory system is depicted in Diagrams I, II and III. Figure 5.1.1. shows the layers and the microscopical structures of an artery and a vein.

In this brief anatomy, arteries and veins are described from rostral to caudal with regard to their topographical position to the aorta and the vena cava. The abdominal vessels are shown in Figure 5.1.2.

5.2. Terms applied to define spatial relationships

In anatomy, the basis to define all spatial relationships, is the imaginary median plane, which runs from the head to the tail. This divides the animal into two equal (right and left) halves. "Medial" and "lateral" are terms which show the relationship to the median plane, meaning towards and away from the median plane respectively.

Another imaginary plane used is the sagittal plane, which runs parallel to the median plane. This plane also divides the animal into left and right sections but they are not necessarily equal. There can be many sagittal planes possible to imagine but by definition there can only be one median plane. The transverse plane lies perpendicularly to the median plane, and divides the animal into a *rostral* and a *caudal* part. These planes in turn are traversed by the coronal plane which divides the body into a *ventral* and *dorsal* part. The English term *rostral* is applied to define structures which are situated in the direction of the head, whilst *caudal* refers to the structures situated in the direction of the tail. However, the Latin anatomical terms *rostralis* and *caudalis* are used only to define structures in the head. The terms *cranialis* and *caudalis* are used in the rest of the body.

The terms *proximal* and *distal* stand for the anatomical definition of towards and away from the centre, the median line or point of attachment or origin. These terms are used particularly for structures of the extremities such as the tail, legs and head. Figure 5.2.1. depicts these spatial relationships.

5.3. The circulatory system

The circulatory system (Tractus circulatorius) can be differentiated into a general, or systemic circulation to the body, and the pulmonary circulation to the lungs. The systemic circulation carries oxygenated blood from the heart to tissues and organs, via arteries, and deoxygenated blood back to the heart via veins. The pulmonary circulation carries deoxygenated blood through arteries to the lungs, and oxygenated blood through veins towards the heart. The ramification of the aorta can be divided into the so-called visceral and parietal branches.

The main visceral branches of the thorax and abdomen are:
- the pulmonary arteries (Aa. pulmonales)
- the celiac artery (A. coeliaca)
- the mesenteric arteries (Aa. mesentericae)
- the suprarenal arteries (Aa. suprarenales)
- the renal arteries (Aa. renales)
- the testicular or ovarian arteries (Aa. testicularis sive ovaricae)

The main parietal branches are:
- the intercostal arteries (Aa. intercostales)
- the costoabdominal arteries (Aa. costoabdominales)
- the rostral phrenic arteries (Aa. phrenicae craniales)
- the caudal phrenic arteries (Aa. phrenicae caudales)
- the lumbar arteries (Aa. lumbales)
- the iliolumbar arteries (Aa. iliolumbales)

– the middle caudal arteries (Aa. caudales media)
– the iliac arteries (Aa. iliacae interna et externa)

5.3.1. Arteries of the thorax

The ascending aorta lies dorsally to the pulmonary artery (A. pulmonalis) arising from the left ventricle. Outside the pericardium where the left and right coronary arteries (Aa. coronaria sinistra et dextra) arise, the ascending aorta continues as the aortic arch (Arcus aortae). This gives off three main branches, the anonyme artery (Truncus brachiocephalicus), the left common carotid artery (A. carotis communis sinistra) and the left subclavian artery (A. subclavia sinistra). The aortic arch bends dorsally to the left and passes the trachea on the left side running over the left main bronchus (Bronchus principalis sinister). The aorta descends dorsally to the heart and oesophagus, giving rise to intercostal arteries (Aa. intercostales) and costal arteries (Aa. costoabdominales). Before entering the abdominal cavity through the aortic opening (Hiatus aorticus), the rostral phrenic arteries (Aa. phrenicae craniales) arise from the descending thoracic aorta. From here the thoracic aorta continues as the abdominal aorta (Aorta abdominalis).

5.3.1.1. Coronary arteries (Aa. coronariae)

The coronary arteries originating from the aortic root (just behind the semilunar valves), supply the heart with blood. Besides this blood supply, the heart recieves accessory vessels such as the cardiomediastinal artery. This artery supplies blood to a part of the atria, the rostral vena cava and the pulmonary veins. The left coronary artery (A. coronaria sinistra) branches into the circumflex branch (Ramus circumflexus), which runs to the dorsal part of the left ventricle wall, continuing respectively to the conic region of the right ventricle, and the atrium. The right coronary artery (A. coronaria dextra) passes dorso-caudally to the right ventricle, giving off a branch to the right atrium.

5.3.1.2. Anonyme artery (Truncus brachiocephalicus)

The anonyme artery arises as the first arterial trunk from the aortic arch (Arcus aortae), and runs in an antero-rostral direction. The adjacent vessel, the right common carotid artery (A. carotis communis dextra), runs rostrally and ramifies at the thymic margin into the right internal carotid artery (A. carotis interna dextra) and the right external carotid artery (A. carotis externa dextra), supplying the right side of the neck, the head and brain. At the root of the right common carotid artery, the right subclavian artery (A. subclavia dextra) branches and runs towards the right foreleg.

5.3.1.3. Left common carotid artery (A. carotis communis sinistra)

The left common carotid artery emerges just next to the vertex of the aortic arch (Arcus aortae) before the left subclavian artery (A. subclavia sinistra). It lies rostrally to the left side of the neck and head. From there it ramifies, along with other vessels, into the left internal carotid artery (A. carotis interna sinistra) and the left external carotid artery (A. carotis externa sinistra) both of which supply the head and brain of the animal.

5.3.1.4. Left subclavian artery (A. subclavia sinistra)
The left subclavian artery is rather long compared with the right subclavian artery. This vessel bends in the direction of the left foreleg giving off two branches, i.e. the costocervical trunk (Truncus costocervicalis) and the internal thoracic artery (A. thoracica interna). From the costocervical trunk the profound cervical artery (A. cervicalis profunda) arises, which divides into the right muscular arteries and the caudal thyroid artery (A. thyroidea caudalis). The internal thoracic artery originating from the left subclavian artery ramifies into several smaller vessels. One of which, the left bronchoesophageal artery (A. broncho-esophagea) divides into branches towards the trachea, bronchus (Ramus bronchialis) and oesophagus (Ramus esophageus).

5.3.1.5. Pulmonary trunk (Truncus pulmonalis)
The pulmonary trunk originating from the right ventricle, divides into a left and a right branch. The left branch which runs dorsally to the aortic arch (Arcus aortae) and the rostral vena cava, ramifies into several arteries towards the different lobes of the left lung. The right branch however passes the beginning of the aortic arch ventrally as a single vessel towards the right lung which consists of one lobe.

5.3.1.6. Botallic duct (Ductus arteriosus)
Prior to birth this shunt between the pulmonary trunk (Truncus pulmonalis) and ascending thoracic aorta (Aorta ascendens) is responsible for short-circuiting the blood of the foetus, together with the opening of the septum between the left and right atrium. After birth the Botallic duct is obliterated and replaced by connective tissue, and is subsequently called the arterial ligament (Ligamentum arteriosum).

5.3.2. Veins of the thorax

The three largest veins of the body are the rostral venae cavae (Vv. cavae craniales), and the caudal vena cava (V. cava caudalis) situated respectively rostrally and caudally to the heart. At various intervals, veins are equiped with valves which, in combination with other physiological circumstances, force the blood to flow in cardial direction. From the right lung four large pulmonary veins (Vv. pulmonales) emerge from the different lobes and fuse with the only vein of the left lung to form one main branch. This enters the heart in the dorsal part of the left atrium.

5.3.2.1. Rostral vena cava (V. cava cranialis)
The rostral vena cava is formed by the confluence of the internal jugular vein (V.

jugularis interna) and the subclavian vein (V. subclavia) and is double. The right rostral vena cava (V. cava rostralis dextra) is rather short, and runs directly towards the anterior part of the right atrium. The left rostral vena cava (V. cava rostralis sinistra) runs dorsally to the aortic arch (Arcus aortae) alongside the left auricle, receiving parietal branches. The vessel continues dorsally confluencing with the caudal vena cava (V. cava caudalis). Finally the vein enters the right atrium of the heart.

5.3.2.2. Jugular veins (Vv. jugulares interna et externa)

These paired veins drain blood mainly from the head, neck and shoulders in the direction of the heart. The external jugular vein (V. jugularis externa) receives blood from the linguofacial vein (V. linguofacialis) and the maxillary vein (V. maxillaris). Before the vessel unites with the subclavian vein (V. subclavia) it receives blood from the cephalic vein and the axillary veins. The internal jugular vein (V. jugularis interna) confluences with the subclavian vein in the thoracic cavity.

5.3.2.3. Subclavian vein (V. subclavia)

The subclavian vein unites as a paired vessel with the external jugular vein (V. jugularis externa) carrying blood from the foreleg region to the heart. The subclavian vein and the jugular vein confluence with the rostral vena cava (V. cava cranialis).

5.3.3. Arteries of the abdomen

The abdominal aorta (Aorta abdominalis) runs via the aortic opening (Hiatus aortae) of the diaphragm, to the pelvic region. Here it bifurcates into the iliac arteries (Aa. iliacae interna et externa) in the direction of both hind legs.

The aortic opening is positioned between the left lateral and the left medial crus of the diaphragm and ends near the rostral part of the second lumbar vertebra. The aorta lies alongside the spinal column, somewhat dorsally to the caudal vena cava.

5.3.3.1. Caudal phrenic artery (A. phrenica caudalis)

The first branch arising from the abdominal aorta (Aorta abdominalis) is the caudal phrenic artery. It divides into several branches as it approaches the diaphragm, phrenic nerve (Nervus phrenicus) and the left suprarenal gland. This artery may consist of three branches arising directly from the aorta, two of which run directly to the diaphragm, whilst the third ramifies to the suprarenal gland.

5.3.3.2. Celiac artery (A. celiaca)

Sections 5.3.3.2. to 5.3.3.4. are mainly based on findings of Boekelaar (1985), which describe best our own observations.

This unpaired artery, branching from the aorta, ramifies to the splanchnic organs of the ventral epigastric region of the abdomen. From its origin the celiac artery forms a rostral semicircular arch, situated ventrally to the diaphragm. After approximately one centimetre, several arteries emerge from this junction which is situated dorsally to the portal vein, i.e. the common hepatic artery (A. hepatica), the left gastric artery (A. gastrica sinistra), and the splenic artery (A. lienalis).

5.3.3.2.1. Common hepatic artery (A. hepatica)

The common hepatic artery is closely attached to the portal vein (Vena portae) and arises from the right side of the caeliac artery (A. celiaca). It runs in a latero-ventral direction towards the liver. It bifurcates forming the hepatic artery proper (very small), and the gastroduodenal artery (A. gastroduodenalis) which is the continuation of the common hepatic artery. The hepatic branch runs rostrally towards the liver hilus and ramifies into the hepato-oesophageal arteries and lobar hepatic branch. The gastroduodenal artery runs dorsally to the portal vein in the direction of the proximal duodenum and the stomach. It ramifies into the right gastric artery (A. gastrica dextra), the rostral pancreaticoduodenal artery (A. pancreaticoduodenalis cranialis) and the right gastroepiploic artery (A. gastroepiploica dextra).

Originating from the rostral pancreaticoduodenal artery, duodenal and pancreatic branches (Rami pancreatici) arise, along with several other branches leading to the common bile duct (Ductus choledochus) (Boekelaar, 1985). Furthermore, the pancreaticoduodenal branches anastomose with the ascending duodenal branch of the caudal pancreaticoduodenal artery (A. pancreaticoduodenalis caudalis), which ramifies from the rostral mesenteric artery (A. mesenterica cranialis).

The right gastric artery gives rise to arteries leading towards the stomach and duodenum. Frequently it anastomoses with the branch of the left gastric artery (A. gastrica sinistra) which runs along the lesser curvature of the stomach (Boekelaar, 1985). The third branch of the gastroduodenal artery, the gastroepiploic artery, gives rise to the pyloric, gastric, and epiploic branches. These branches supply blood to the stomach, pancreas, greater omentum, pylorus and duodenum. They anastomose with branches of the left epiploic artery which arises from the splenic artery (A. lienalis).

5.3.3.2.2. Left gastric artery (A. gastrica sinistra)

The left gastric artery, which is the vessel adjacent to the caeliac artery (A. celiaca), runs latero-dorsally in portal direction and via the gastrophrenic ligament, finally towards the stomach. The oesophageal branches, fundic branches, the ventral gastric branch and subsequently the dorsal gastric branch arise from this vessel (Boekelaar, 1985).

5.3.3.2.3. Splenic artery (A. lienalis)

The splenic artery is embedded in the splenic segment of the pancreas, and ramifies in the direction of the spleen. The first branch, the gastrosplenic artery (A. gastrolienalis) divides into short gastric and splenic branches (Greene, 1963; Hebel and Stromberg, 1986). According to Boekelaar (1985) there is only one short gastric artery. Subsequently, pancreatic and splenic branches and the left epiploic artery (A. epiploica sinistra) originate from the junction of the splenic and gastrosplenic arteries. The splenic artery runs to the pancreas, the omentum (which is connected to the spleen) and to the greater curvature of the stomach respectively.

5.3.3.3. Rostral mesenteric artery (A. mesenterica cranialis)

The rostral mesenteric artery arises caudally from the celiac artery (A. celiaca) as an unpaired vessel, and runs in a ventral direction. It gives rise to small pancreatic branches (Rami pancreatici), to the middle colic artery (A. colica media), the right colic artery (A. colica dextra), the caudal pancreaticoduodenal artery (A. pancreaticoduodenalis caudalis), the jejunal arteries (Aa. jejunales) and the ileocaecocolic artery.

5.3.3.3.1. Middle colic artery (A. colica media)

This artery, originating from the upper part of the rostral mesenteric artery (A. mesenterica cranialis), ramifies near the margin of the transverse colon into two branches. The left branch runs towards the proximal part of the descending colon. Subsequently, it anastomoses with the ascending branch of the left colic artery (A. colica sinistra). The right colic artery (A. colica dextra) runs to the proximal part of the ascending colon as well and anastomoses with the ascending branch of the ileocaecocolic artery (see 5.3.3.3.).

5.3.3.3.2. Right colic artery (A. colica dextra)

This artery originates from the rostral mesenteric artery (A. mesenterica cranialis) and runs into the mesocolon towards the ascending part of the colon. The vessel ramifies on the intestinal margin into both an ascending and a descending branch. Subsequently, the ascending branch runs parallel to the colic branch of the middle colic artery (A. colica media) supplying both the ascending and the transverse colon. The right descending colic artery runs to the colon, anastomosing with the ileocaecocolic artery (see 5.3.3.3.).

5.3.3.3.3. Caudal pancreaticoduodenal artery (A. pancreaticoduodenalis caudalis)

The caudal pancreaticoduodenal artery arises from the caudal part of the rostral mesenteric artery (A. mesenterica cranialis) just before the right colic artery (A. colica dextra). Branches lead to the distal part of the ascending duodenum. The vessel continues towards the mesoduodenum and to the descending part of the duodenum. There the vessel ramifies to the duodenal and jejunal segment of the pancreas, and to the common bile duct (Ductus choledochus) respectively.

5.3.3.3.4. Jejunal arteries (Aa. jejunales)

From the rostral mesenteric artery (A. mesenterica cranialis) anything from between twelve up to sixteen arteries branch off, running via the mesentery towards the jejunal and ileal parts of the gut. On the mesenteric border of the bowel they ramify into many anastomoses (the so-called arcades) providing blood to the small intestine.

5.3.3.4. Caudal mesenteric artery (A. mesenterica caudalis)

The caudal mesenteric artery usually arises from the right common iliac artery (Aa. iliaca interna et externa). It can however arise from the caudal abdominal aorta (Aorta abdominalis caudalis) or its bifurcation. The vessel branches shortly after its origin into the rostral rectal artery (A. rectalis cranialis) and the left colic artery (A. colica sinistra). The left descending colic branch runs into the mesentery of the descending colon, confluencing with the left branch of the middle colic artery (A. colica media).

5.3.3.5. Right renal and suprarenal arteries (A. renalis dextra et Aa. suprarenales dextrae)

The right renal artery (A. renalis dextra), the origin of which is situated somewhat caudal to, or opposite to the rostral mesenteric artery (A. mesenterica cranialis), passes transverso-dorsally to the caudal vena cava (V. cava caudalis). It then runs towards the kidney hilus and bifurcates into dorsal and ventral branches. The main branches of the renal arteries have shunts between the cortex and the medulla. Before entering the kidney, these segmental arteries subdivide into smaller branches at the ventral part of the right renal vein (V. renalis dextra). From this region, the dorsal arterial branch leading towards the kidney gives rise to the uretic artery (A. uretica), which runs along the ureter in a caudal direction. Approximately halfway along the renal artery, the right testicular artery (A. testicularis) or ovaric artery (A. ovarica) and the right suprarenal artery (A. suprarenalis dextra) arise. The latter vessel can also rise from the aorta passing transverso-dorsally to the caudal vena cava (V. cava caudalis) or from the right phrenic artery (A. phrenica dextra).

5.3.3.6. Left renal and suprarenal arteries (A. renalis sinistra et Aa. suprarenales sinistrae)

The left renal artery (A. renalis sinistra) arises from the aorta, situated caudally to the right renal artery (A. renalis dextra). It runs in a caudo-lateral direction towards the kidney hilus. Halfway along, the artery branches into the left suprarenal artery (A. suprarenalis sinistra) and the testicular artery (A. testicularis) or ovaric artery (A. ovarica). The left renal artery runs dorsally to the left renal vein (V. renalis sinistra) towards the kidney hilus and is attached closely to this vein. The left suprarenal gland also receives a branch of the left caudal phrenic artery (A. phrenica caudalis sinistra).

5.3.3.7. Testicular or ovarian arteries (Aa. testicularis sive ovarica)

The paired testicular artery (A. testicularis) of the male rat emerges from the aorta. As described above, both the right and the left testicular arteries can also rise from the renal arteries (Aa. renales). Each vessel runs obliquely downwards, crossing the ventral surface of the ureters, passing through the inguinal canal to the scrotum. There the epididymal artery (A. epididymalis) branches off.

The paired ovarian artery (A. ovarica) of the female rat arises from the aorta and runs slightly obliquely in a caudal direction to the ovaries. Just before reaching the ovaries, the vessel divides into the tubal artery (Ramus tubarius) and the ovarian and uterine branch (Ramus uterinus), going to the oviduct, ovary and uterus, respectively.

5.3.3.8. Iliolumbar and lumbar arteries (Aa. iliolumbales et lumbales)

The paired iliolumbar artery (A. iliolumbalis) arises from the abdominal aorta (Aorta abdominalis) just caudally to the testicular or ovarian arteries (Aa. testiculares sive ovaricae). The localization of this artery varies considerably and can appear anywhere from the margin caudal to the testicular or ovaric arteries, to appearing just proximal to the bifurcation of the iliac arteries. Throughout the extensive length, the abdominal aorta gives rise to the dorsal lumbar arteries (Aa. lumbales dorsales), which supply the vertebral column, the muscles of the lumbar region and the spinal cord.

5.3.3.9. Common iliac arteries (Aa. iliacae interna et externa)

Both common iliac arteries separate just below the caudal mesenteric artery (A. mesenterica caudalis) running obliquely downwards. The vessels leave the abdominal cavity via the inguinal dorsal ligament. As they go towards the extremities, they bifurcate into the internal iliac arteries (Aa. iliacae internae), while the main trunks continue as femoral arteries (Aa. femorales). The femoral artery continues as the popliteal artery (A. poplitea) towards the foot, and empties into the dorsal metatarsal arteries (Aa. metatarsea). The internal iliac arteries also give rise to the muscular arteries (Aa. musculares), the rostral gluteal artery (A. glutea rostralis), the umbilical artery (A. umbilicalis) and finally the pudendoepigastric trunk (Truncus pudendoepigastricus).

5.3.3.10. Median caudal artery (A. caudalis mediana)

The median caudal artery is one of the terminal branches of the aorta (Aorta abdominalis). It is unpaired and continues downwards into the tail. From it the paired lateral caudal artery (A. caudalis lateralis) arises supplying the tail throughout its complete length.

5.3.4. *Veins of the abdomen*

Only the largest veins along with some non-concomitant veins are described here. The concomitant branches are depicted in the schematic survey of the arterial circulatory system (Diagrams I, II and III).

5.3.4.1. Caudal vena cava (V. cava caudalis)

The caudal vena cava is formed by the confluence of the iliac veins (Vv. ilacae interna et externa) receiving blood from the lower extremities and the pelvic region. This vein runs ventro-laterally along the aorta. It crosses the diaphragm dorsally to the liver and enters the thoracic cavity.

5.3.4.2. Hepatic and caudal phrenic veins (Vv. hepaticae et Vv. phrenicae caudales)

The hepatic veins (Vv. hepaticae) are unpaired. They are positioned proximally to the liver and run directly into the caudal vena cava (V. cava caudalis). Occasionally the caudal phrenic veins (Vv. phrenicae caudales), which collect blood from the diaphragm, contribute to the hepatic vein (V. hepatica). Mostly, however, they run directly into the caudal vena cava.

5.3.4.3. Portal system

The portal system includes all veins collecting blood from the alimentary tract (Canalis alimentarius), the spleen, pancreas and common bile duct (Ductus choledochus). From these, visceral blood is conveyed into the liver by the portal vein (V. portae). Within the liver, this vein ramifies like an artery emptying into the capillary network, before entering the general circulation via the hepatic veins (Vv. hepaticae). From there the blood is conveyed to the caudal vena cava (V. cava caudalis).

5.3.4.3.1. Portal vein (V. portae)

The portal vein is formed by the confluence of the rostral mesenteric vein (V. mesenterica rostralis), the splenic vein (V. lienalis) and the gastroduodenal vein (V. gastroduodenalis). The hepatic artery proper is attached very closely to the portal vein. The portal vein runs from the proximal duodenum, and just outside the entrance to the liver the vessel bifurcates into a left and right hepatic trunk (Truncus hepaticae sinistra et dextra) going towards the various liver lobes.

5.3.4.3.2. Rostral mesenteric vein (V. mesenterica cranialis)

The rostral mesenteric vein is formed by its tributaries receiving blood from the jejunum, the duodenal part of the pancreas, the caudal pancreaticoduodenal vein (V. pancreaticoduodenalis caudalis) and the adjacent caudal mesenteric vein (V. mesenterica caudalis). The efferent blood stream from the biliary system, the duodenal part of the pancreas and from the corresponding part of the duodenum runs via the middle pancreaticoduodenal vein towards the portal vein (V. portae). The middle colic vein (V. colica media) enters the mesenteric vein (V. mesenterica) on the left dorsolateral side. The rostral mesenteric vein further receives tributaries from the right gastric vein (V. gastrica dextra) and the gastroduodenal vein (V. gastroduodenalis).

5.3.4.3.3. Gastroduodenal vein (V. gastroduodenalis)

The gastroduodenal vein is formed by the confluence of the right gastroepiploic vein (V. gastroepiploica dextra), the pancreaticoduodenal vein (V. pancreaticoduodenalis) and the pyloric vein (V. pylorica). It receives blood from the greater curvature of the stomach, the duodenum, the pancreas and the pylorus respectively.

5.3.4.3.4. Splenic vein (V. lienalis)

The splenic vein is formed by the fusion of the left gastroepiploic vein (V. gastroepiploica sinistra), the short gastric vein (V. gastrica), the coronary vein (Greene, 1963), and the pancreatic vein (V. pancreatica). These veins receive blood from the stomach, the omentum, the oesophagus, and the spleen, while the pancreatic branch receives blood from the margin of the pancreas along the dorsal layer of the greater omentum.

5.3.4.4. Renal and testicular or ovarian veins (Vv. renales et testiculares sive ovaricae)
The renal vein (V. renalis) and the testicular vein (V. testicularis) are paired. Proximal to the iliolumbar vein (V. iliolumbalis), the right renal vein enters the vena cava on the lateral side. The left renal vein (V. renalis sinistra) is positioned somewhat caudally to the right renal vein (V. renalis dextra). The renal vien receives blood from the left suprarenal gland and from testicular branches. Sometimes, the latter vessel follows the testicular artery (A. testicularis) obliquely to the caudal vena cava (V. cava caudalis). The right renal vein (V. renalis dextra) is usually separated from the right renal artery (A. renalis dextra) and receives venous blood from the right suprarenal gland via the caudal suprarenal vein (V. suprarenalis caudalis). The same pattern as described for the testicular veins, applies to the ovarian veins (Vv. ovaricae). One should be aware of differences in the origin of blood vessels in this specific region.

5.3.4.5. Iliolumbar and lumbar veins (Vv. iliolumbales et lumbales)
On its trajectory from the iliac bifurcation towards the renal veins, the vena cava receives blood from the iliolumbar veins (Vv. iliombales) and occasionally from the testicular or ovarian veins (Vv. testiculares sive ovaricae). Throughout its length the caudal vena cava (V. cava caudalis) receives blood from the dorsal lumbar veins (Vv. lumbales I–VII). These tributaries collect blood from the spinal cord as well as from the vertebral column.

5.3.4.6. Iliac and femoral veins (Vv. iliacae et femorales)
The iliac veins (Vv. iliacae interna et externa) are the most caudal tributaries of the vena cava receiving blood from the hind legs through the femoral veins (Vv. femorales).

5.4. The thoracic viscera

Unlike the splanchnic organs the thoracic viscera are surrounded by a fairly strong construction consisting of the ribs, the sternum, the clavicles, the thoracic part of the vertebral column and muscles. This firm framework protects the thorax from being compressed too easily, thereby maintaining heart and lung functions. The thorax begins at the thymic margin and is defined caudally by the diaphragm. The diaphragm divides the trunk of the rat into a thoracic and an abdominal cavity. Its muscular activity along with the thoracic muscles and the various bones enlarges and reduces the thoracic cavity to enable inspiration and expiration respectively. The thoracic cavity is subdivided by membranous pouches, such as the pericardium and the pleura, which contain the heart and lungs respectively.

5.4.1. The heart (Cor)

The heart lies to the left of the mediastinum in the ventral part of the thorax, and is enclosed by a double walled pouchy membrane, the pericard, which is fixed to the sternum by the sternopericardial ligament. Rostro-ventrally this ligament is connected to the thymic lobes. The pericard totally envelops the heart and serves amongst other things the hydration of this organ. The apex of the heart, pointing somewhat to the left in the direction of the diaphragm, is in close contact with the median lobe of the left lung. The heart consists of a left and right ventricle with their respective atria with auricles. The left and right part of the heart are separated by a fairly thick curved septum.

5.4.2. The thymus (Thymus)

The thymic gland consists of two lobes situated antero-rostrally to the heart, and covers the caudal part of the trachea, the rostral venae cavae (Vv. cavae craniales) and the arteries which emerge from the aortic arch (Arcus aortae). This gland is fully grown after about three months and is clearly recognizable because of its whitish colour. In human beings, this gland disappears upon maturity, in contrast to the rat where the thymus remains throughout its entire life.

5.4.3. The respiratory system (Apparatus respiratorius)

The respiratory system consists amongst other things of the pharynx, the larynx, the trachea, the bronchi, and the left and right lung. Air enters the system via the nasal cavities. The pharynx is divided into the nasopharynx, just above the palatum, and the oropharynx whose cavity is situated behind the buccal cavity. In the latter part of the pharynx lies the division between the respiratory system and the digestive tract. The trachea which runs from rostral to caudal, divides into a left and right main bronchus, which further ramifies into smaller bronchi and bronchioli. The left lung consists of one lobe. Its total volume is somewhat smaller than that of the right lung. The right lung has four lobes namely a rostral, a median, a caudate, and an accessory lobe which is subdivided.

5.4.4. The oesophagus (Esophagus)

The oesophagus resembles a straight tube which runs from the pharyngeal area towards the hiatus oesophagicus of the diaphragm. The abdominal part of the oesophagus is fairly short. In rest, the lumen of the oesophagus is firmly closed prohibiting reflux. The oesophageal wall consists of circulary and longitudinal muscle layers which possess a peristaltic function for the transport of food.

5.5. The abdominal viscera

The abdominal cavity is surrounded by flexible muscle layers of which the inside wall is covered by the peritoneal membrane. This membrane covers all abdominal organs and keeps them in position. The muscle layers of the abdominal wall consist mainly of the internal and the external abdominal muscles, and the rectus abdominal muscle. The left and the right part are symmetric and meet at the linea alba which is practically bloodless and can easily be divided to open the abdomen.

5.5.1. The liver (Hepar)

The liver is divided into four lobes. The largest one, the median lobe, is positioned ventrally. It covers the left lateral lobe as well as the right lateral and caudate lobes. The liver is held onto the diaphragm by several ligaments, and fits rostrally around the oesophagus. The rat liver has no gall bladder but bile ducts exist throughout it. The common bile duct consists of several junctions and tributaries, receiving bile directly from the liver lobes. The bile, flowing through the common bile duct, enters the duodenum through Oddi's sphincter, which can close the duct. The bile is five times more concentrated than that of mice who do have a gall bladder.

5.5.2. The stomach (Ventriculus)

The stomach is positioned in the left upper part of the abdomen just below the diaphragm. At approximately the middle of the lesser curvature, the stomach is connected to the oesophagus. From this point the stomach is divided into three parts, the cardiac, the pyloric and the fundic. The caudal, pouch shaped part of the stomach forms the greater curvature, to which the head of the pancreas is connected along with a part of the omentum. The pylorus, which is situated to the right side of the stomach, demarcates the entrance to the duodenum.

5.5.3. The spleen (Lien)

This organ is situated in the dorso-lateral part of the abdomen slightly rostral to the left kidney. The distal part of the spleen points mainly ventrally whilst its greater part is directed dorsally. The hilus of the spleen is in close contact with the fundus of the stomach, and follows it alongside its greater curvature (depending upon the mobility of the gastrolienal ligament). The omentum is fixed onto the hilus of the spleen. The enlarging of the spleen is directly correlated to the amount of blood contained by the sinusoids of this reservoir.

5.5.4. The pancreas (Pancreas)

This whitish grey diffuse glandular organ which consists of a right lobe, a left lobe, a head and a body, has internal and external secretion. It lies in the rostro-dorsal part of the abdomen strangled between the duodenum, the proximal part of the jejunum and the transverse colon. The pancreas contains numerous acini, in between which are the islets of Langerhans which produce insulin. The gland has a great number of pancreatic ducts which can greatly differ between rats within the same strain (Castaing et al., 1980). The lobular gland has a pronounced tree shaped structure. The outlets of most pancreatic ducts are directed towards the common bile duct. Some of these ducts however are directed towards the spleen, and in several cases are directly open to the duodenum (Richards et al., 1964; Hebel and Stromberg, 1986). The pancreatic ducts fuse more or less with the smaller ducts of the distal part, thereby forming the common bile duct, which finally enters the duodenum through the sphincter of Oddi, approximately three centimetres from the pylorus.

5.5.5. The small intestine

The length of the small intestine is about seven times the length of the body of the rat (without the tail). It is positioned in "garland like" loops throughout the abdomen. They are fixed by peritoneal folds (the mesentery). The arterial and venous blood vessels of the gut are attached closely to each other, running through the mesentery to and from the intestinal border. The arterial branches divide just before the intestine into branches forming arcades alongside the intestinal margin. The small intestine consists of three parts:

– The first part (the duodenum) consists of a loop of approximately ten centimetres in length. It runs ventro-transversely towards the right lateral abdominal wall and subsequently from the dorsal to the median plane curving as the transverse duodenum ending at the margin of the transverse colon.

– The second part (the jejunum) consists of several loops and forms the longest part of the intestine. The segments can be recognized macroscopically by their blood supply. The exact transition from one part of the small bowel into another, however, can best be defined both macroscopically and microscopically by measuring the diameter, blood supply and formation of Peyer's patches on the one hand, as well as by determining changes in cell structure of the intestine on the other.

– The third part (the ileum) consists of one loop according to its blood supply which is provided by the ileocecal artery. The transition of the jejunum and ileum is marked by the triangular ileocecal ligament. The terminal ileum segment narrows at the end and is connected to the caecum. The orifice of the ileum bulges into the lumen of the caecum and is closed by a muscular sphincter, which works as a ventil. The jejunum and ileum are attached to the dorsal abdominal wall by an extensive fold of the peritoneum, the so-called mesentery, which allows flexible movements of each loop.

5.5.6. The caecum (Cecum)

After opening the abdomen, this large part of the alimentary tract is immediately visible. It can be situated in different regions of the abdomen due to its mobile nature. Normally the caecum is situated ventrally in the left caudal part of the abdominal cavity. As a kind of diverticulum, it is divided into a base, a body and an apical part. Because the caecum is only fixed onto the proximal part of the colon, and by the triangular ligament to the distal part of the ileum, it is very mobile. For the transition of the caecum to the adjacent part of the colon, almost the same can be stated as for the transition of the ileum into the caecum (see below).

5.5.7. The colon (Colon)

This large intestine can be divided into a rather short and a relatively longer part, the colon and the rectum respectively. They can be subdivided into the ascending, transverse and descending colon. The colon is approximately one sixth of the length of the small intestine. The colon emerges from the caecum close to its outlet. At the entrance of the colon a fold of mucous membrane prevents the immediate penetration of food into the colon. After a period of digestion, the peristaltic movements of the caecum are reversed and the food is driven into the colon.
The three parts of the colon are:
– The first part (the ascending colon) ascends slightly in a ventral direction followed directly by a caudal curve. In the pelvic region the colon runs obliquely towards the right latero-dorsal side of the abdominal cavity. Subsequently, it ascends to the duodenojejunal transition on the margin of the transverse colon.
– The second part (the transverse colon) is attached securely to the duodenojejunal part of the small intestine forming a sort of half link of a chain. After this loop, the colon descends alongside the tranverse segment of the duodenum from ventral to dorsal.
– The third part (the descending colon) starts from the rostro-dorsal side of the left kidney, going towards the rectum and is attached to the mesentery at the margin of the colon where the mesenterial lymph nodes are situated.

5.5.8. The rectum (Rectum)

The rectum is the terminal part of the colon, and has a length of approximately eight centimetres. It penetrates the pelvic region and runs dorso-caudally to the terminal ileal segment and ends in the anus. In this part of the digestive tract, digestion is virtually complete, water absorption takes place and a semi solid mass known as faeces, is formed.

5.5.9. The kidney (Ren)

The renal excretory system consists of two kidneys which are positioned retroperitoneally at the dorsal wall of the abdomen. The renal artery, the vein, and the ureter emerge from the hilus of the kidney. The ureters are long thin transparent passages, which transport urine to the bladder, and run obliquely downwards to the urinary bladder.

References

Boekelaar, A.B. (1985) The extrinsic innervation of the stomach and other upper abdominal organs in the rat. Thesis, University of Amsterdam, the Netherlands.

Castaing, D., Houssin, D., and Bismuth, H. (1980) Hepatic and portal surgery in the rat. Masson: Paris, New York, Barcelona and Milan.

Greene, E.L. (1963) Anatomy of the rat. Hafner, New York.

Hebel, R., and Stromberg, M.W. (1986) Anatomy and embryology of the laboratory rat. BioMed Verlag, Birgit Hebel, D-8031 Wörthsee, FRG.

Lambert, R. (1965) Surgery of the digestive system in the rat. Charles C. Thomas Publisher: Springfield, Ill., USA.

Nomina Anatomica Veterinaria (NAV) third edition; Nomina Histologica (NH) second edition (1983). Ithaca, New York.

Richards, Ch., Fitzerald, J., Carol, B., Rosenstock, L., and Lipkin, L. (1964) Segmental division of the rat pancreas for experimental procedures. Lab. Invest. 13: 1303 1321.

Rowett, H.G.Q. (1965) The rat as a small mammal. John Murray, Fifty Albemarle street London.

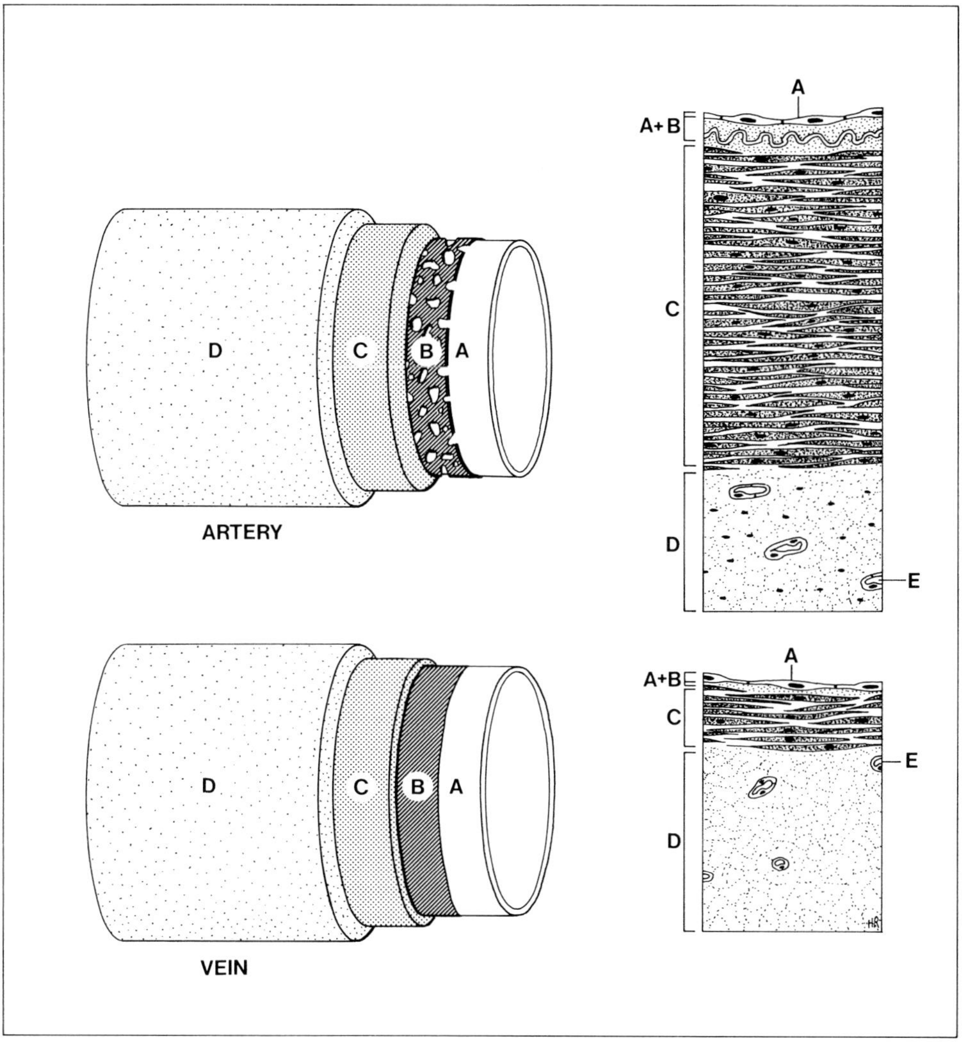

Figure 5.1.1. Structure of an artery and a vein.
Layers of a medium-sized artery (muscular artery) and a vein (left). Comparison of the microscopical structures of the corresponding vessels (right).
A. Endothelium.
B. Internal elastic limiting membrane (membrana elastica interna for the artery and the rete elasticum for the vein).
A + B. Internal tunic [intima] (tunica interna).
C. Middle tunic (tunica media; smooth muscle cells and elastic membranes).
D. Adventitial tunic [adventitia] (tunica externa; elastic connective tissue with elastic fibres).
E. Vasa vasorum (small arteries).
(Modified after: Junqueira L.C., Carneiro J., Contopoulos A. Basic Histology, 2nd ed. Lange Medical Publications, 1977.)

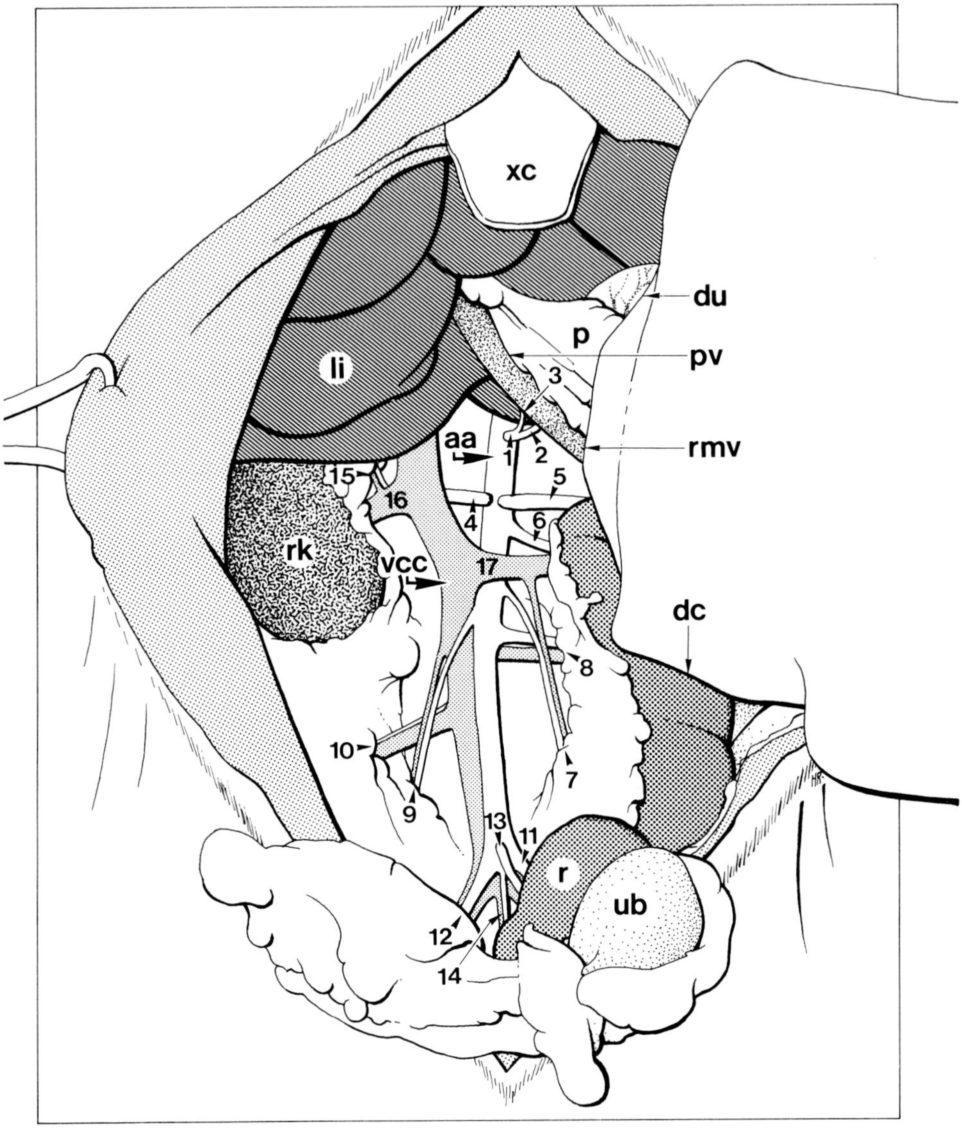

Figure 5.1.2. Topography of the main arteries and veins of the abdominal cavity.
In this ventral aspect of the abdominal cavity of a male rat most of the intestines are drawn to the left side of the animal (to the right as viewed by the surgeon), packed in moistened gauze, while fat deposits are partly removed. (Continued on next page.)

Figure 5.1.2 continued.

aa	Abdominal aorta
dc	Descending colon
du	Duodenum
li	Liver
p	Pancreas
pv	Portal vein
r	Rectum
rk	Right kidney
rmv	Rostral mesenteric vein
ub	Urinary bladder
vcc	Vena cava caudalis

1 Celiac artery
2 Celac artery
3 Common hepatic artery
4 Right renal artery
5 Rostral mesenteric artery
6 Left renal artery
7 Left testicular artery and vein
8 Left iliolumbar artery and vein
9 Right testicular artery and vein
10 Right iliolumbar artery and vein
11 Left common iliac artery and vein
12 Right common iliac artery and vein
13 Caudal mesenteric artery
14 Median caudal artery and vein
15 Right suprarenal artery and vein
16 Right renal vein
17 Left renal vein

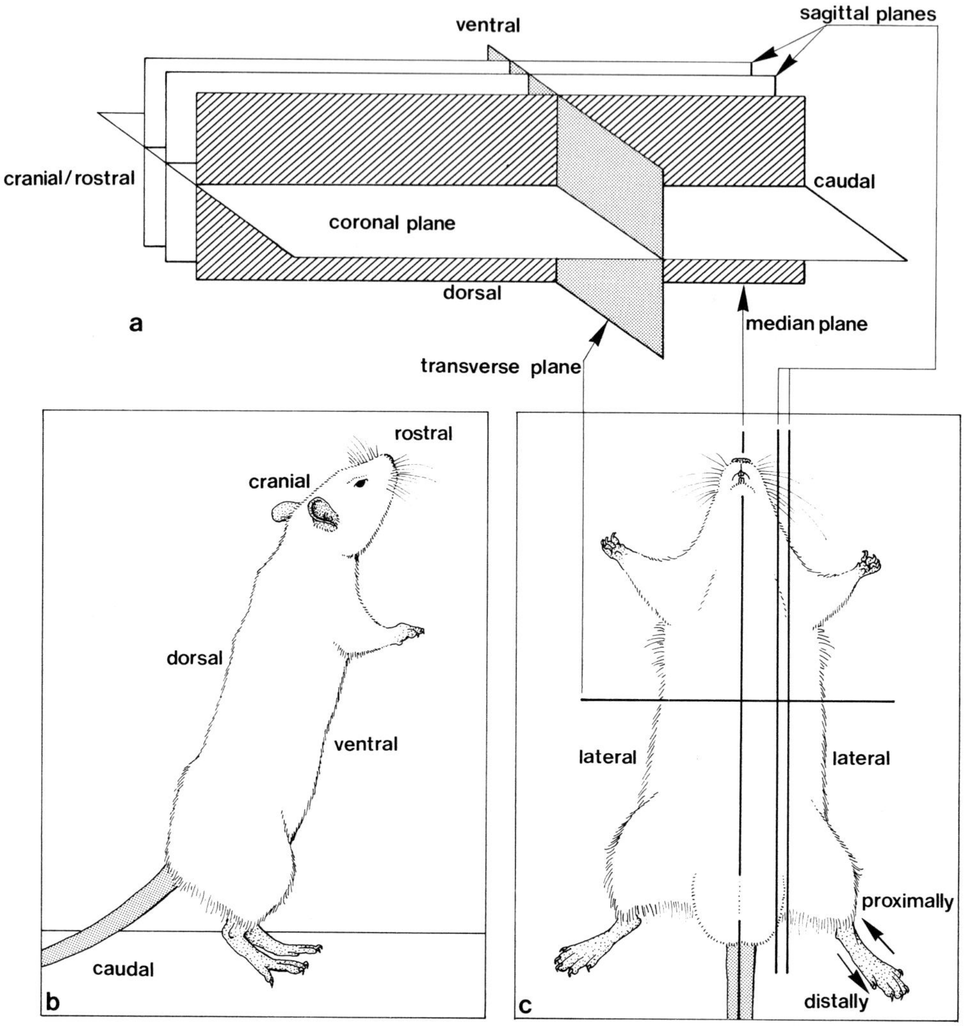

Figure 5.2.1. The spacial relationships.

DIAGRAM I

Branches of the thoracic and abdominal aorta (these vessels are only partially described in the text)

THORACIC AORTA

- ***right and left coronary artery**
  - interventricular artery
    - ventricular branch
    - atrial branch
    - accessory arteries
    - circumflex branch

- ***innominate artery**
  - right subclavian artery
    - vertebral artery
    - superficial cervical artery
      - ascending cervical artery
      - deltoideal artery
      - thoracoacromial artery
    - suprascapular artery
      - right prescapular artery

    - lateral thoracic artery
      - dorsal thoracic branch
      - ventral thoracic branch

    - rostral humeral circumflex artery
    - caudal humeral circumflex artery
    - subscapular artery
      - circumflex scapular arteries
      - thoracodorsal artery

    - brachial artery
      - deep brachial arteries
      - collateral ulnar artery
      - superficial radial artery
      - transversal cubital artery
      - recurrent ulnar artery
      - ulnar artery
        - right palmar artery
      - median artery
        - right dorsal median artery
        - right palmar artery

- ***right internal and external common carotid artery**
  - pterygopalatinal artery
    - right pterygoideal artery
      - pharyngeal artery
      - pterygoideal artery
    - right palatinal artery
      - ophthalmic artery
      - dorsal alveolar maxillar artery
      - right muscular artery
      - lacrimal artery
        - descending palatinal artery
        - sphenopalatinal artery
        - infraorbital artery
          - right alveolar artery
          - right nasal artery
    - rostral cerebral artery
      - medial cerebral artery
      - rostral communicating artery
    - choroidal artery

- ***left internal and external common carotid artery**
  - caudal cerebral artery
    - caudal communicating artery
  - occipital artery
  - thyroidal artery
  - pharyngeal artery
  - muscular artery
  - lingual artery
    - deep lingual branches
  - ascending palatinal artery
  - facial artery

right glandular artery
submental artery
ventral masseteric artery
labial mandibular arteries
angular oris artery
labial maxillary artery
right muscular-anastomotical arteries
lateral nasal arteries
angular ocular arteries
caudal auricular artery
caudal masseteric artery
rostral auricular artery
maxillary artery
alveolar mandibular artery
right mental artery
pterygoideal artery
right pterygoideal artery
deep temporal artery
right masseteric artery
right buccinator artery

superficial temporal artery
right masseteric artery
right temporal artery
transverse facial artery
palpebral artery

***left subclavian artery**
costocervical trunk
deep cervical artery
right muscular branches
caudal thyreoidal branches
dorsal intercostal artery
left bronchial artery
internal thoracic artery
thymic artery
mediastinal artery
bronchoesophageal trunk
right tracheal branch
left broncheal branch
esophageal branch
right pericardial artery
right sternal artery
right perforating artery
musculophrenic artery
rostral epigastric artery

vertebral artery
basilar artery
left medullar artery
caudal cerebellar artery
rostral cerebellar artery
superficial cervical artery
ascending cervical artery
deltoidal artery
suprascapular artery
left prescapular artery

***axillary artery**
thoracodorsal artery
lateral thoracic artery
left dorsal thoracic artery
left ventral thoracic artery

circumflexo-subscapular trunk
rostral humeral circumflex artery
caudal humeral circumflex artery

subscapular artery
thoracodorsal branch
circumflexascapular branches

***brachial artery**
deep brachial artery
superficial brachial artery

superficial radial artery
collateral ulnar artery
transverse cubital artery
recurrent ulnar artery
ulnar artery
right palmar artery
interosseal arteries
right dorsal ulnar artery

median artery
right palmar artery
dorsal median artery

***intercostal arteries**
right dorsal intercostal branches
left spinal branches
ventral costoabdominal branches
costoabdominal artery

***rostral phrenic artery**

ABDOMINAL AORTA

***rostral phrenic arteries**

***celiac artery**
common hepatic artery
hepatic artery proper
hepatoesophageal artery
lobar hepatic branches

gastroduodenal artery
right gastric artery
rostral pancreaticoduodenal artery
duodenal branches
pancreatic branches
common bile duct branches
gastroepiploic artery
pyloric branch
gastric branches
epiploic branch

left gastric artery
esophageal branches
fundic branch
ventral gastric branch
dorsal gastric branch

splenic artery
gastrosplenic artery
short gastric artery
splenic branches
pancreatic branches
splenic branches
left epiploic artery

***rostral mesenteric artery**
pancreatic branches
middle colic artery
right colic branch
left colic branch
right colic artery
ascending branch
descending branch
caudal pancreaticoduodenal artery
jejunal branch
duodenal branches
pancreatic branches

***right renal artery**
right suprarenal artery

***left renal artery**
left suprarenal artery
internal testicular artery
epididymal branch

***ovarian artery**
tubal branch
ovaric branch
uteric branch

***iliolumbar artery**
iliac branches
lumbar branches

***caudal mesenteric artery**
left colic artery
rostral rectal artery

***common iliac artery**
internal iliac artery

  - muscular branch
- rostral gluteal branch
  - rostral gluteal branch
  - caudal gluteal branch
- umbilical artery (male)
  - deferential artery
  - prostatic branch
  - rostral vesical branch
  - ureteric branch
- umbilical artery (female)
  - uterinal branch
  - vaginal branch
    - uretic branch
- internal pudendal artery (male)
  - caudal gluteal branch
  - penile branch
    - urethral branch
    - dorsal penile branch
    - deep penile branch
- internal pudendal artery (female)
  - clitoral branch
    - urethral branch
    - dorsal clitoral branch
    - deep clitoral branch
  - lateral femoral circumflex artery
  - medial femoral circumflex artery
  - obturator artery

- pudendoepigastric trunk
  - caudal epigastric artery
    - dorsal epigastric branch
    - ventral epigastric branch
  - external pudendal artery
    - dorsal pudendal branch
    - ventral pudendal branch

- external iliac artery
  - femoral artery
    - superficial circumflex ilial artery
    - deep femoral artery
    - superficial epigastric artery
    - descending genus artery
      - muscular branch
      - articular branch
    - saphenal artery
      - medial tarsal artery
      - communical artery
      - plantar arteries
      - metatarsal plantar arteries
    - popliteal artery
      - caudal femoral artery
      - caudal tibial artery
      - rostral tibial artery
        - dorsal pedal artery
          - dorsal metatarsal arteries

DIAGRAM II

Branches of the portal vein (these vessels are only partially described in the text)

PORTAL SYSTEM

***left hepatic trunk**

***right hepatic trunk**

***portal vein**
- gastroduodenal vein
  - pyloric vein
    - rostral pancreaticoduodenal vein
  - rostral pancreaticoduodenal vein
  - right gastroepiploic vein
- splenic vein
  - left gastric vein
  - pancreatic veins
  - left gastroepiploic vein
    - short gastric vein
- coronary vein
    - esophageal branch

rostral mesenteric vein
- dorsal jejunal veins
- ventral pancreaticoduodenal vein
- middle pancreaticoduodenal vein
  - caudal pancreatic branches
  - biliary vein
  - duodenal branches
- right colic vein
- middle colic vein
- ileocecocolical veins

caudal mesenteric vein
- left colic vein
- rostral rectal vein

***concomitant branches**

DIAGRAM III

Branches of the rostral and caudal venae cavae (these vessels are only partially described in the text)

ROSTRAL VENA CAVA

*__right innominate vein__
- right anterior caval vein
  - rostral intercostal vein
  - internal mammary vein
  - right subclavian vein
  - internal jugular vein
  - external jugular vein
    - lingo-facial vein
    - maxillary vein

*__left innominate vein__
- left anterior caval vein
  - azygos vein
    - internal costal veins
      - phrenic vein
  - internal thoracic vein
  - left subclavian vein
    - axillary vein
  - left internal jugular vein
    - caudal thyroidal vein

*__external jugular vein__
- lingo-facial vein
- maxillary facial vein
- posterior external jugular vein
  - cephalic vein
  - anterior jugular vein
    - transverse cervical vein
    - transverse scapular vein
    - superficial cervical vein

*__concomitant branches__

CAUDAL VENA CAVA

*__right rostral phrenic vein__
- right rostral suprarenal vein

*__hepatic veins__
- caudal phrenic vein

*__left renal vein__
- left suprarenal vein
  - internal testicular vein (male)
- left caudal phrenic vein
- uretic vein
- left ovarian vein (female)

*__right renal vein__
- right caudal suprarenal vein
- uretic vein

*__right internal testicular vein__
- epididymal branch
- pampiniform plexus

*__left internal testicular vein__
- epididymal branch
- pampiniform plexus

*__ovarian vein__
- uteric branches

*__iliolumbar vein__
- lumbar branch
- iliac branch

*__common iliac veins__
- external iliac vein
- medial femoral circumflex

*__concomitant branches__

Manual of Microsurgery on the Laboratory Rat, Part I
Van Dongen, Remie, Rensema and Van Wunnik (eds)
© *1990 Elsevier Science Publishers B.V. (Biomedical Division)*

CHAPTER 6

Anaesthesia of the laboratory rat

R. REMIE, A. P.M.G. BERTENS, J.J. VAN DONGEN, J.W. RENSEMA
and G.H.J. VAN WUNNIK

6.1. Introduction

The anaesthetic management of experimental animals deserves a good deal of attention. Both ethically and legally one must reduce the perception of pain and minimize discomfort felt by the animal. There are also other factors to be considered when selecting the anaesthetic. The chosen anaesthetic should cause minimum interference to the experiment and the interpretation of results. Another important factor is the nature and the duration of the surgical procedure to be performed. Operations which interfere with liver function, such as partial or total hepatectomy, portacaval anastomosis, or orthotopic liver transplantation, should not be performed under an anaesthetic that has to be cleared from the circulation by the liver. Here you would be advised to use enflurane or isoflurane anaesthesia, as both are largely expelled via the lungs, with only a very small portion of the drugs being metabolized by the liver.

Today there is a vast range of good anaesthetics available, to be used to obtain adequate analgesia (a temporary abolition or diminution of pain perception), restraint, sedation and in some cases a muscular relaxation and a (para)sympathetic reflex inhibition.

It is not possible to go into anaesthetic principles in this manual in depth. The investigator (microsurgeon) is, however, referred to the outstanding books in this area by C.J. Green (1979) and P.A. Flecknell (1987).

6.2. Pre-operative care

Since anaesthesia causes a disturbance of the normal physiology and most operations put the animal under severe strain, it is essential that the animals are healthy. Chronic respiratory diseases introduce an especially high anaesthetic risk. In order to minimize the risk of losing animals after hours of exacting surgery the use of "specified pathogen-free" (SPF) animals (see Chapter 2) is strongly recommended. Besides the animal's health there are other biological factors which must be taken into account, e.g. variations in weight and age, differences between strains, sex, nutrition, acclimatization, endocrinological status, and even circadian rhythms which may influence the dose-response ratio in the experimental animal. Animals which are frequently handled and gently stroked are much easier to anaesthetize.

In several species, for example dog, cat, ferret, pig etc., preanaesthetic fasting is necessary to reduce vomiting. Since vomiting does not occur in rats, fasting is not necessary. However, fasting for a period of 12–24 hours prior to surgery on the digestive system is recommended, so that the stomach and the intestines are as empty as possible. It is wise to give the animals a glucose solution, to protect them against hypoglycaemia. Any changes in the metabolic state of the animal must be noted, as it may influence your experiment, especially when liver surgery is performed.

Pre-anaesthetic medication

Flecknell (1987), in his book about anaesthesia of the laboratory animal, gives seven reasons for pre-anaesthetic medication:

1. It reduces fear and apprehension, and aids stress-free introduction of the anaesthesia.
2. It reduces the amount of other anaesthetic agents required to induce general anaesthesia, thus decreasing the unwanted side effects of these agents.
3. It makes the introduction of anaesthesia smoother.
4. It aids towards smoother recovery from the anaesthesia.
5. It reduces salivary and bronchial secretion which might obstruct the airways.
6. It blocks the vaso-vagal reflex (bradycardia).
7. It reduces post-operative pain.

Depending upon the skills of the laboratory staff, it should be possible to administer intraperitoneal (i.p.), intramuscular (i.m.) or subcutaneous (s.c.) injections, without causing too much discomfort to the animal. The i.p. and the s.c. injections are recommended as they cause less pain to the animal. In rats pre-anaesthetic sedation is not usually required. However, if the anaesthetic is to be administered intravenously (i.v.) sedation is recommended (see also Chapter 7.2).

To achieve chemical restraint in rats, it is best to use fentanyl-fluanisone (Hypnorm) at a dosage of 0.3–0.5 ml/kg, i.p., of the undiluted solution containing 0.315 mg fentanylcitrate (equivalent to 0.2 mg fentanyl) and 10 mg fluanisone/ml. This produces a neuroleptanaesthesia with poor muscle relaxation. The action of Hypnorm can be reversed by the morphine antagonist naloxone (0.1 mg/kg, i.v.). This can be of use when respiration is depressed and cyanosis develops, or when recovery must be accelerated. It is better, however, to use buprenorphine (Temgesic) which is also used to reduce post-operative pain. Using the correct dosage Hypnorm will produce in about 5 minutes an analgesia and sedation which will last for 20–30 minutes. This neuroleptanaesthesia allows small superficial surgery such as cardiac puncture.

Diazepam (Valium) or midazolam (Dormicum) induce good sedation and muscle relaxation at a dosage of 4 mg/kg, i.p. or s.c.

Ketamine (25–60 mg/kg, i.m.) induces deep sedation with poor muscle relaxation and only superficial analgesia.

To reduce excessive saliva production, bronchial secretion and contraction, and to protect the heart against parasympathetic (vagal) inhibition, it is useful to administer atropine at a dosage of 0.05–0.1 mg/kg i.p. or s.c.

6.3. General anaesthesia

Injectable agents

The combination of 0.3–1.0 ml/kg (i.p.) Hypnorm (depending upon the required duration) and 3.0–5.0 mg/kg diazepam (Valium) or midazolam (Dormicum) will produce profound analgesia and sufficient muscle relaxation to allow intra-abdominal and intra-thoracic surgery for from 15 to over 30 minutes. Additional doses of Hypnorm (0.1 ml/kg, i.p.) can be given to prolong the anaesthetic period. A very sophisticated way of administering the above mentioned anaesthetic combination of fentanyl/fluanisone/midazolam, is by mixing one part of midazolam with two parts of water and one part of Hypnorm. This is called the FFM-mixture and gives, at a dosage of 3.4 ml/kg (i.p.), a medium to long term anaesthesia. Combination of FFM with atropine (0.05–0.1 mg/kg, i.p. or s.c.) is expedient.

The combination of ketamine (25–60 mg/kg, i.p.) and xylazine (2.5 mg/kg, i.p.) provides about 30 minutes of surgical anaesthesia, and must be used in combination with atropine. Additional doses of ketamine (20–40 mg/kg) can be given every 10–20 minutes to prolong anaesthesia.

Alphaxolone-alphadolone (10–12 mg/kg, i.v.) produces a medium surgical anaesthesia of short duration, approximately 5–12 minutes, with a rapid onset of action (approximately 20 seconds). If the bolus injection is followed by an intravenous infusion of 0.2 mg/kg/min, a prolonged period of anaesthesia can be induced. Rats are in general fully recovered after about one hour. Due to the unpredictable responses in rats, alphaxolone-alphadolone should not be given i.p. or i.m.

Despite the fact that pentobarbitone is probably the most commonly used laboratory animal anaesthetic, the high variability in response of rats to barbiturates, makes its use here less reliable. The use of pentobarbitone is therefore best avoided as safer and more effective agents are available. Moreover, at a dosage of 30–60 mg/kg i.p. severe respiratory depressions are brought about and the mortality rate is high.

Another commonly used anaesthetic is urethane, which induces a long lasting stable anaesthesia with low cardiovascular and respiratory system depression. However, urethane is carcinogenic, making it potentially dangerous to the user. Moreover, animals which have been anaesthetized with urethane should not be allowed to recover.

Injectable anaesthetics which are expelled from the circulation by the liver are contra-indicated during hepatic surgery, as the recovery period can be severely prolonged.

Inhalation anaesthetics

The induction of anaesthesia in rats, is most conveniently done by inhalation anaesthesia, using an anaesthetic chamber made of inert transparent material such as perspex. Anaesthetic vapour should preferably be supplied from an anaesthetic machine (Figure 6.3.1.). Unfortunately, however, it is common practice to anaesthetize rats in a glass chamber containing cotton wool which is moistened with liquid anaesthetic. The direct contact of the animal with the vaporizing liquid is highly unpleasant causing freezing of the skin and irritation of the mucous membranes. A further disadvantage is the unpredictably high concentration of the anaesthetic.

Following induction, anaesthesia should be maintained by placing the animal in front of a small face mask connected to the anaesthetic machine (Figure 6.3.2.).

Open methods for laboratory rat anaesthesia are widely used because they are relatively simple and inexpensive. Here, however, a lot of anaesthetic agent is wasted, and high concentrations of unused anaesthetic may be formed in the environment. As there is a great difference in concentration of anaesthetic gas, it is also hard to maintain a stable and profound surgical anaesthesia.

Many of these drawbacks are eliminated when an anaesthetic machine is used. The total gas flow from the anaesthetic machine should at least be 2.5–3 times the minute volume of the rat ($\pm$0.22 l/min), i.e. 550–660 ml/min.

Endotracheal intubation of the rat allows for assisted ventilation when necessary (see section 6.5.). After some practice, intubation is easy to perform and this technique is strongly recommended when repeated or prolonged administration of anaesthetic gases or artificial respiration with a mechanical ventilator is indicated (intrathoracic surgery). Long-term anaesthesia can also be induced via an injectable anaesthetic, followed by intubation and maintenance via an inhalation anaesthetic.

In every instance it is very important to provide the breathing circuit with a waste anaesthetic gas scavenging system (Figure 6.3.2.). Halothane with N_2O and O_2 is an excellent agent, with an induction time of 2 to 3 minutes and a smooth recovery time of between 5 to 10 minutes, depending upon the duration of the anaesthesia. N_2O and O_2 (2:1 or 1:1) are delivered at a total rate of flow of 600–800 ml/min, and the halothane concentration is adjusted according to its effect from between 1–2%. During the induction of the anaesthesia the halothane concentration can be raised to 4%, but must be reduced as soon as possible.

The halogenated methyl-ethyl ethers like isoflurane, enflurane and methoxyflurane can also be used, especially during liver surgery. Their specific characteristics are reviewed by Wade and Stevens (1981). For further information, the reader is referred to Flecknell (1987) and Green (1979).

Ether (diethyl-ether) is one of the most popular volatile anaesthetic agents. It is a very good analgesic, it gives excellent muscle relaxation and it is inexpensive. However, it has several drawbacks one of which being the considerable amount of excitation during induction. Furthermore ether is unpleasant for the animal, because of its irritant properties which affect the mucosal lining of the mouth and the respiratory tract. This irritation is mostly followed by bronchial and salivary secretion and in some cases respiratory infections may develop. Ether also stimulates the sympathetic nervous system, which leads to increased catecholamine levels in rats. Ether is highly flammable and forms explosive mixtures with both oxygen and air. In traditional anaesthetic chambers ("ether jars"), ether can form toxic compounds (peroxides), which can cause severe respiratory depression.

6.4. Management during anaesthesia

Following induction of anaesthesia we have to maintain anaesthesia of the animal for a certain length and depth required for the operation, whilst keeping the physiological state of the animal as near normal as possible.

Depth of anaesthesia

Anaesthesia is applied to block the perception of pain, therefore the absence of response to a painful stimulus is by definition essential. In the rat, pinching of the tail or the interdigital skin (pedal reflex) is a useful test to determine the level of surgical anaesthesia. Changes of colour in rats is best seen at the ears and feet (only for albino rats) and the mucosa of the mouth. If they become cyanotic or extremely pale it shows a low oxygen level in the blood, mostly caused by bad circulation. Rate and depth of respiration as well as the colour of the liver and pulsation of blood vessels (during abdominal surgery) also supply useful information concerning anaesthesial depth.

Temperature

Since the central heat-regulating mechanism is depressed during anaesthesia, small animals like rats lose a great deal of heat at their body surface and from their respiratory tract, causing a rapid fall in temperature. If no special precautions are taken, the body temperature can, depending on the anaesthetic, fall within 20 minutes to 33° C, and after one hour temperatures below 30° C can be reached. This hypothermia often causes untimely death of the animal. Therefore temperature should be monitored and maintained within the physiological range. Thermostatically controlled heated pads (Figure 6.4.1.) are commercially available and must be used even during short time anaesthesia, because hypothermia develops very rapidly in rats and is a frequent cause of anaesthetic death. Care must, however, be taken not to burn the animal (pad temperature < 41° C).

In order to avoid heat loss via the respiratory tract during inhalation anaesthesia, the anaesthetic gases must be warmed and humidified (Figure 6.3.1.).

Fluid balance

Hypovolaemia causes cardiovascular failure eventually leading to untimely death of the animal. Especially during prolonged abdominal and thoracical surgery fluid loss can be excessive. A further loss of water occurs through evaporation from the respiratory tract. As already mentioned above, warming and humidification of the anaesthetic gases is essential. As a routine during abdominal surgery, the intestines must be moistened every now and then, using warm (35° C) saline solution. If the distortion of the fluid balance is due to severe blood loss (more than 10% of the circulating volume), then replacement with whole blood obtained from a donor animal is necessary. The total amount of circulating blood in the rat is about 6 ml/100 g body weight. After a long-term operation or after a laparotomy 2–4 ml of a 0.9% NaCl (saline) solution must be injected i.p. or s.c. (not more than 1.5 ml at one place s.c.).

6.5. Endotracheal intubation

In combination with an anaesthetic circuit, endotracheal intubation allows for easy control of ventilation, and the possibility to assist the ventilation when necessary.

Intubation may be performed using an otoscope (Tran and Lawson, 1986) or a purpose made laryngoscope. In our hands, the method described below is very reliable. It requires little effort to master and uses simple readily available equipment.

After induction of anaesthesia using halothane/N_2O/O_2, alphaxalone-alphadolone (Saffan, 8–10 mg/kg, i.v.) or 2.5 ml/kg of the FFM-mixture is administered and the rat is placed on a special holder or on any other inclined plane. The jaws are opened wide using an eye lid retractor or part of a large paperclip (Figure 6.5.1.). The neck of the animal must be illuminated with a powerful light-source (Figure 6.5.2.). The light penetrating the tissues will illuminate the larynx, and the focal cords can be located (Figure 6.5.3.). The tube (Figure 6.5.4.) must then be brought via the pharynx alongside the epiglottis, through the laryngeal opening into the trachea, towards the bifurcation (Figure 6.5.5.). Endotracheal tubes for use in the rat are best made from intravenous plastic catheters (Hemalock, Angiocath or Surflo, 14, 16 or 18G). Figure 6.5.4. shows a Hemalock arterial stick (General Electric), with a silicon ring 2 cm from the tip. This ring prevents the tube from being pushed out, as it will be fixed behind the focal cords allowing no gas to escape. Figure 6.5.6. shows how the animal is gently picked up from the special holder, in order not to pull out the tube. Subsequently, the animal is attached to the mechanical ventilator (Figure 6.5.7.).

After some practice it may be possible to omit the Saffan or FFM anaesthesia and only use halothane/N_2O/O_2.

6.6. *Controlled ventilation*

Respiration is often depressed by anaesthetics, causing hypercapnia (elevated level of CO_2), respiratory acidosis and hypoxia. Both depth and frequency of ventilation are of vital importance, and it may sometimes be necessary to assist the spontaneous ventilation. During operations in which the thoracic cavity is opened, controlled ventilation is a requisite.

Mechanical ventilators allow an accurate adjustment of:
1. Inspiration/expiration ratio
2. Pressure build up in the airways
3. Volume of delivered anaesthetic gas
4. Frequency

Respiration data for the rat are:

Inspiration/expiration ratio	1:2
Maximal pressure	2 kPa
Tidal volume (approximate)	0.0062 × bodyweight in gram
Respiratory frequency	70–150/min

The tidal volume is the volume of gas which is drawn into the respiratory tract with every breath. Multiplication of the tidal volume and the frequency gives us the minute volume. The tidal volume can be calculated in rats with a body weight of more than 250 g, with the above mentioned formula. For animals weighing less than 250 g, the multiplication factor is 0.0067.

The "Amsterdam infant ventilator MK 3" (Figure 6.6.1.), originally designed for pediatric anaesthesia, is very well suited as a mechanical ventilator for rats. It has a low dead space, especially when used with an adapted Luer fitting. The so-called intermittent positive pressure ventilation (I.P.P.V.) should be employed at a carefully calculated rate, and a tidal volume calculated with the above given formula. The I.P.P.V. can be combined with a "positive end expiratory pressure" (P.E.E.P.) for the maintenance of a residual pressure, which maintains an alveolar distension thus preventing pulmonary oedema.

6.7. *Anaesthesia in pregnant rats*

Pregnant rats require special care when anaesthetized. Hypotension can be dangerous to the foetuses because of reduced placental blood flow. Bad maternal respiration can cause hypercapnia, which in turn can result in a fatal respiratory acidosis in the foetuses. It is therefore advisable to carry out endotracheal intubation and assist ventilation. Virtually all anaesthetics cross the placenta, and provide some degree of anaesthesia in the foetuses allowing surgical procedures to be performed. When the mother is sufficiently deeply anaesthetized, preferably using a volatile anaesthetic like halothane/N_2O/O_2 (1:1), which allows a good oxygenation, the foetuses will also have reached an acceptable level of analgesia.

It is extremely stressful immediately prior to parturition to move the animal. Therefore one must not transport animals to the operating theatre in the awaken state, and pre-anaesthetic medication should preferably be given within the animal house.

For induction, the combination Hypnorm/midazolam in conjunction with atropine is preferred. After induction, general anaesthesia should be maintained using N_2O/O_2/halothane. If this type of anaesthesia is not available, then FFM (i.p.) should be used.

The normal duration of pregnancy is between 20 and 22 days but this can be increased to 24 days when for example barbiturates are used to induce anaesthesia for the operation. Use of other anaesthetics such as the combination Hypnorm/midazolam in conjunction with atropine, has not been seen to prolong the pregnancy.

After the operation the mother animal must be transported before awakening and replaced exactly on the same spot within the animal house.

6.8. Post-operative care

Recovery

The room in which the animals are to recover must be warm (27–30° C) and quiet. This temperature can be achieved by placing the rat's cage on a heating pad, in a room where the temperature is between 21 and 25° C. If the animal is allowed to recover in its own cage with wood-shavings as bedding, it is wise to cover the bedding with tissue paper, which is less irritant and less dangerous to the recovering animal (airway obstruction).

Inhospitable recovery conditions such as a cold or noisy environment, will cause a lot of stress for the animal. This can lead to enhanced levels of catecholamines and corticosteroids (up to four times the control value) if allowed to continue for several hours up to half a day. These enhanced levels can drastically interfere with the results obtained from these animals. One has to be aware of these stress-induced rises in corticosteroid levels, especially during transplantation research.

Management of post-operative pain

Pain in rats is often accompanied by immobility. For example after a laparotomy the back of the animal may be arched to reduce tension on the abdominal muscles. As it is not always easy for the research worker to recognize signs of pain (Soma, 1987), it is good practice to administer analgesics for 24–72 hours post-operatively (Flecknell, 1987; Spinelli, 1987). The long-acting, potent, partial morphine antagonist buprenorphine to be administered at a dosage of 0.1–0.5 mg/kg s.c., two times in the first 24 hours after the operation, is the drug of choice in rats. Buprenorphine can also be used to reverse respiratory depression after Hypnorm anaesthesia.

6.9. Euthanasia

The act of euthanasia involves the killing of an animal with a minimum of physical and mental suffering. Rats are best euthanized using a moistened 65% CO_2/O_2 gas mixture. Unconsciousness is induced very quickly, peacefully and painlessly within 45 sec of exposure. Subsequently, the CO_2 percentage should be raised to 100% and the animal should be left for 20 minutes, to make sure that it is dead.

Another recommended method of rat euthanasia is a rapid intravenous or intrathoracic injection with pentobarbitone (100 mg/kg).

References

Flecknell, P. A. (1987) Laboratory animal anaesthesia: an introduction for research workers and technicians. Academic Press, London.

Green, C. J. (1979) Animal anaesthesia. Laboratory animals LTD, London.

Soma, L. R. (1987) Assessment of animal pain in experimental animals. Lab. Animal Sci. Special Issue January 1987.

Spinelli, J. S. (1987) Reducing pain in laboratory animals. Lab. Animal Sci. Special Issue January 1987.

Tran, D. Q. and Lawson, D. (1986) Endotracheal intubation and manual ventilation of the rat. Laboratory Animal Sci. 36: 540–541.

Wade, J. G. and Stevens, W. C. (1981) Isoflurane: An anesthetic for the eighties? Anesth. and Analg., 60: 666–682.

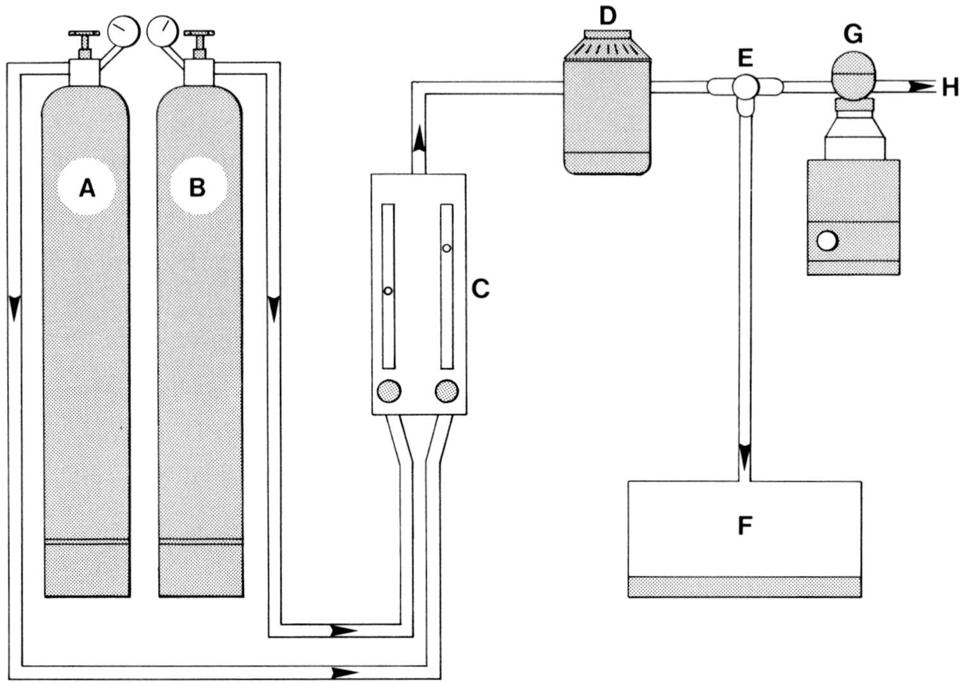

Figure 6.3.1. Schematic presentation of the anaesthetic machine.
A. N_2O-cylinder.
B. O_2-cylinder.
C. Flowmeter block (Rotameter).
D. Vaporiser.
E. Three-way valve.
F. Anaesthetic chamber.
G. Humidifier (heater).
H. Connection to the face mask or the mechanical ventilator.

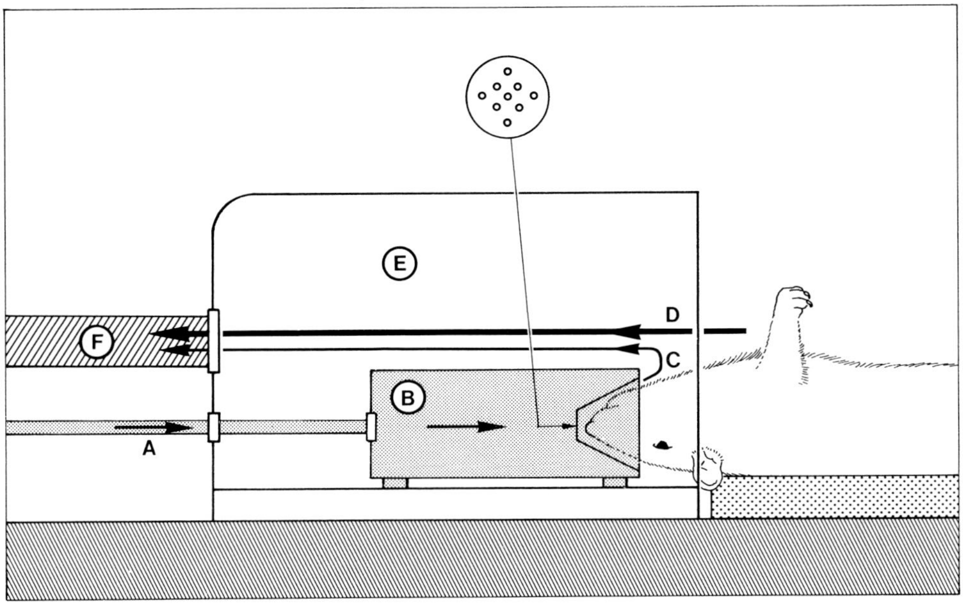

Figure 6.3.2. Breathing circuit with a waste anaesthetic gas scavenging system.
A. N_2O/O_2/Halothane gas flow.
B. The face mask.
C. Waste anaesthetic and exhaled gases.
D. Air flow.
E. Scavenger.
F. Exhaust.

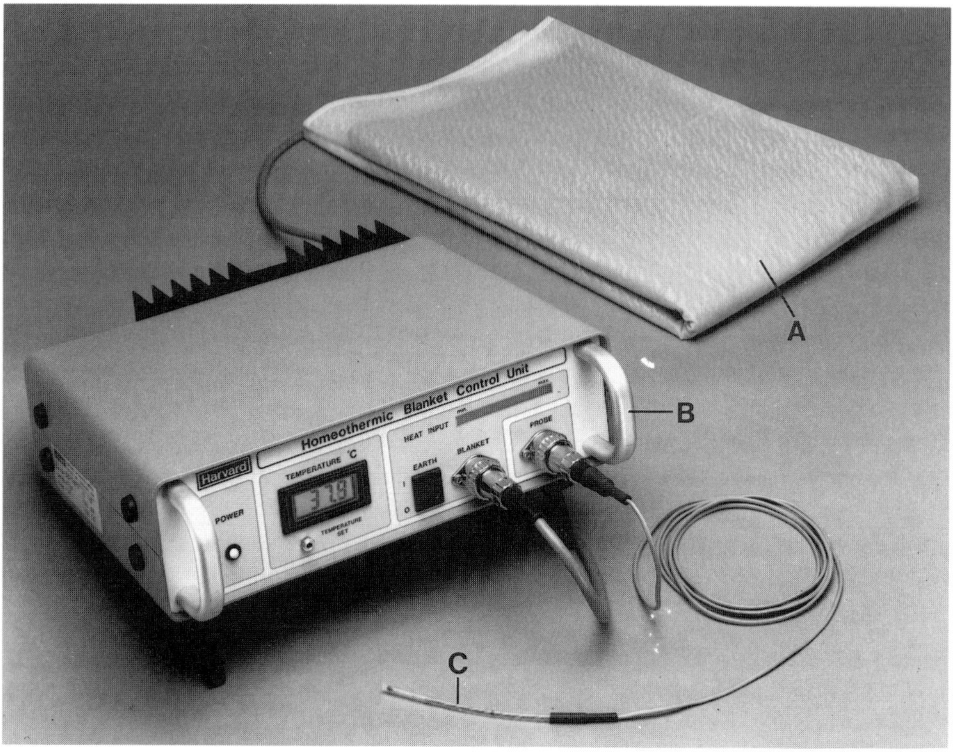

Figure 6.4.1. Homeothermic blanket system.
A. The blanket.
B. The control unit.
C. The thermistor probe.

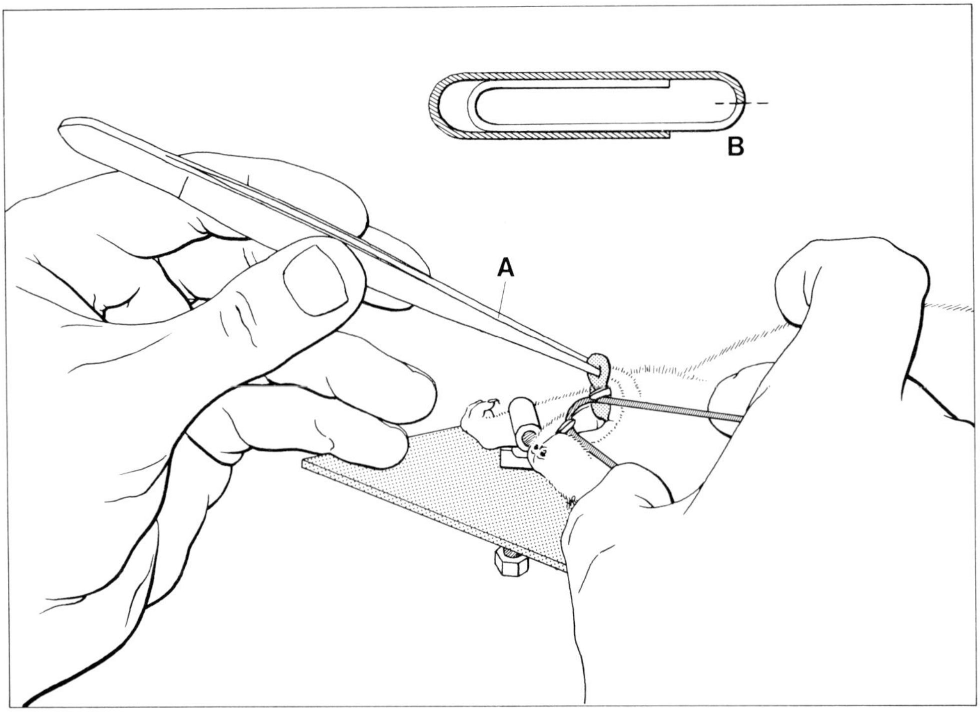

Figure 6.5.1. Endotracheal intubation (I).
The tongue is slightly retracted with surgical forceps and a part of a large paperclip is pushed between the incisors.
A. Surgical forceps.
B. Large paperclip, of which the shaded part is used.

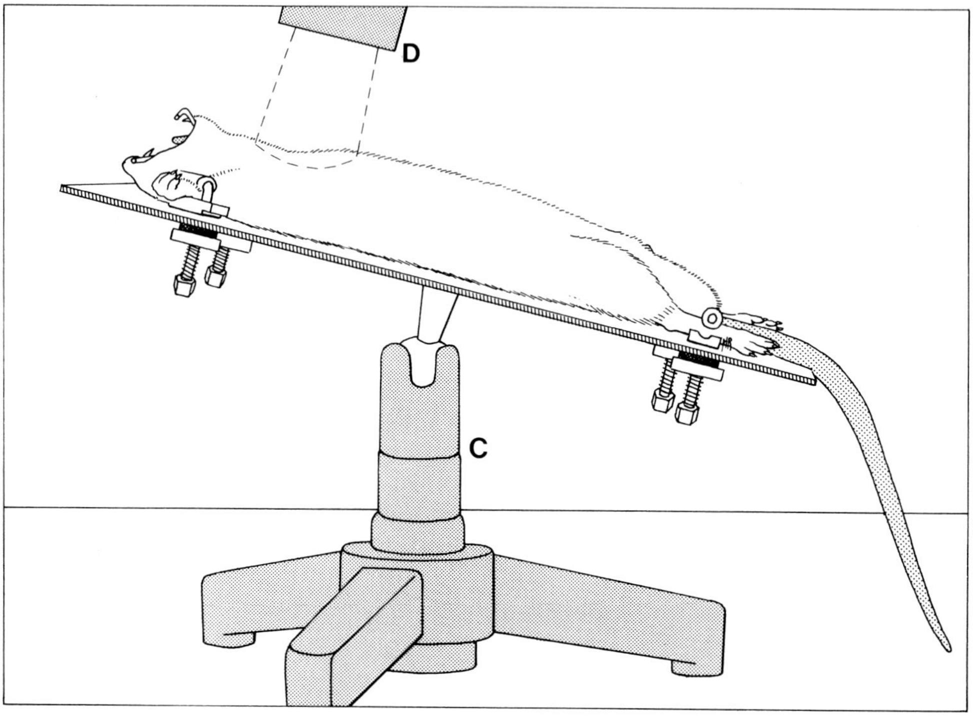

Figure 6.5.2. Endotracheal intubation (II).
Transillumination of the neck gives good visability of the vocal cords.
C. Adjustable small operation table.
D. Light source.

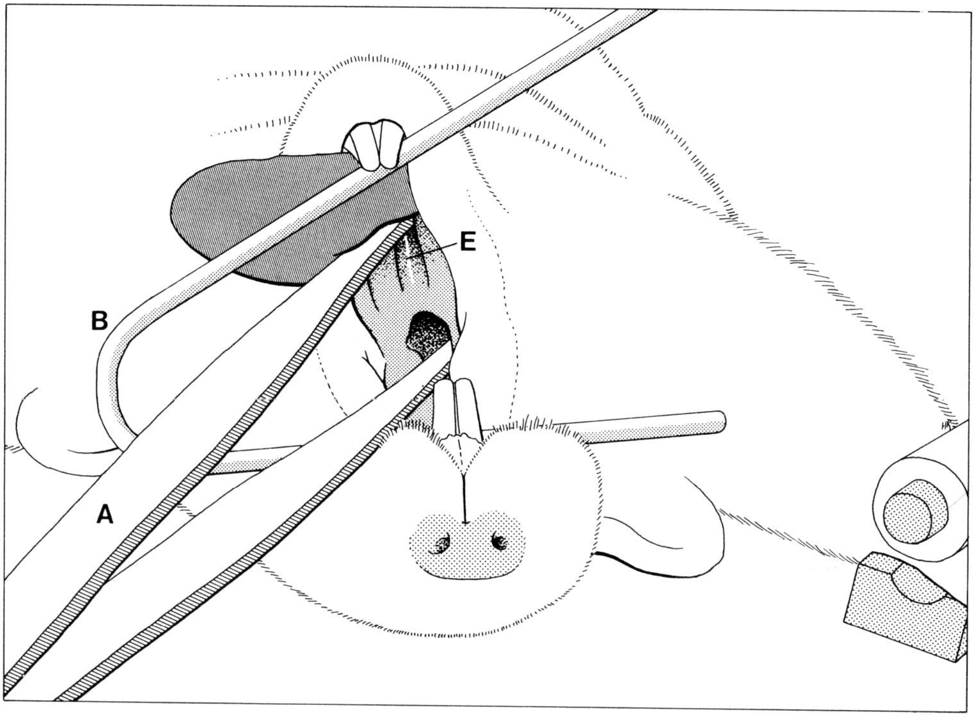

Figure 6.5.3. Endotracheal intubation (III).
View of the laryngeal cavity. The tongue has been pushed up by a pair of forceps. The vocal cords are opened and closed during respiration. When they are open, a clear light-red spot can be seen against the dark-red background.
A. Surgical forceps.
B. Modified paperclip.
E. Area where the vocal cords are located.

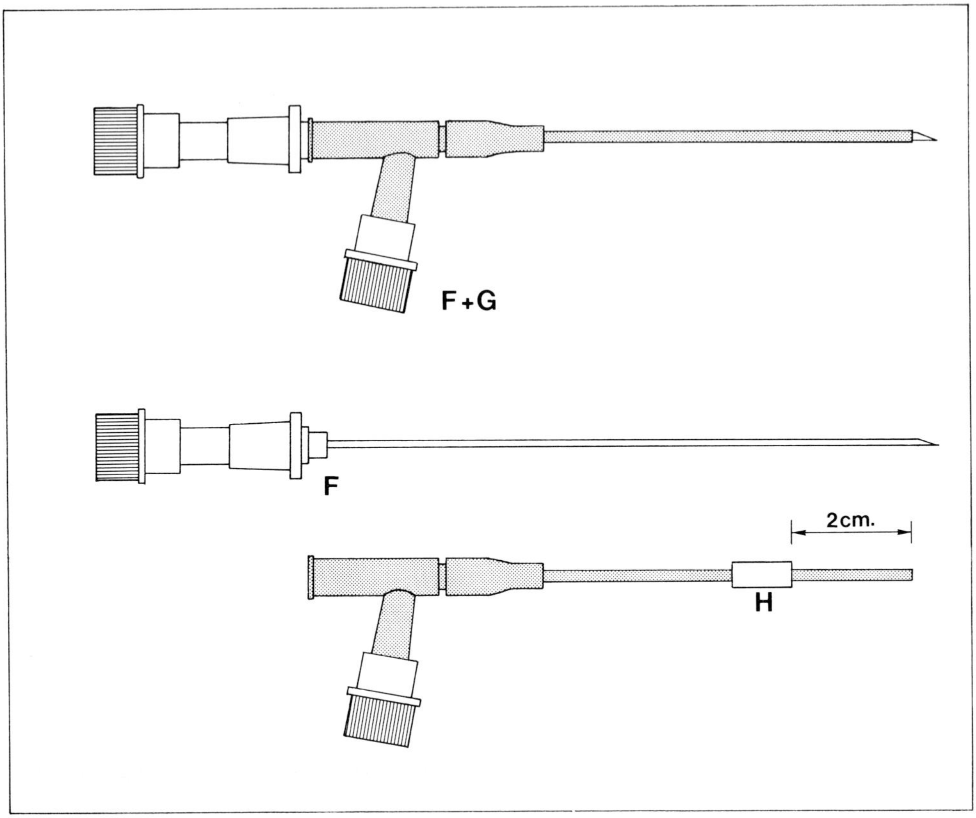

Figure 6.5.4. Endotracheal intubation (IV).
Drawing of the Hemalock arterial stick (General Electric), which is used as a tube for endotracheal intubation (F+G). Before insertion into the trachea, the needle (F) is removed and a small piece of silicon tubing (H) is put around the tube to prevent leakage of anaesthetic gas.

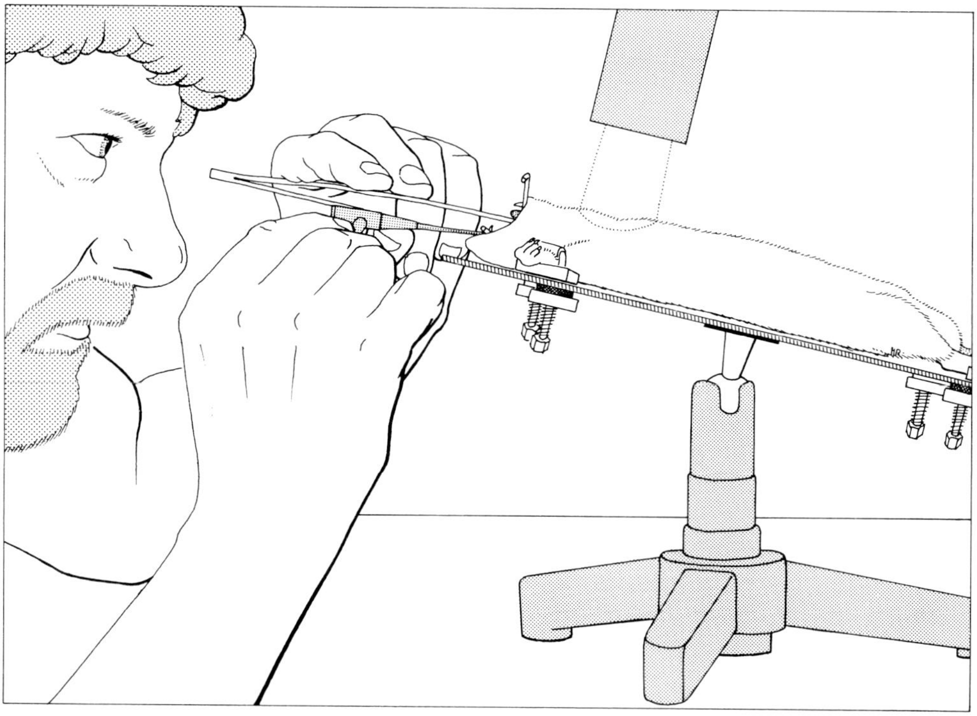

Figure 6.5.5. Endotracheal intubation (V).
The eye of the microsurgeon is in line with the forceps and the animal. The tube is gently pushed into the trachea without damaging the vocal cords.

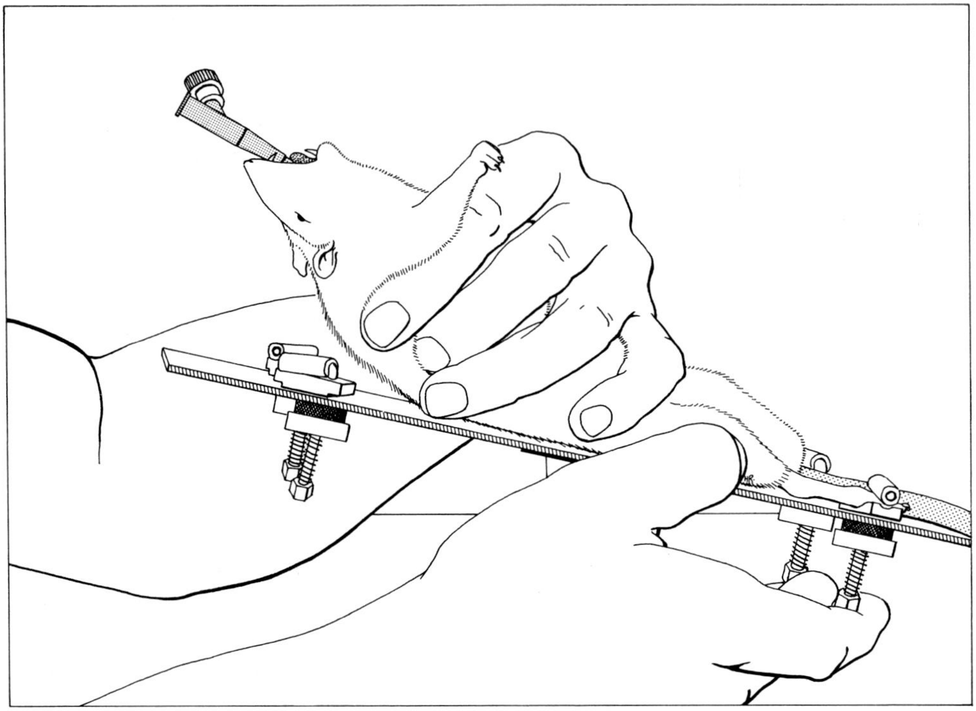

Figure 6.5.6. Endotracheal intubation (VI).
The intubated animal should be removed carefully from the intubation-table.

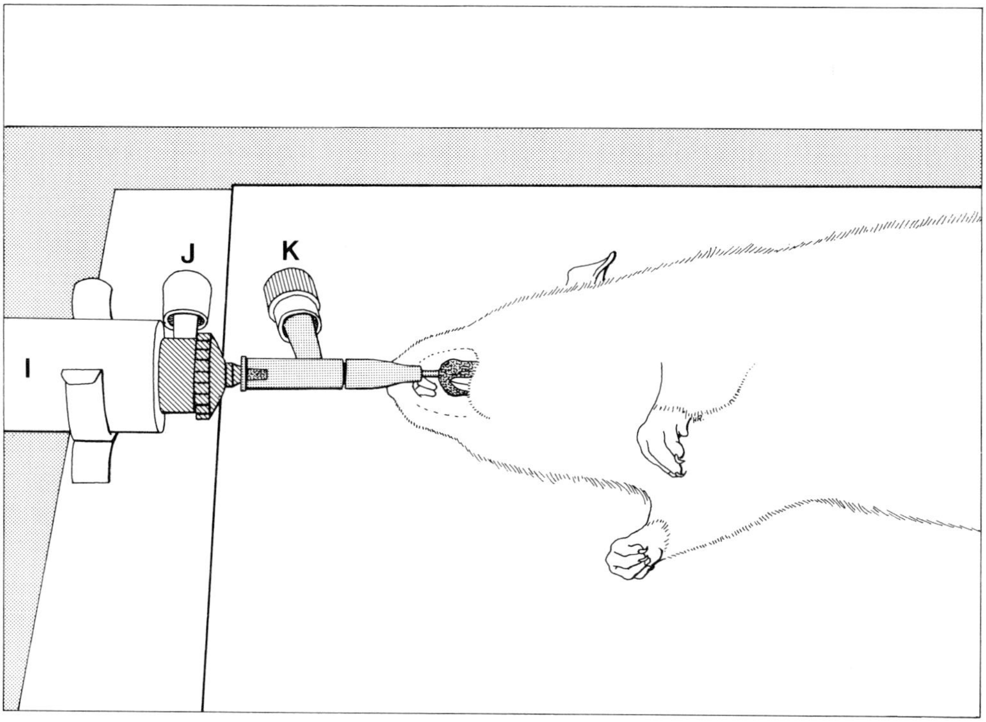

Figure 6.5.7. Endotracheal intubation (VII).
The endotracheal tube is connected via a low dead-volume adapter to the anaesthetic circuit. The sidepiece (K) is normally closed, but can be opened to remove mucus from the endotracheal tube.

I. Connector of the anaesthetic machine.
J. Low dead-volume connector.
K. Sidepiece.

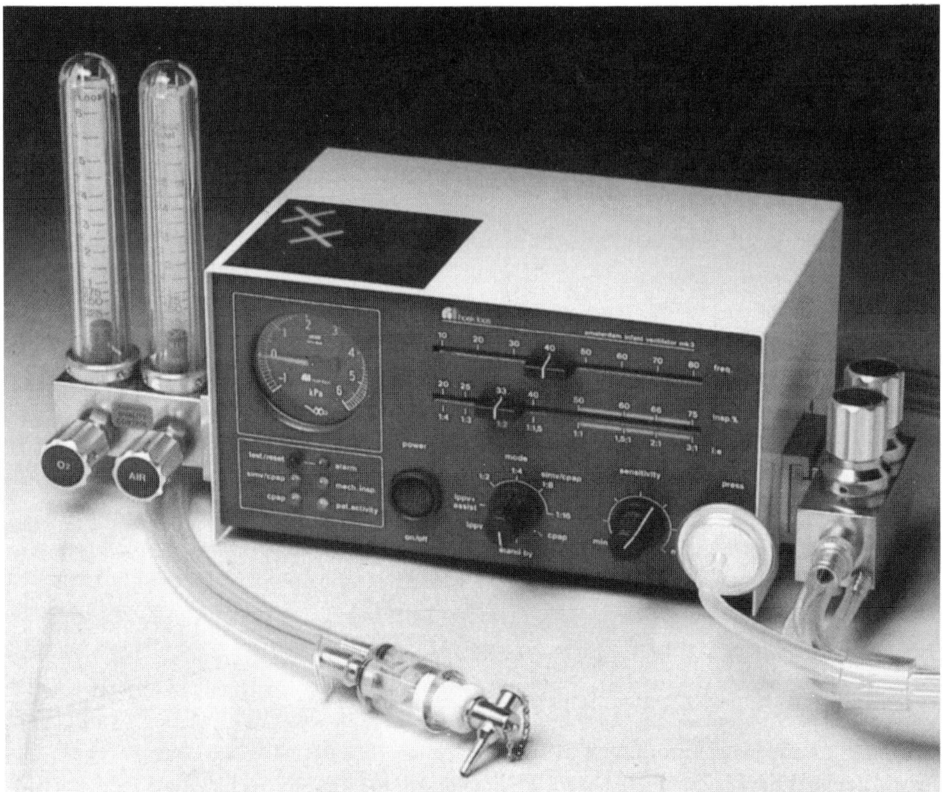

Figure 6.6.1. The mechanical ventilator.

Manual of Microsurgery on the Laboratory Rat, Part I
Van Dongen, Remie, Rensema and Van Wunnik (eds)
© 1990 Elsevier Science Publishers B.V. (Biomedical Division)

CHAPTER 7

General techniques

R. REMIE, J.J. VAN DONGEN, J.W. RENSEMA and
G.H.J. VAN WUNNIK

7.1. Introduction

In this chapter you will find general information about rat experiments, and about some special equipment used during surgery or afterwards. For easy reference, some procedures which are repeatedly used in operation techniques are described here. In the respective chapters reference is made to this chapter.

7.2. Injections and other administerings

Practical considerations
Drugs or other compounds which are water-soluble should preferably be dissolved in sterile saline solution (0.9% NaCl weight/volume (w/v)) or in distilled water for injection (aqua ad injectabilita) for all the different routes of administration. Less soluble compounds need a more complex solvent like 50% (volume/volume (v/v)) dimethylsulphoxide (DMSO) in saline or other combinations.

For insoluble compounds a homogeneous suspension is required. A 10% (w/v) of gum arabic is suitable, as is a 0.5% (w/v) of gum tragacanth, or a 0.5–4% (w/v) of carboxymethyl-cellulose (CMC).

In case the compound is only lipid-soluble, various types of oil can be used. Vegetable oils such as olive-, maize- and arachis oil are preferred to mineral oils like paraffin oil. If fat-soluble compounds are to be injected intravenously, this can be best administered as an emulsion using a proper emulsifier (lecithin or gum arabic).

Injection volumes

Injection volumes are of course limited and will depend mainly on the route of administration. Table I summerizes the safe injection volumes for the most common routes of administration in a rat of 250 g.

TABLE I

Intravenous (i.v.)	1.0 ml
Intraperitoneal (i.p.)	5.0 ml
Intramuscular (i.m.)	0.25 ml
Subcutaneous (s.c.)	2.0 ml
Intragastric (i.g.)*	5.0 ml

*The maximum volume to be injected depends upon the degree of stomach filling.

Rate of injection

In general all injections must be administered slowly, and one must pay attention to the state of the animal's respiration during the injection.

Injections by the i.p., s.c. and i.g. routes can be carried out more quickly. Factors that may influence the rate of injection are, for example, the physiological/pharmacological effect of the compound, its concentration, and the pH of the solution to be injected. Rats can tolerate quite a wide range of pH (from pH 4.5–8.0), but to let the blood buffer the pH difference, one must inject very slowly.

If possible all fluids to be injected should be at room temperature (or even warmer).

Needle size

Hypodermic needles are made of stainless steel and have a plastic hub of differing colours. Needles are made in different sizes and lengths, and are usually categorized by a gauge (G) number. The plastic hub colour refers to a coding for the diameter of the needle. This is shown in Table II which shows gauge number (British Standard), corresponding diameter in mm and the colour. As a general rule, one must use the needle with the smallest diameter that is compatible with the nature (viscosity or particle size) of the compound to be administered. Needles are inexpensive and should be disposed of after use. A blunt needle causes much more pain to the animal than a sharp one, and also makes the injection more difficult. It goes without saying that the thinner the needle, the lesser the pain inflicted.

For i.v., i.p., i.m., and s.c. injections (see Table I) of aqueous solutions, a 25G or smaller needle is recommended. For viscous solutions a larger diameter of up to 21G may be necessary.

TABLE II

The most frequently used hypodermic needles

G–No.	DIAM. (mm)	COLOUR	G–No.	DIAM. (mm)	COLOUR
30	0.30		21	0.80	Green
29	0.35		20	0.90	Yellow
28	0.38		19	1.00	Cream
27	0.42	Grey	18	1.20	Pink
26	0.45	Brown	17	1.40	
25	0.50	Orange	16	1.70	
24	0.55	Purple	15	1.80	
23	0.60	Blue	14	2.10	
22	0.70	Black			

Intravenous injections

– The tail vein injection.

The two ventro-lateral veins of the rat's tail can be used. Prior to the insertion of a 25G needle, the tail should be immersed for two minutes in hot water (40° C) or held under a heating lamp, to dilate the veins. To ensure good venous filling and a higher percentage of successful injections, an assistant must apply pressure at the root of the tail using his fingers. The veins are immediately beneath the skin and must be entered at a shallow angle (Figure 7.2.1.). Pulling the tail during injection must be avoided because the caudal vertebra will occlude the veins possibly causing damage to the vessel.

– The dorsal penile vein injection.

This vein provides an excellent route for intravenous administration. The penis is pushed out by gently pressing its base, and should be held at the glans penis with the thumb and the index finger (Figure 7.2.2.). The penile vein is easily seen and entered with a 25G needle.

– The dorsal metatarsal vein injection.

This vein can be seen after clipping the dorsal surface of the foot and swabbing it with alcohol. Figure 7.2.3. shows how to put pressure on the vein using the index and the middle finger, whilst holding the toes with the ring finger and the thumb. The vein is easily seen and can be entered with a 25G or a smaller needle. The thumb can be used as a steadying support, as the needle is pushed into the vein.

Intraperitoneal injection

Figure 7.2.4. shows how the rat is held with its head slightly down. It is important to keep the head of the animal down during the injection, as this will help to prevent the needle from entering the gastro-intestinal tract, which would move down in the direction of the diaphragm.

The needle must be inserted into the left caudal area of the abdomen as viewed by the surgeon. This is the best place for this injection as there are no vital organs except for the small intestine in this area (Figure 7.2.5.). In the right caudal area of the abdomen is the caecum and in the middle the urinary bladder which could be punctured. Use, if possible, a short 25G needle and enter the abdomen with a short thrust. Slight aspiration (20 μl) will tell you if you punctured a vein or if your needle has entered the intestine.

Intramuscular injection
The region of the biceps femoris, the semitendinosus, and the gluteus superficialis are the most frequently used muscles for i.m. injections. Figure 7.2.6. shows an injection in the caput pelvis of the biceps femoris (Figure 7.2.7.). A short 25G needle should be used, taking care not to insert it too deeply, to avoid causing any damage to the underlying nerves. Figure 7.2.6. also shows how the rear limb is stretched during the injection. Short aspiration causing a vacuum ensures that the needle is not pushed into a blood vessel.

Subcutaneous injection
Restrain the animal by grasping the skin of the scruff of the neck as shown in Figure 7.2.8. The needle (25G or smaller) should be positioned in a horizontal plane and should be pushed in over its total length. This is not the only place suitable for s.c. injection. Figure 7.2.9. shows an alternative, which can be used if the animal has a chronically implanted cannula. If this place is chosen for the injection the animal should be anaesthetized, or at least have its head covered with a piece of cloth.

Oral administration
Oral or intragastric administration is usually carried out using a 16 or 18G, 7–11 cm long blunt needle with a bulb at the end, to prevent the needle from damaging the oesophagus or entering the laryngeal opening into the trachea. Figure 7.2.10. shows how the animal is held firmly by the skin of the neck and back, and the position in which the needle is brought down along the palatine into the oesophagus. Note that the head is immobilized and is in line with the back.

When drugs have to be administered orally to animals with implanted cannula(e), it is more practical to use minimal anaesthetic, such as Halothane/N_2O/O_2 (see Chapter 6.3.), thereby reducing the possibility of rupturing the cannula(e) when holding the animal as described above. An alternative method for intragastric administration in these animals is by gastric intubation, using a polyethylene (PE) catheter (0.75 ID $\times$ 1.45 OD) marked at a distance of approximately 10 cm. Figure 7.2.11. shows how the animal is held by an assistant and how the PE catheter is inserted.

7.3. Shaving the animal

As already mentioned in Chapter 3.6, rats have very thin hairs, which are best removed with an electrical clipper. The Favorita II (Aesculap, GT 104) is a very reliable and efficient clipper when used with a cutterhead of 1/20 mm clipping height. Figures 7.3.1. and 7.3.2. show how the anaesthetized animal should be held to be shaved, prior to abdominal surgery and implantation of a permanent jugular vein cannula. Figure 7.3.3. shows how the head is shorn.

7.4. Preparation of cannulae and other materials

Most cannulae used in the rat are made of silicon rubber. Silicon tubing is very flexible, causes little or no immunity problems, and can easily be sterilized. As a routine we use Silastic Tubing (Dow Corning) which is available in various sizes. Table III shows the length of the catheters, the diameter used for each cannula and the positioning of the silicon rings which are wrapped around the tubing.

TABLE III

CANNULA TYPE	LENGTH (cm)	I.D. × O.D. (mm)	RINGS (cm from tip)	TIP (I.D. × O.D.) (mm)
Heart cannula	10	0.51 × 0.94	4.2	
Bile cannula (prox.)	18	0.51 × 0.94	0.7 and 5	
Bile cannula (dist.)	18	0.51 × 0.94	0.7 and 5	0.30 × 0.64
Thoracic duct cannula	18	0.51 × 0.94	0.7 and 5	
Iliolumbar cannula	18	0.51 × 0.94	0.7 and 5	0.30 × 0.64
Portal vein cannula	18	0.51 × 0.94	0.7 and 5	
Renal vein cannula	18	0.51 × 0.94	0.7 and 5	
Gut cannula	15	1.57 × 2.41	0.7 and 4.5	

The heart cannula

10 cm length of tubing are required with one squarely cut end and one cut at a 45° angle. Using a felt-tipped pen, a little dot is marked on 42 mm from the squarely cut end of the tubing (the tip). Using a 20G sharpened blunt needle (hole puncturer, Figure 7.4.1.), the tip must be perforated squarely, 1.5 mm from the end. This perforation prevents the cannula from being sucked against the wall of the vena cava during blood sampling. Subsequently, a silicon ring should be wrapped around the cannula at the previously marked place, using a 20G needle pushed into the silicon glue (Figure 7.4.2.). The cannula should then be gently rotated between the thumb and the index finger of both hands, and the silicon ring is allowed to dry.

The bile cannula
The proximal bile cannula, the one that will be inserted into the common bile duct in the direction of the liver, is 18 cm long and has one square cut and one bevelled end. Silicon rings should be wrapped around the cannula at 7 mm and at 5 cm distance from the bevelled end, as described above.

The distal bile cannula, which will be inserted into the common bile duct in the direction of the gut, is also 18 cm long and has one square cut and one bevelled end. Due to the decreasing diameter of the common bile duct in the direction of the gut, the distal cannula must have a smaller tip-diameter (Figure 7.4.3.) For this reason the square cut end of the cannula should be immersed in ether, causing the tubing to dilate. When the tubing is wide enough, a 13 mm piece of small diameter Silastic tubing is inserted. Subsequently, two silicon rings are wrapped around the cannula, one at the joint of the two tubes and another 5 cm from the first. The tip should then be cut at a 45° angle, 7 mm from the first silicon ring.

The thoracic duct, renal vein and portal vein cannulae
These three cannulae resemble the proximal bile cannula, with however a tip modification. Figure 7.4.3. shows the two perforations that should be made in the tip of the cannula using a 20G hole puncturer as described above (heart cannula).

The iliolumbar cannula
The iliolumbar artery cannula is the same as the distal bile cannula. The length of the tip can be adapted at your own discretion.

The gut cannula
This cannula is the largest of all, and resembles the one shown in Figure 7.4.3. The perforations are made with a 18G hole puncturer, and the silicon rings are at 7 mm and at 4.5 cm from the tip respectively.

Preparation of a button used for the portacaval anastomosis
The button is made using a specially made copper mould in which two holes are drilled (Figure 7.4.4.). A piece of teflon tubing with an internal diameter of 1.6 mm and an external diameter of 2.3 mm is inserted into hole A, and is cut to its final length (6.5 mm). Subsequently, this piece of tubing is pushed over a metal pin with a diameter of 1.6 mm. The pin is fixed in a lathe, and a groove of 0.04 mm is made at 0.5 mm from the edge. Finally, the button is replaced into the mould (hole B) and is cut to its final form (Figure 7.4.5.). For dimensions see Figure 7.4.6.

Preparation of a swivel
Swivels must be used when for example infusions are given to a freely moving animal, or when fluids like bile are collected over a longer period of time. Several types of swivels have been described (Thomas and Mayer, 1968; Strubbe, 1974; Darracq et

al., 1980). We routinely use a modification of the one described by Darracq. This swivel is made of a 1 ml syringe and two hypodermic needles as shown in Figure 7.4.7. The swivel as described by Strubbe is extremely useful for the infusion of fluids, as it has a very low dead-volume.

Preparation of a small stainless steel L-shaped adapter
Before a cannula can be fixed to the skull, it must be connected to a stainless steel needle bent to a 90° angle (L-shaped adapter). From a 20G needle the point is removed, and the surface should be polished with emery paper. Using the device shown in Figure 7.4.8. the needle is bent to a 90° angle. As shown in the same Figure, the L-shaped adapter has one short and one longer end.

The experimental cage
Rats equiped with cannulae must be housed separately to keep them from gnawing at the polyethylene caps which seal the cannulae. The cage depicted in Figure 7.4.9. was originally designed at the Department of Animal Physiology of the Groningen University and has been adapted at the University Centre of Pharmacy in Groningen, the Netherlands. The cage itself is made of transparent material, such as PVC or Lexan, and all the other parts are made of stainless steel, making it suitable for mechanized cleaning.

7.5. Sutures and suture techniques

Sutures
Since the introduction in 1957 of the micro needle, swadged on a 7–0 silk suture, the development of micro sutures has accelerated. The two main factors in the development of micro sutures have been the material used, and the needles.

Both resorbable (polydioxanone, polyglycolic acid, and polylactic acid or combination thereof) and non-resorbable materials are used today. In microvascular surgery a great deal of experience has been gained with silk, polypropylene, nylon and polyester. The use of resorbable micro sutures, however, are still under investigation. Today the suture materials are of high quality, they cause no reactions, they pull easily through tissue and can be knotted securely. Most manifacturers of suture material provide a complete assortment of sutures for microsurgery, ranging from 7–0 (55 μm) to 12–0 (8 μm).

Alongside the sutures, the needle size has also diminished. Sutures used in microsurgery have to be atraumatic, and needles must be round-bodied with a flattened end to allow better control. The most frequently used arch length for the needle is 3/8. You must never use cutting needles in microvascular surgery. Figure 7.5.1. shows a needle, and the parameters by which it is described.

Apart from the micro sutures there is an overwhelming supply of macro sutures, both resorbable and non-resorbable, with all types of needles. For long-term strength a non-resorbable suture is a requisite. A resorbable suture is appropriate for short-term strength and for internal use. The rate of reabsorption must, however, be considered, and must correspond with the healing rate of the tissue.

Besides the eyeless swaged-on needles, eyed needles (french or split) may be used as well. Figure 7.5.2. shows how the needle, held by the needle holder, is quickly threaded.

The properties of suture materials are discussed briefly in the following paragraphs.

Braided or monofilament

Braided sutures handle well, and have a higher coefficient of friction than monofilament sutures. The knots therefore are less likely to slip. These sutures, however, do not pull through the tissue as smoothly as monofilament sutures do. Moreover, braided materials have interstices that can harbour micro organisms, which can cause local infections.

Resorbable suture materials

Plain catgut (prepared from the intestines of sheep) elicits a foreign-body response, and is rather rapidly digested and absorbed by tissue enzymes (± 8 days). Treatment of the surface of catgut with chromic acid makes the suture more resistant to these tissue enzymes. The digestion time is hereby prolonged to up to ± 25 days, proportional to the degree of chromicizing.

Synthetic suture materials such as polyglactin 910, polyglycolic acid and polydioxanone are hydrolysed, and the degradation products cause no significant tissue reaction. The resorption time of polyglactin 910 is about 70 days and that of polydioxanone about 190 days. Their tensile strength, however, is lost much more quickly, in approximately 30 and 50 days respectively.

Non-resorbable suture materials

The non-resorbable suture materials include for example silk, nylon, polyethyleneterephthalate, polypropylene, polytetrafluoroethylene and stainless steel wire. Silk is commonly used for skin and ligatures, due to its excellent handling properties. It can, however, cause local tissue reactions.

Polyethyleneterephthalate is a braided material with a very high tensile strength. The monofilament plastics are of an intermediate strength, they handle poorly, but they do pull easily through tissue.

In this manual we will state the appropriate type of suture that we used for each operation.

Macro suturing and knot tying

Several suture patterns are used in surgery on laboratory rats, for closure of muscle and skin layers.

Figure 7.5.3.A shows the interrupted suture which is used for closing small wounds. Figure 7.5.3.B shows the simple over-and-over continuous suture, which is probably the one chosen for the majority of general closure procedures. It is simple and quick to perform but has one disadvantage, in that should the suture be cut or broken shortly after the operation, the whole incision is rendered open. This, however, rarely happens if proper technique is applied.

A somewhat more complicated suture is shown in Figure 7.5.3.C and is called the interrupted horizontal mattress suture. This suture pattern is used for seromuscular layers (Halsted stitch). Figure 7.5.3.D shows a subcuticular suture, which can be used for closure of the abdominal skin, but it is rarely applied.

The basic knot in surgery is the square or reef knot (Figure 7.5.3.$E_{1,2}$). It is essential that the first tie lies flat; if it does not, a square knot will slip like a granny knot. Many surgeons routinely tie three loops as a precaution. If using multiple knots, it is not so important to use square knots.

If you turn the thread twice around the needle holder, the friction of the first loop will be improved. This can be advantageous especially when using monofilament plastics. Subsequently, the knot should be completed with a single loop as depicted in Figure 7.5.3.F.

If you lack experience, practise these suture patterns on a rubber glove.

Micro suturing and knot tying

The technique of micro suturing is basically the same as the macro suture technique, except that in microsurgery we only use the interrupted and the continuous sutures. Due to the need of an operating microscope there are additional problems, including the vulnerability of the suture material, and the unintended movements.

Initially, purely holding the needle is very difficult as it jumps around and even when you finally succeed in holding it, it seems to point in any direction other than the one required. The best way to handle a suture is by picking the thread up with your left hand, using straight jewellers forceps, approximately 2 cm from the needle. Dangle the needle until it just comes to rest on the surface below. Now you can turn the needle in whichever direction you require. Hold the needle with a needle holder or angulated forceps, 2/3 around the circumference.

When you commence a suture, make sure that the needle is set up in the needle holder in such a way that it is right in line with the direction required. When you insert the needle into the tissue, the needle tip should point horizontally (Figure 7.5.4.) to avoid an unwanted "through-stitch" or puncturing a blood vessel. The needle should pass the opposite vessel wall as illustrated in Figure 7.5.5. (for further details see part 7.6., anastomosis). Until you gain experience you should make sutures from the top right to the bottom left, in an incision which runs from the top left to the bottom right. This is the most natural and easiest direction for right-handed surgeons. After some practice, you can turn your object and try various sutures on different incisions, leading to the most difficult, which is the vertical incision. This exercise will teach you how to rotate your instruments, and how to flex or extend your wrist in order to let the needle pass through the tissue in the right direction.

Tying a knot looks very simple when you see it being done by an expert, however, it can be very frustrating in the beginning of your microsurgical career. Acland (1980) divided the procedure for tying a knot into four separate actions:

1. Picking up the thread with the right-hand forceps.
2. Making a loop on the tip of the left-hand forceps (Figure 7.5.6.(1)).
3. Picking up the short end of the thread with the right-hand forceps.
4. Pulling the loop off from the right-hand forceps and tightening the knot (Figure 7.5.6.(2)).

Figures 7.5.6.(3) and (4) show how the knot is completed. You should practice these procedures, using a rubber glove, in which you have made an incision. The fingers of a glove can also be used to practise an end-to-end anastomosis.

7.6. Anastomosis

End-to-end anastomosis (termino-terminal anastomosis)

Before starting with the anastomosis, both vessel ends must be free from blood or blood clots. This is best achieved by intraluminal irrigation, with a diluted heparin solution (10 IU/ml). The stay- or corner sutures can be placed in several ways. The most simple technique is placing the second stay suture at 180° from the first, "the symmetric biangulation". Eccentric or asymmetric biangulation was suggested by Cobbett (1967). Figure 7.6.1. shows the positioning of the first two sutures, which are placed at "10 o'clock" and at "2 o'clock". By doing this you can ensure that you do not grasp the opposite side of the vessel by mistake. Moreover, you will avoid making a through-stitch. Note that the distance between the place of insertion and the edge of the vessel is approximately 0.25–0.35 mm. The size of the bite may be varied according to the diameter of the vessel, the thickness of the vascular wall, and the size of the suture and needle. If you have trouble seeing the colourless, translucent vessel, place a piece of blue plastic beneath the vessel to gain a better view of the fine details of the vessel end. Once these (stay or corner) sutures have been made and tied, there must be some tension put on their ends in order to flatten the vessel wall and expose the anastomosis using small bulldog clamps.

When passing the needle through the vessel wall, do not take the full thickness of the tissue between the jaws of your forceps as this will cause a great deal of damage. The correct way of passing the needle through is by lifting the vessel wall at the adventitia (see Chapter 5), or by placing the left-hand forceps on the underside of the tissue (Figure 7.5.3.) and gently pushing the vessel wall up, which is then easily penetrated.

Subsequently, the needle should pass perpendicularly through the other side of the vessel wall. Again do not take the entire thickness of the vessel, but take the adventitia, or use the forceps to give some support to the top side of the vessel just beyond and beside the place where the needle should emerge (Figure 7.5.4.). As soon as the needle holder reaches the tissue, the needle must be released and can be grasped at the other side.

When pulling the needle through the tissues, you must let it follow its own curvature. If you do not let it follow its curvature, the stitch holes will become unnecessarily enlarged. After you have pulled the needle through, the thread must be pulled through in the entry-exit line direction, to reduce the damage caused to the tissue by angulation of the thread at both the entry and the exit hole. The next suture is placed at "12 o'clock" (in the middle of the stay sutures) and tied. If you succeed in dividing the circumference of the vessel into equal parts, and you make sure that the other end of the vessel matches, the edges can be brought together evenly, achieving the optimal result. If you do not, the anastomosis is destined to be crude and distorted, and stenosis will make it unsuccessful.

After you have finished the anterior wall (this is the front wall), rotate the vessel as shown in Figure 7.6.2. This can be done either by rotating the clamps, or by rotating only the sutures. Now the anterior wall has become posterior (this is the back wall). Subsequently, place a central suture in the original "6 o'clock" position. The next sutures should be placed between "6 o'clock" and "2 o'clock", and between "6 o'clock" and "10 o'clock", while the "6 o'clock" suture is placed under some tension. Depending on the diameter of the vessel between 6 and 12 sutures should be placed equidistantly. The distance between stitches must be approximately 0.35 to 0.4 mm. For example a 1–mm artery requires between 6 and 8 stitches.

In microsurgery, vessel approximators are frequently used. They are available with and without cleats to hold the stay sutures. A piece of Silastic tubing (2 mm in diameter) will ideally serve as a substitute blood vessel as you begin to master the end-to-end anastomosis technique in experimental microsurgery.

End-to-side anastomosis (termino-lateral anastomosis)

After making a hole in the vessel wall, which corresponds to the internal diameter of the vessel that will be used for the anastomosis, the stay sutures should be placed at "9 o'clock" and at "3 o'clock" and are then tied (Figure 7.6.3.). When you use a continuous suture technique, you must leave one end (the one without the needle) a little longer than the other and use it to put some tension on the anastomosis. The other end with the needle is used for suturing. If the vessel cannot be turned over for direct visualization of the posterior wall, the posterior wall should be sutured first from the inside (Figure 7.6.3.A.).

In case the vessel can be turned over, the anterior wall should be sutured first. Then, after turning over the vessel, which allows the anterior wall to become posterior, the posterior wall can be inspected from the inside. This is then followed by another anterior wall suture, completing the anastomosis (Figure 7.6.3.B.).

When you use the interrupted technique, the sutures should be placed as indicated in Figure 7.6.1.

Here again, a piece of Silastic tubing will serve ideally as a substitute blood vessel, while mastering this technique.

Techniques for veins and arteries

As already indicated above, the technique used for the anastomosis depends on a number of circumstances. Some general rules that may be of use are listed below.

Interrupted sutures are preferable when:

- the external vessel diameter is smaller than 2 mm
- performing end-to-end anastomosis between arteries
- performing end-to-end anastomosis between an artery and a vein
- vessel diameters are different
- using 9–0 or smaller sutures

If you strictly adhere to these rules, it would mean that almost every anastomosis in the rat would be made using the interrupted technique. However, there are some exceptions.

Continuous or running sutures are preferable in the rat when:

- transplanting organs (both the artery and the vein)
- performing end-to-end anastomosis between large veins
- performing end-to-end anastomosis in the gut

Advantages of a continuous suture are:

- a shorter ischaemic time for the organ to be transplanted, as no time consuming knots have to be tied
- haemostasis is achieved more rapidly because the vessel ends are sealed together better
- less tissue irritation is caused by the knots
- a better endothelialization
- easier to learn and master

Disadvantages of a continuous suture are:

- when the suture is pulled too tight, a purse-string effect will cause stenosis
- if the suture breaks, the whole procedure has to be repeated

One of the severest complications in microvascular surgery is thrombosis at the suture line. Thrombosis, however, is mainly caused by improper technique. Some of the main mistakes are listed below:

- traumatic suture technique
- a damaged intima

– a through-stitch
– inverted adventitia

7.7. Opening and closure of the abdominal wall

When the abdominal wall has been shaven and disinfected (Figure 7.7.1.), the rat is turned in a supine position and is secured to the operating table with tape. A midline incision is made from the level of the pubic bones (symphysis pubis) to the xiphoid cartilage, as shown in Figure 7.7.2., using a sharp-blunt pair of scissors. Note that the skin is slightly elevated to avoid unwanted damage to the underlying tissues (Figures 7.7.3. and 7.7.4.). Subsequently, the abdominal muscles are lifted as shown in Figure 7.7.5. and a small transverse incision is made. The tissue is spread (Figure 7.7.6.) to allow air to enter the peritoneal cavity. The abdomen is then opened by making an incision, over the linea alba towards the sternum (Figure 7.7.7.) up to the distal part of the fourth sternebra, thus exposing the xiphoid process. A small incision should then be made in the connective tissue on the left side of the xiphoid cartilage, which is the right side as viewed by the surgeon (Figure 7.7.8.). The operation which is to follow this laparotomy utilizes this small lateral incision to allow easy retraction and fixation of the left lateral lobe of the liver, together with the intestines.

The abdominal wall is closed in two layers. The first layer is the abdominal muscle (m. obliquus internus abdominis, m. obliquus externus abdominis and the m. rectus abdominis), which is closed using a continuous suture technique with a resorbable 4–0 suture as illustrated in Figures 7.7.9., 7.7.10., and 7.7.11. For ease and speed when making the suture, special attention should be payed to the position and the movement of the fingers and the forceps (Figures 7.7.11. and 7.7.12.). Figures 7.7.13., 7.7.14., and 7.7.15. show how the knot is tied in three stages. The second layer is the skin, which is closed using running suture technique with either a 4–0 resorbable or non-resorbable suture making use of the same method (Figure 7.7.16.).

7.8. Subcutaneous tunnelling of cannulae

As with the permanent jugular vein cannula, which runs subcutaneously from the neck to the crown of the head (see Chapter 8), cannulae can also be subcutaneously passed with ease from the abdomen to the crown of the head. Before you pass the cannula(e) to the head, you must have sutured the total abdominal muscle layer and the abdominal skin, leaving only about 1 cm open. Use artery forceps to secure the suture during the tunnelling procedure. Figures 7.8.1. and 7.8.2. show how the animal is held and how a slender needle holder (e.g. Ryder) is pushed subcutaneously through the connective tissue to a distance of about 8 to 10 cm. Subsequently, the point of the needle holder is turned towards the opening in the abdominal skin (Figures 7.8.3. and 7.8.4.) and is pushed out (Figure 7.8.5.). During this procedure the point of the needle holder should be as near to the skin as possible, as this will prevent it from entering any muscle layer. The cannula(e) are then grasped (Figure 7.8.6.) and pulled through to emerge at the crown of the head. Figure 7.8.7. shows how the animal must be held after the cannula(e) have been pulled through to the head. The reason behind this is to stretch the animal allowing the cannula(e) to find its/their own position without being under any tension. Finally the abdominal skin should be closed completely.

7.9. Fixation of cannulae

Preparation of the crown of the head

The head of the animal should be shaven and disinfected with a chlorhexidine solution. An incision of approximately one centimetre should be made in the crown of the head. This will provide enough space to mount three stainless steel screws (1.0 mm in diameter and 4.2 mm in length) in the crown of the skull which are used for additional anchoring. The membranous tissue should be removed, using curved jewellers forceps, and the bregma (the point on the top of the skull where the coronal and sagittal sutures meet) is then exposed. With a 3/0-round dental drill, three holes should be made, two on the left and one on the right of the bregma (Figure 7.9.1.). The stainless steel dental drill should be loosely held between the thumb and fore finger to allow rotating movements. To ensure that the underlying tissues like the dura, the rostral sagittal sinus or the transverse sinus are not punctured, the conical end of the drill is covered with a piece of polyethylene (PE) tubing leaving about 2 mm of the tip uncovered (Figure 7.9.1.). If you have access to a mechanical drill, this procedure can be carried out very quickly. The screws are fitted into the holes using specially prepared surgical forceps and a small screwdriver (Figures 7.9.2., 7.9.3., and 7.9.4.). They are tightened to such an extent, that approximately 2 mm is left between the skull and the head of the screws.

Connection of the L-shaped adapter

Prior to fixation the cannula has to be slid over the short end of the L- shaped adapter (Figure 7.9.5.). To serve this purpose you may use some diethyl-ether to make the Silastic even more supple and the cannula will slide smoothly over the stainless steel tubing.

Some catheters should now be flushed with saline (0.5 ml) and filled with a 60% polyvinylpyrolidone (MW 10.000) solution in saline with 500 IU/ml heparine (PVP-solution), which will be indicated in the respective chapters. The long end of the L-shaped stainless steel adapter should be closed with a piece of heat sealed PE-tubing (Figure 7.9.5.).

Subsequently, the cannula together with the angled adapter must be fixed to the skull with acrylic glue. Make sure the glue flows under the heads of the screws and that it is wrapped around the verticle part of the adapter as this will prevent any movement (Figure 7.9.6.). After closure of the skin with two sutures, the final result should look like Figure 7.9.7. Figures 7.9.8., 7.9.9., and 7.9.10. show several combinations of cannulae on the crown of the head.

Whenever a cannula is filled with PVP-solution you must be aware of the fact that there sometimes may be an interaction between the PVP-solution and the methylmethacrylate which forms an insoluble precipitate. Therefore you must flush the cannula and refill it with PVP-solution one day after the operation, during your routine check of the animal's condition.

7.10. Blood sampling

Cardiac puncture

In order to collect a large quantity of blood, one can perform a cardiac puncture. If you wish to re-use the animal you can, depending on the weight of the animal, collect up to 5 ml; otherwise you can collect up to 10 ml, if the animal is to be lost. If the animal is to be re-used it should be anaesthetized with halothane/N_2O/O_2, otherwise a neuroleptanaesthesia with Hypnorm or FFM can be used.

A new 20G needle and a 10 ml syringe (Luer-type without a lock) filled with 100 μl heparin (500 IU/ml) or citrate solution are required. Locate the point of maximal palpitation of the heart by placing the index finger over the fourth intercostal space as shown in Figure 7.10.1. The needle (without the syringe) should be inserted just through the skin into the intercostal muscles, next to the index finger at a 45° angle to the coronal plane (Figure 7.10.2.). With a short thrust the needle should be pushed into the heart and blood will flow out immediately. Subsequently, attach the syringe to the needle without changing its position, and blood can be withdrawn from the animal (Figure 7.10.3.). The removal of a maximum of 5 ml of blood by cardiac puncture can be repeated weekly in the same animal for several months.

Although the blood volume is rapidly restored (within 24 hours), other constituents of the blood may require a much longer time to return to normal values.

Taking blood samples from the heart catheter (permanent jugular vein cannula)

– Sampling procedures

Sampling of blood from the general circulation takes place as follows: A 40 cm long polyethylene tube (OD 1.45 mm, ID 0.75 mm) filled with saline and stoppered with a small nail, should be attached to the steel tubing at the top of the head. During the sampling procedure, the tube is clamped with curved forceps. A 1 ml syringe is connected to the polyethylene tube and a few drops of blood mixed with PVP-solution are aspirated and discarded. Subsequently, 0.2 ml of saline should be pushed in, to clear the tube. This should then be followed by 2 μl of a heparinized saline solution (500 IU/ml) and a small air bubble should be introduced by opening the tube briefly. More saline should then be injected until the first air bubble has reached the stainless steel tubing. A second air bubble is introduced as a "marker", and injected to a distance of approximately 4 cm. The first air bubble should now be almost at the end of the catheter and will be separated from the circulation by the 2 μl heparin solution (Figure 7.10.4.).

When a sample is taken, the content of the polyethylene tube is aspirated until blood just enters the nozzle of the syringe. A clean syringe is used to take the sample. The first air bubble prevents the blood mixing with the heparin solution, thus ensuring that there is no mixture of blood from the preceding sample with the new sample to be taken. After sampling, the procedure described above must be repeated. At the end of the experiment the polyethylene tubing is removed, and the cannula is refilled with 100 μl of PVP-solution.

This method allows for frequent or even continuous sampling of blood from the general circulation, and also for the administration of drugs as a single dosage or by infusion, using sterile solutions (Steffens, 1969). Animals can be used for several months, if the proper operation and sample technique is applied. If not, fibrogenous tissue will be formed around the tip of the cannula, and the patency will be reduced to several weeks or less.

The sampling procedure can also be applied to other cannulae. However, the distance to which the marker air bubble has to be pushed into the polyethylene tubing must be recalculated, depending on the internal diameter, and the length of the Silastic tubing used for the cannulation of the vessel.

References

Acland, R.D. (1980) Microsurgery practice manual. The C.V. Mosby Company, St. Louis, Toronto, London.

Cobbett, J. (1967) Small vessel anastomosis –a comparison of suture techniques. British Journal of Plastic Surgery, 20: 16–20.

Darracq, C., Conzalez, P., and Balabaud, C. (1980) Double and single swivel joints for infusion and/or body fluid collection of free moving animals. Physiol. and Behav., 25: 327–329.

Steffens, A.B. (1969) A method for frequent sampling of blood and continuous infusion of fluids in the rat without disturbing the animal. Physiol. Behav. 4: 833–836

Strubbe, J.H. (1974) A small swivel joint for infusion of free moving animals. Physiol. and Behav., 12: 317–319.

Thomas, D.W., and Mayer, J. (1968) A simple and inexpensive swivel joint for the infusion of unrestrained animals. Physiol. and Behav., 3: 499–500.

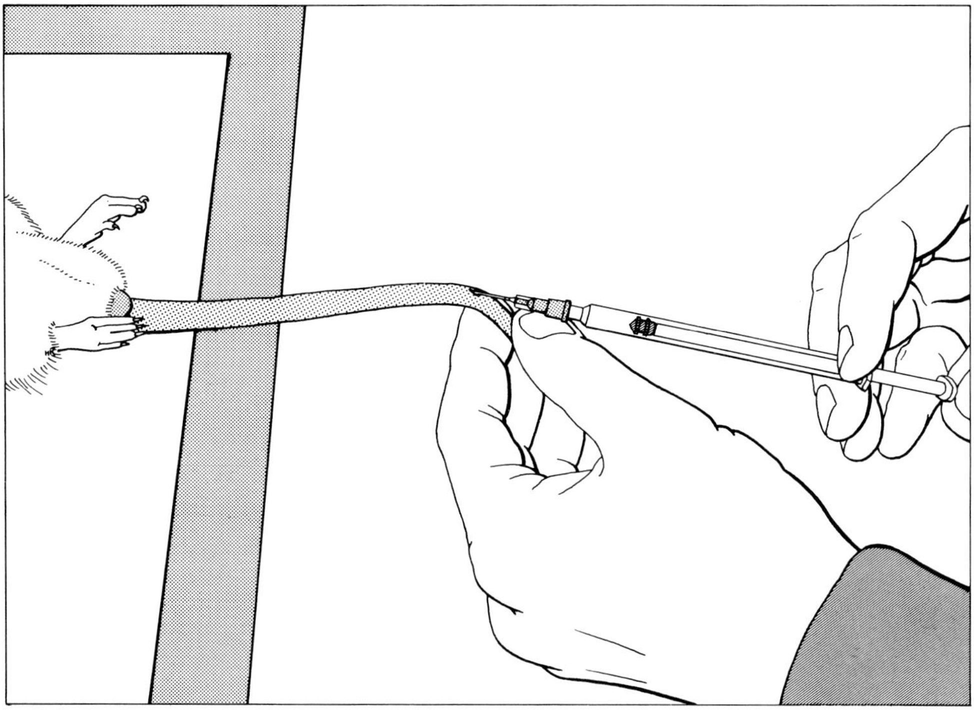

Figure 7.2.1. The tail vein injection.
After the tail is immersed in hot water causing the dilation of the ventro-lateral veins, the most visible vein is chosen for the injection using a 25G needle.

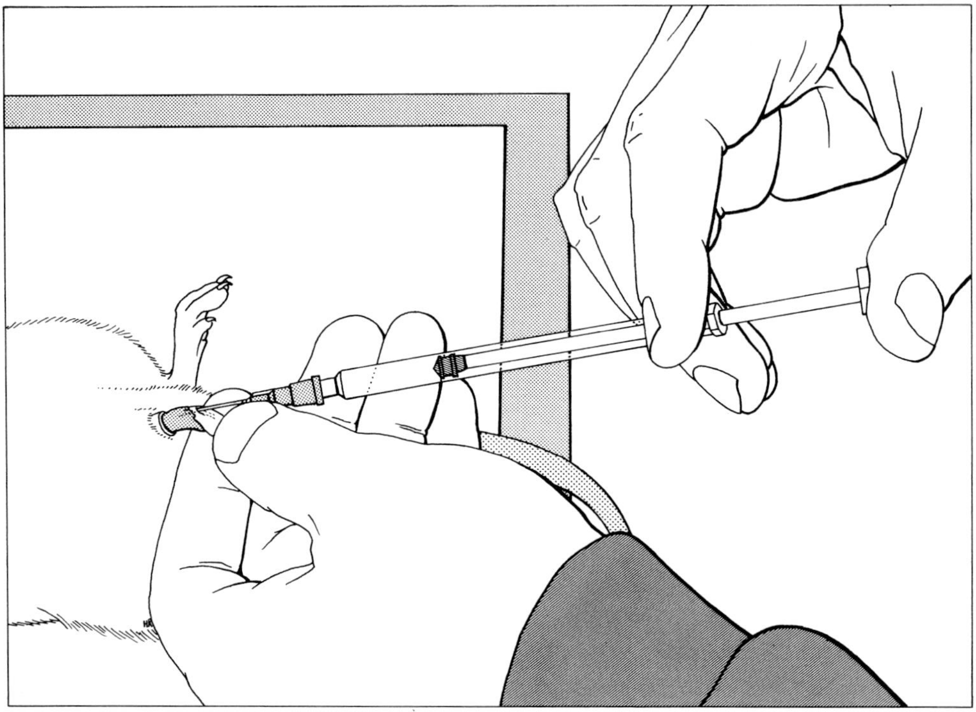

Figure 7.2.2. The penile vein injection.
The penis is extruded, and the glans is held by the thumb and index finger, thereby exposing the penile vein. Only the tip of the 25G needle should be inserted into the vein. Use the left-hand thumb to steady and support the needle.

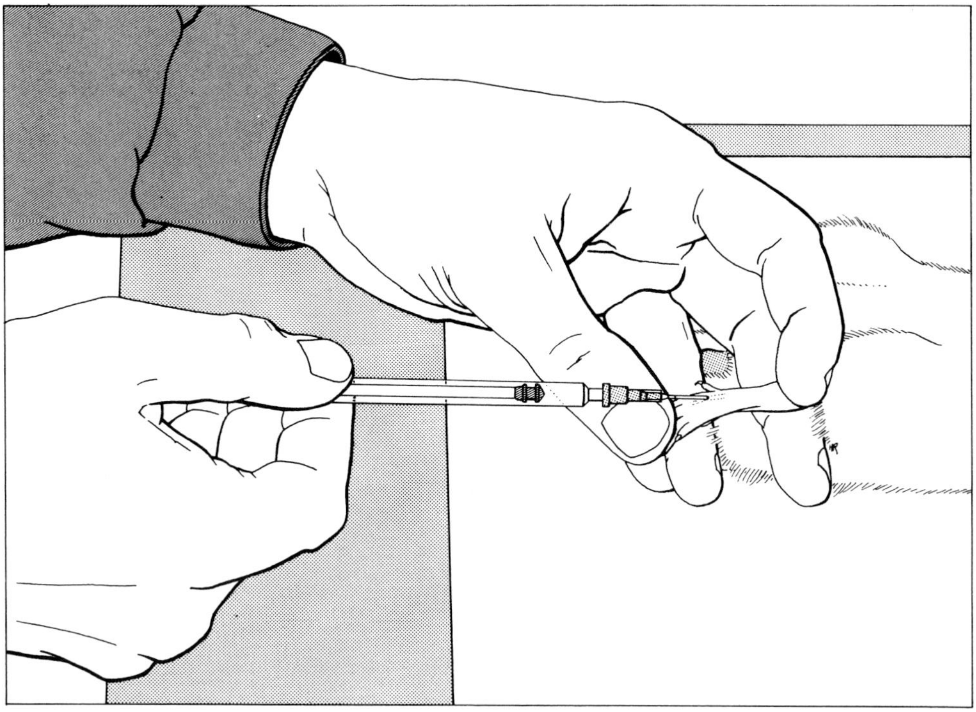

Figure 7.2.3. The dorsal metatarsal vein injection.
Pressure is put on the metatarsal vein and a 25G needle is inserted in a straight line into this vein. After penetration the pressure applied with the left hand index finger should be decreased. Slight aspiration resulting in blood entering the nozzle of the syringe will tell you whether you have entered the vein or not.

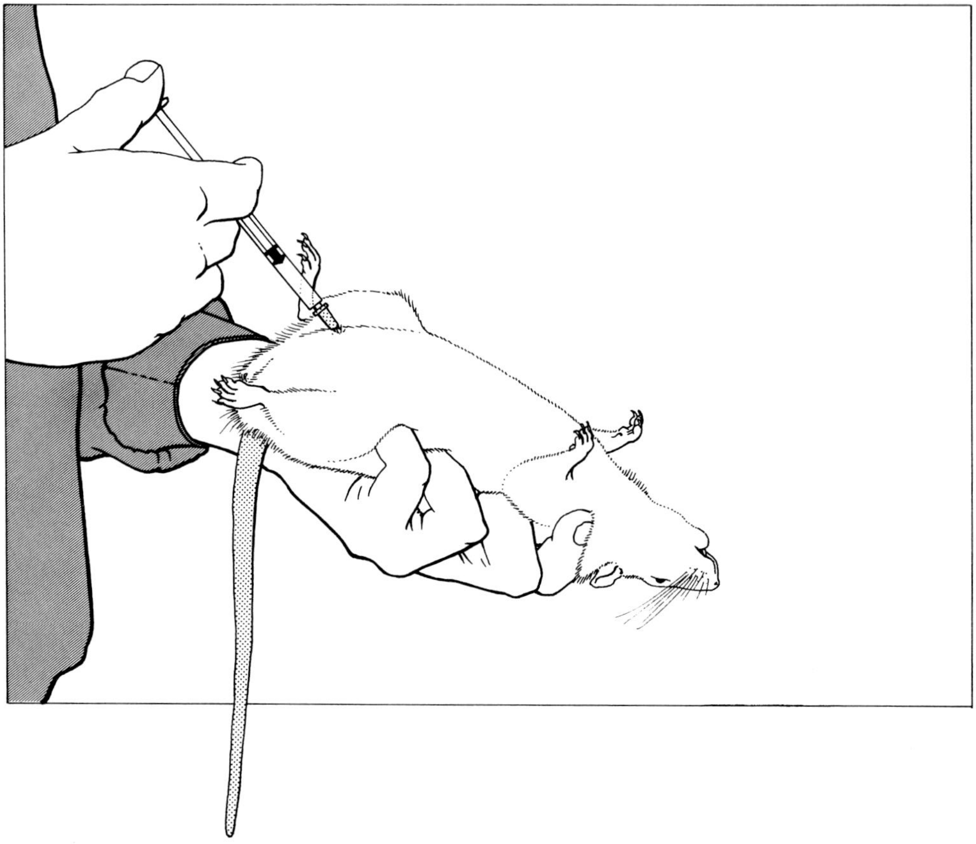

Figure 7.2.4. The intraperitoneal injection.
The animal is firmly held with its head slightly downwards, whilst a 25 G short needle is pushed into the left caudal area of the abdominal cavity, as viewed by the surgeon.

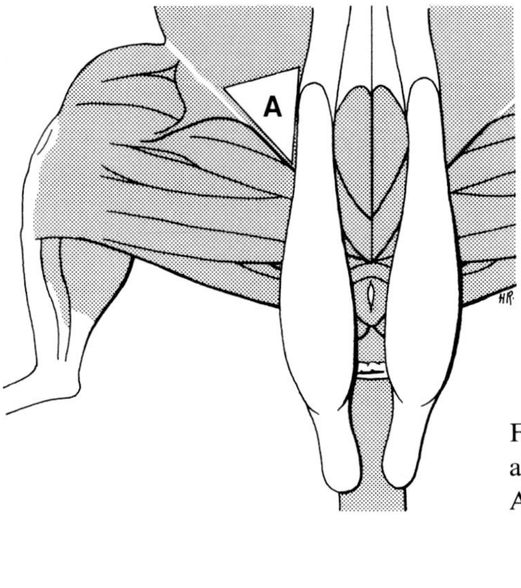

Figure 7.2.5. Detail of the left caudal area of the abdomen.
A. Area of injection.

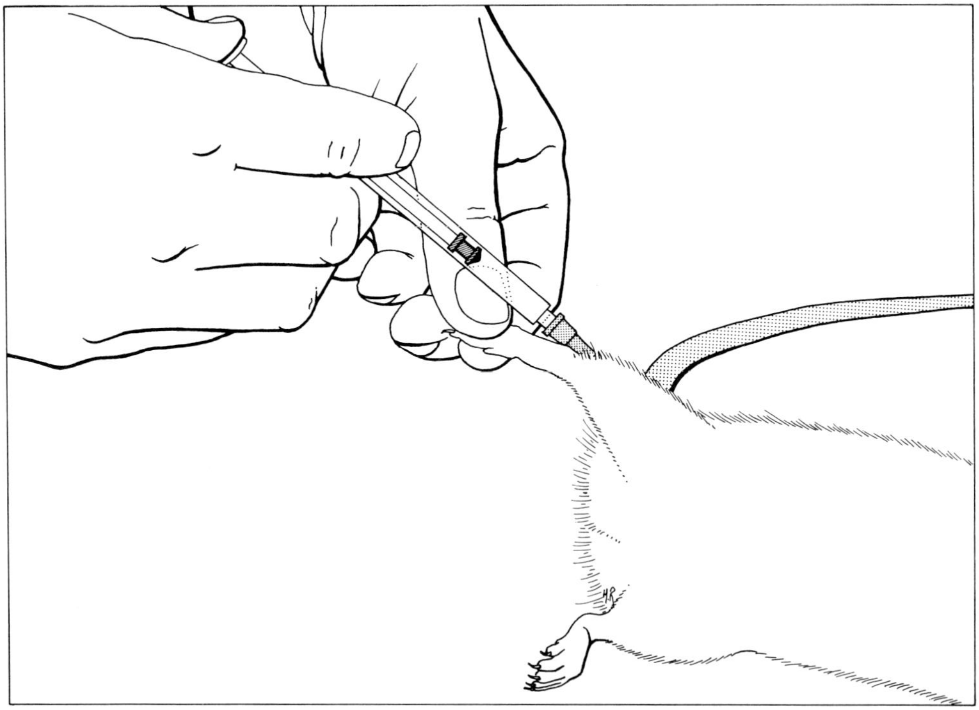

Figure 7.2.6. The intramuscular injection.
Intramuscular injection into the hind leg. A 25G needle is inserted with a short thrust parallel to the bone.

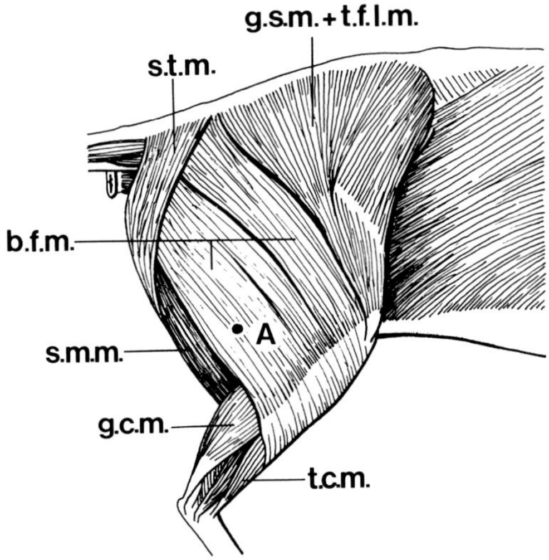

Figure 7.2.7. Site of the intramuscular injectio
A. Site of injection

bfm	Biceps femoris muscle.
stm	Semitendinosus muscle.
gsm	Gluteus superficialis muscle.
tflm	Tensor fasciae latae muscle.
gcm	Gastrocnemius muscle.
smm	Semimembranosus muscle.
tcm	Tibialis cranialis muscle.

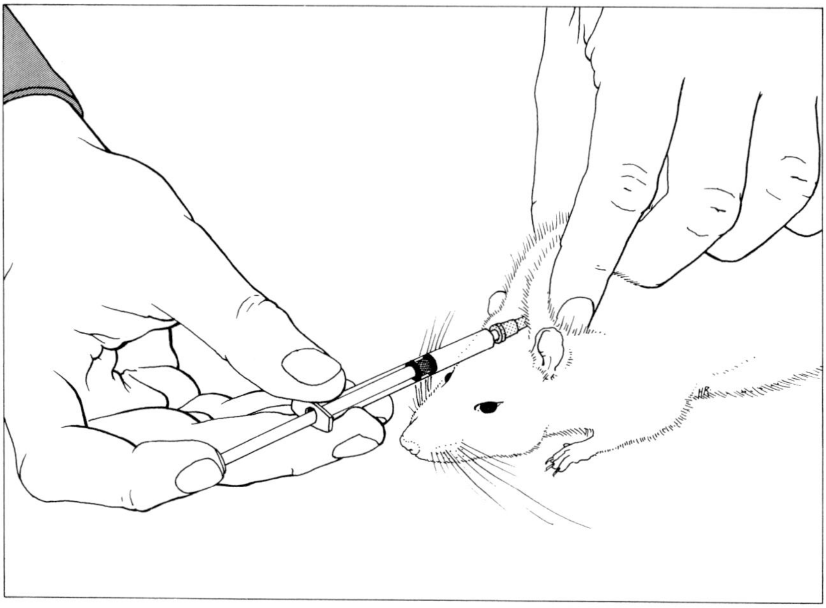

Figure 7.2.8. The subcutaneous injection into the neck.
To avoid backflow of the injected solution through the perforated skin, the needle is totally inserted to ensure a minimum of leakage, especially when larger volumes are to be injected.

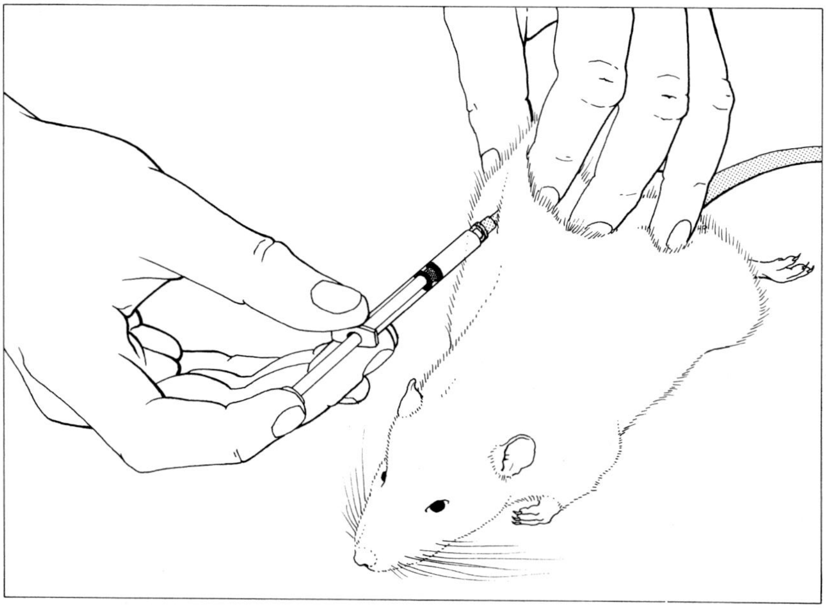

Figure 7.2.9. The subcutaneous injection into the side.
An alternative route for a subcutaneous injection in animals which have been provided with permanent cannulae running in the neck. The animal has to be under light anaesthesia.

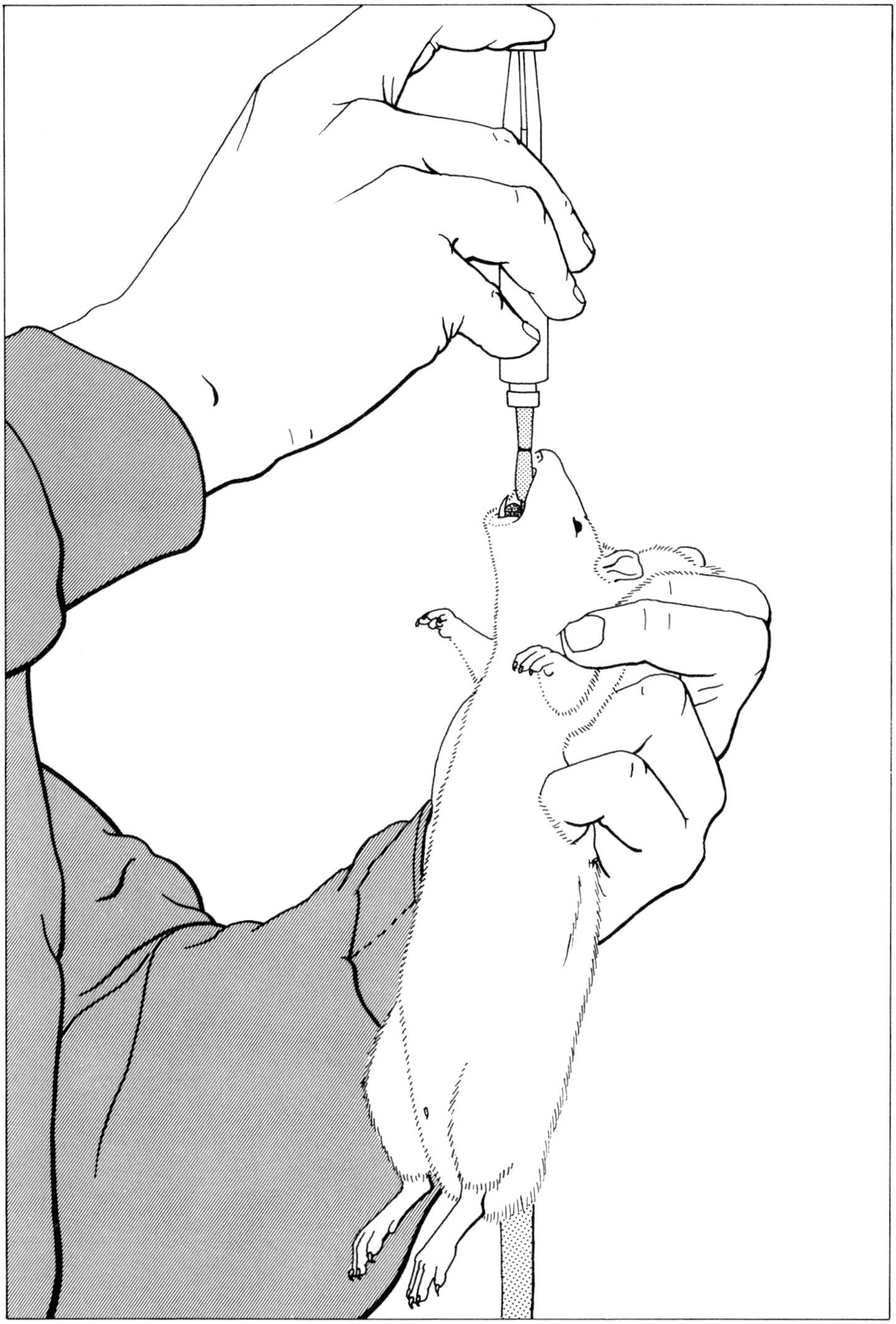

Figure 7.2.10. The intragastric administration.
By holding the skin of the back of the neck firmly, the head will automatically stretch and the mouth will be opened. The blunt oral needle should be completely inserted.

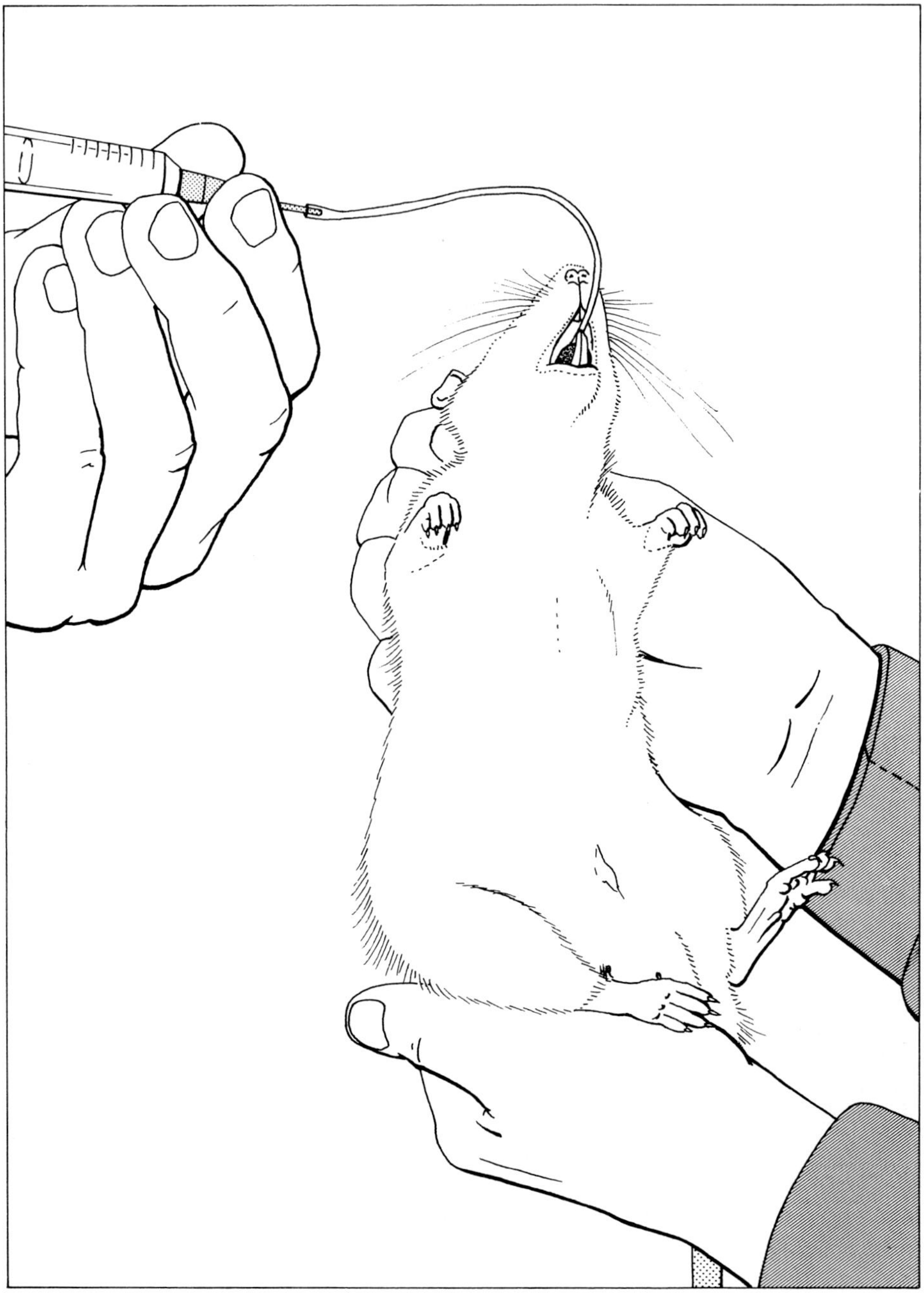

Figure 7.2.11. Intragastric intubation with a polyethylene catheter.
The anaesthetized animal is held by an assistant. The polyethylene tubing is inserted to approximately 10 cm. The animal has to be under light anaesthesia.

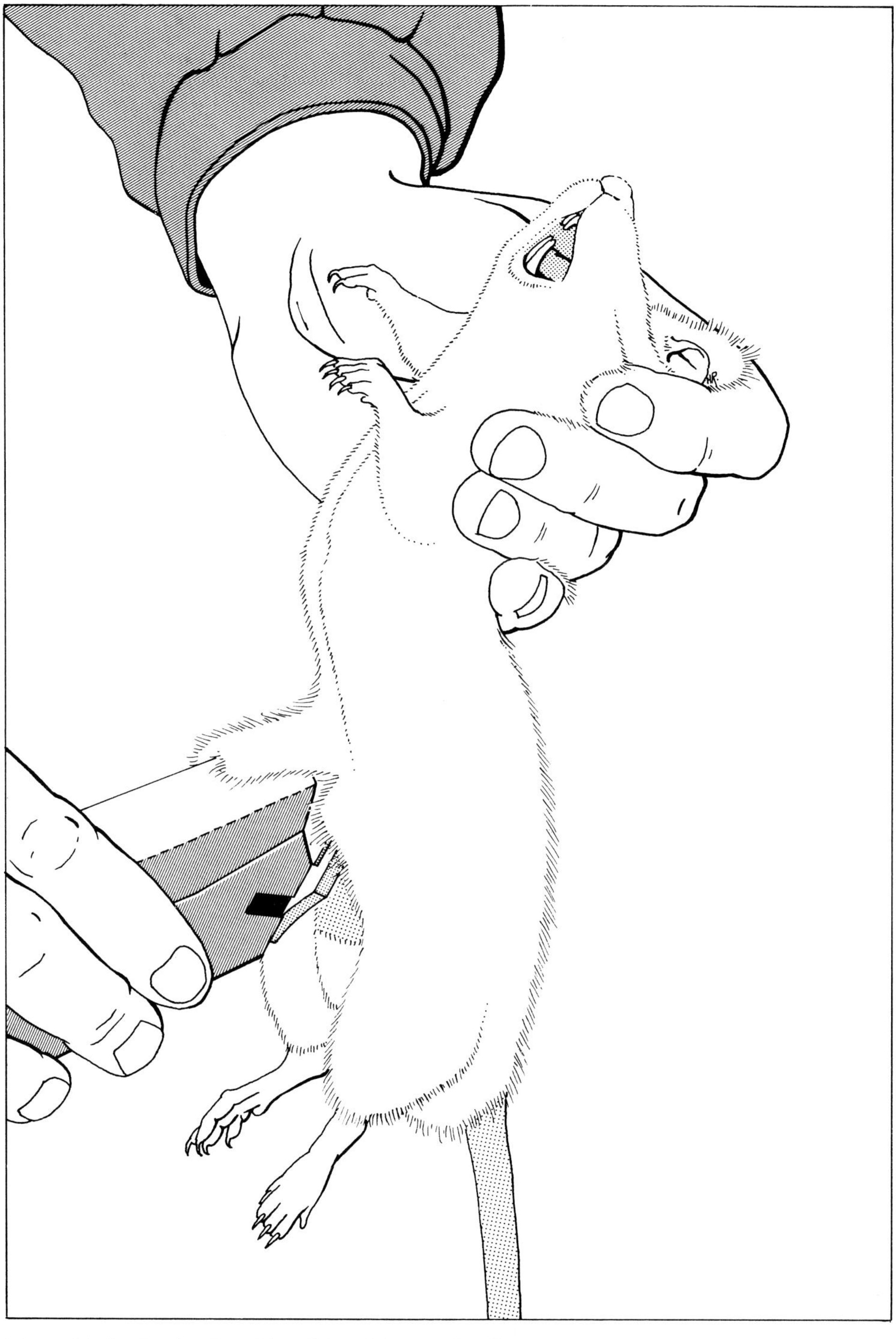

Figure 7.3.1. Shaving the skin of the abdominal wall.
Under anaesthesia the skin of the abdominal wall is shorn. Special care should be taken when shaving the area around the nipples.

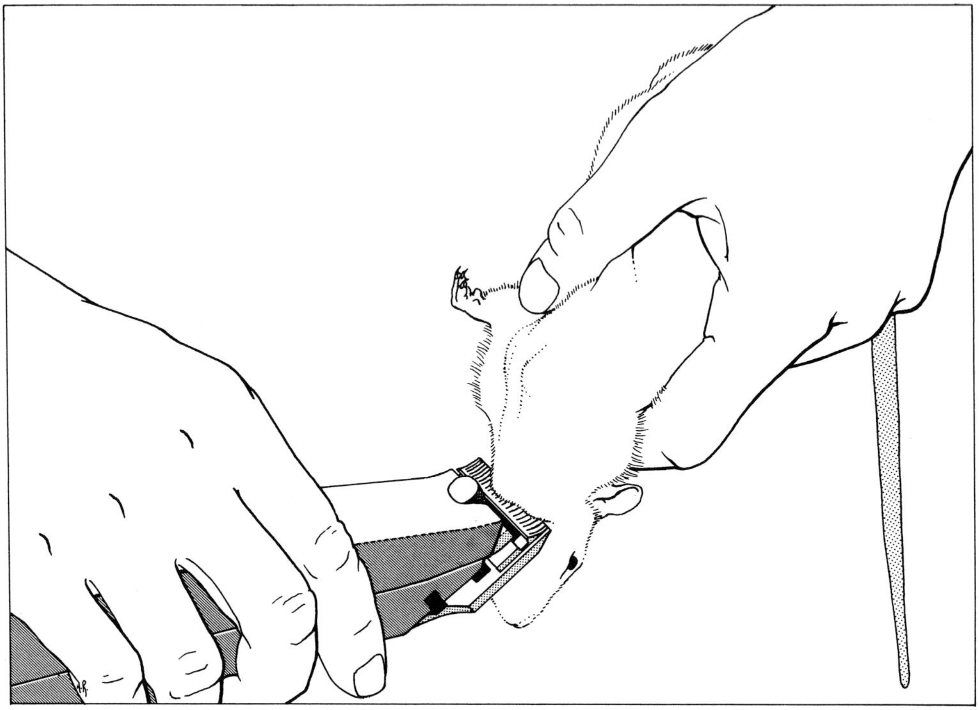

Figure 7.3.2. Shaving the throat.
The anaesthetized animal is held head down, ensuring that the forelegs are clear, while the index finger supports the head.

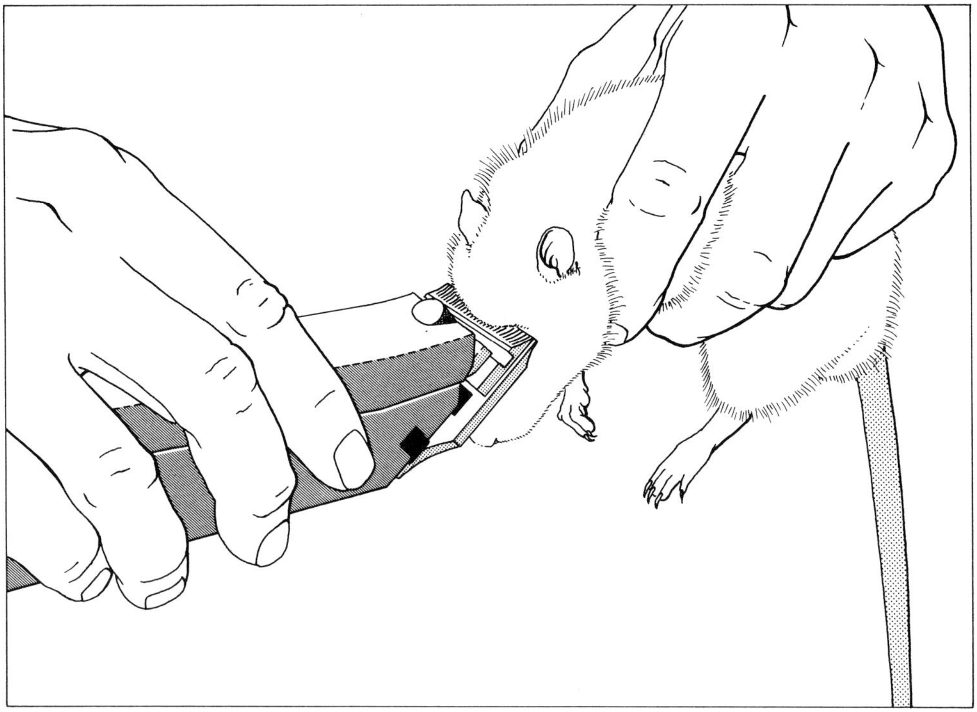

Figure 7.3.3. Shaving the head.
The head of the anaesthetized animal is shorn by gently pushing the head of the rat against the clipper.

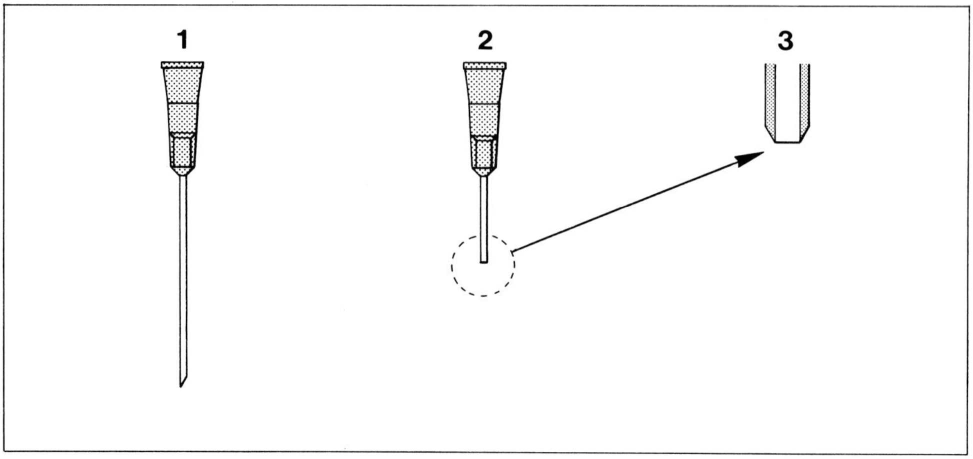

Figure 7.4.1. The hole puncturer.
A 20G needle (1) is cut (2), and sharpened as shown in cross section (3).

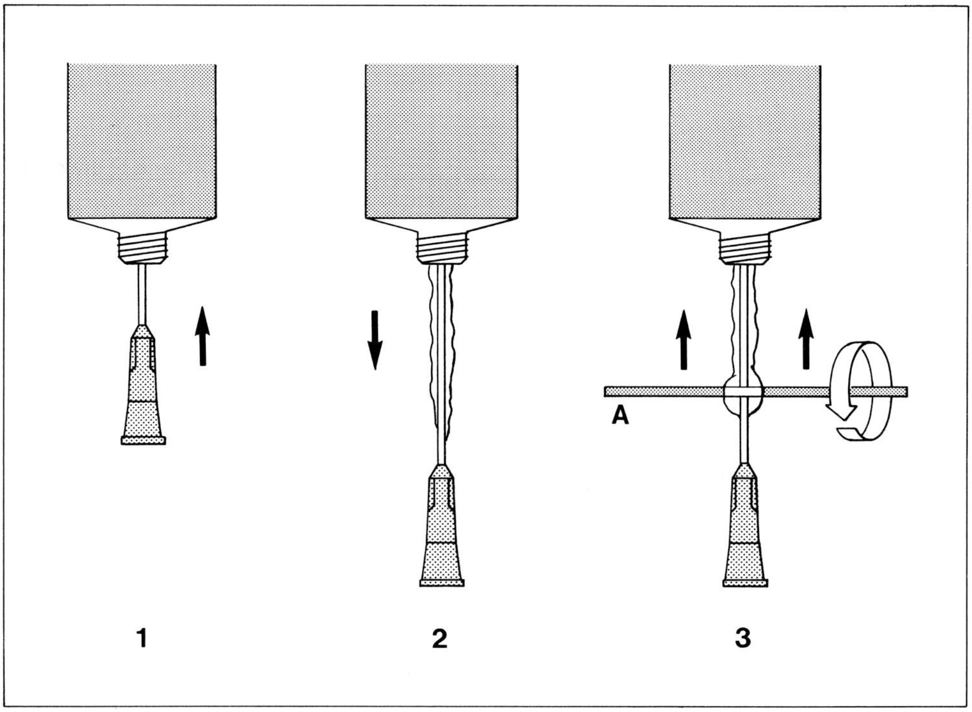

Figure 7.4.2. Preparation of silicon rings.
A 20G needle is inserted into a tube of silicon glue (1) and is withdrawn. Some glue will stick to the shaft of the needle (2). At the previously marked places, silicon glue is wrapped around the cannula (A) by rotating the cannula while moving it in the direction of the tube.

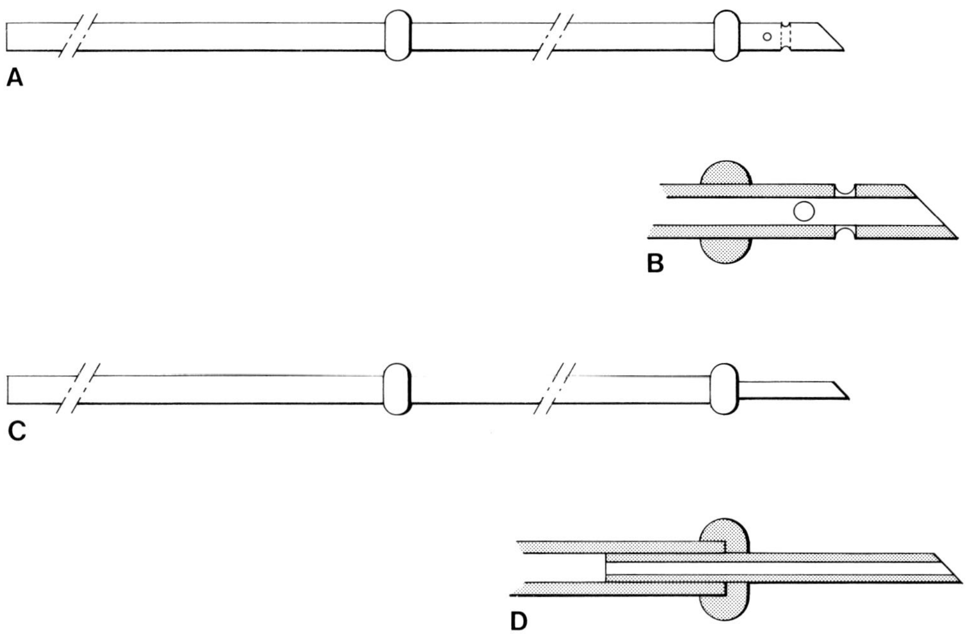

Figure 7.4.3. Examples of cannulae and tips.
Cannula A is an example of the portal cannula, the renal cannula, the thoracic duct cannula and the gut cannula. The gut cannula, however, has a larger diameter (see Table III). Cannula C is an example of the distal bile duct cannula and the iliolumbar cannula. B and D are cross-sections of the cannulae tips showing clearly the perforations, and the small-diameter tip respectively.

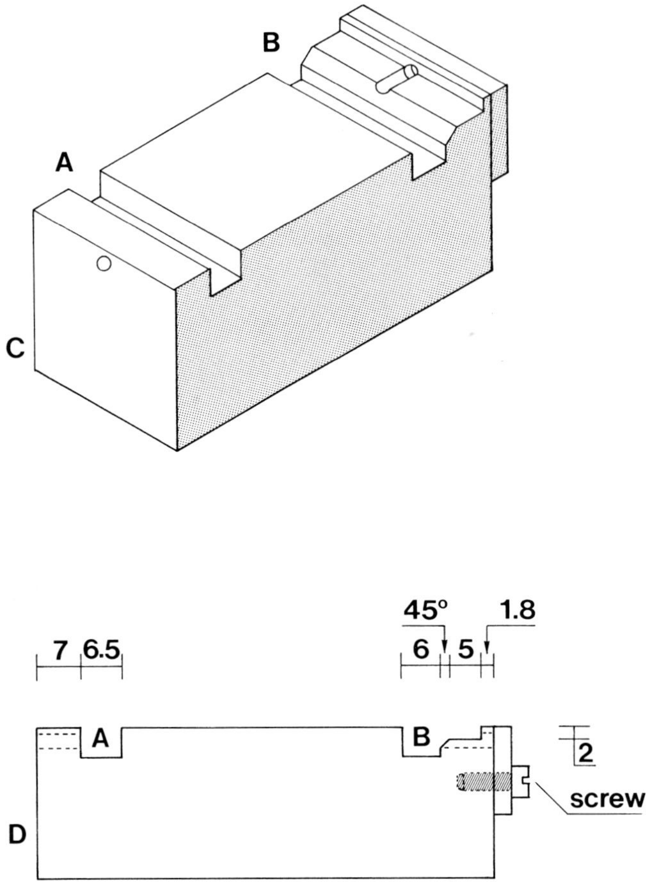

Figure 7.4.4. Preparation of the button.
The button is made of teflon tubing, using a mould (C) in which two grooves (A and B) are milled. D depicts a cross-section of the mould and the relevant dimensions (angles in degrees and distances in millimetres).

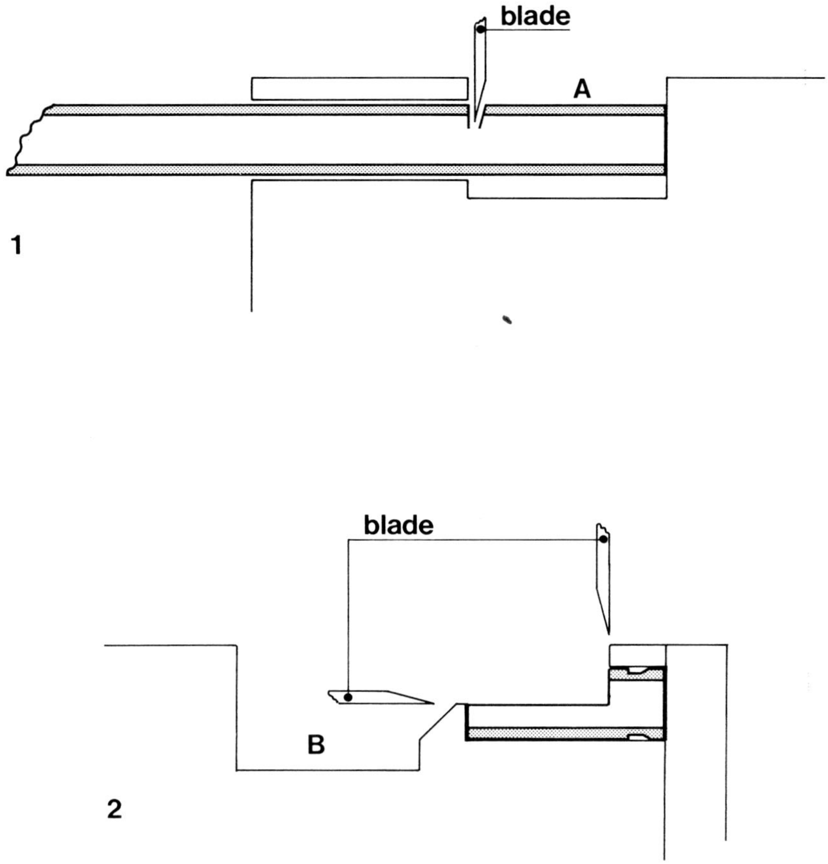

Figure 7.4.5. Details of the preparation of the button.
1. The teflon tubing is cut in groove A of the mould.
2. The button is cut to its final size in groove B of the mould.

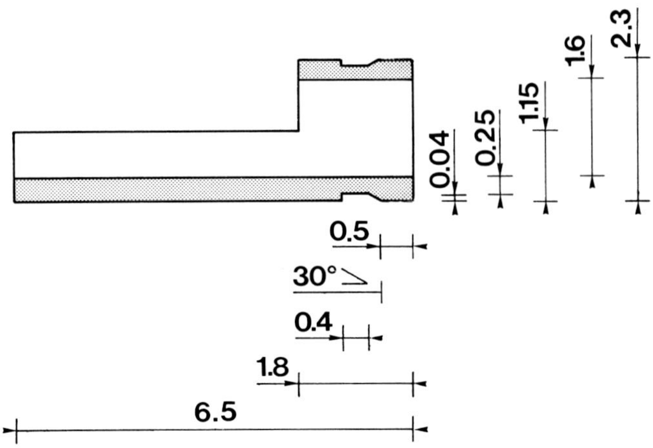

Figure 7.4.6. Dimensions of the button in millimetres.

→

Figure 7.4.7. Preparation of a swivel.
A. The 1 ml syringe is cut at the indicated distance (1), and the plunger is removed. Using a hole puncturer, a hole is made in the centre of the plunger. Two hypodermic needles are cut to size (2 and 3).
B. A small conic piece of perspex (4), having a hole drilled in the centre, which corresponds with the outer diameter of the needle is pushed over the cut needle. The end of the needle should be widened using a centre punch.
C. The syringe together with the plunger are pushed over the needle-part (5). The other prepared needle-part is then pushed onto the syringe (6).
D. A complete swivel attached to polyethylene tubing (7 and 8). The space marked with an asterisk should be filled with high-vacuum grease, to prevent leakage and to allow for easy rotation.

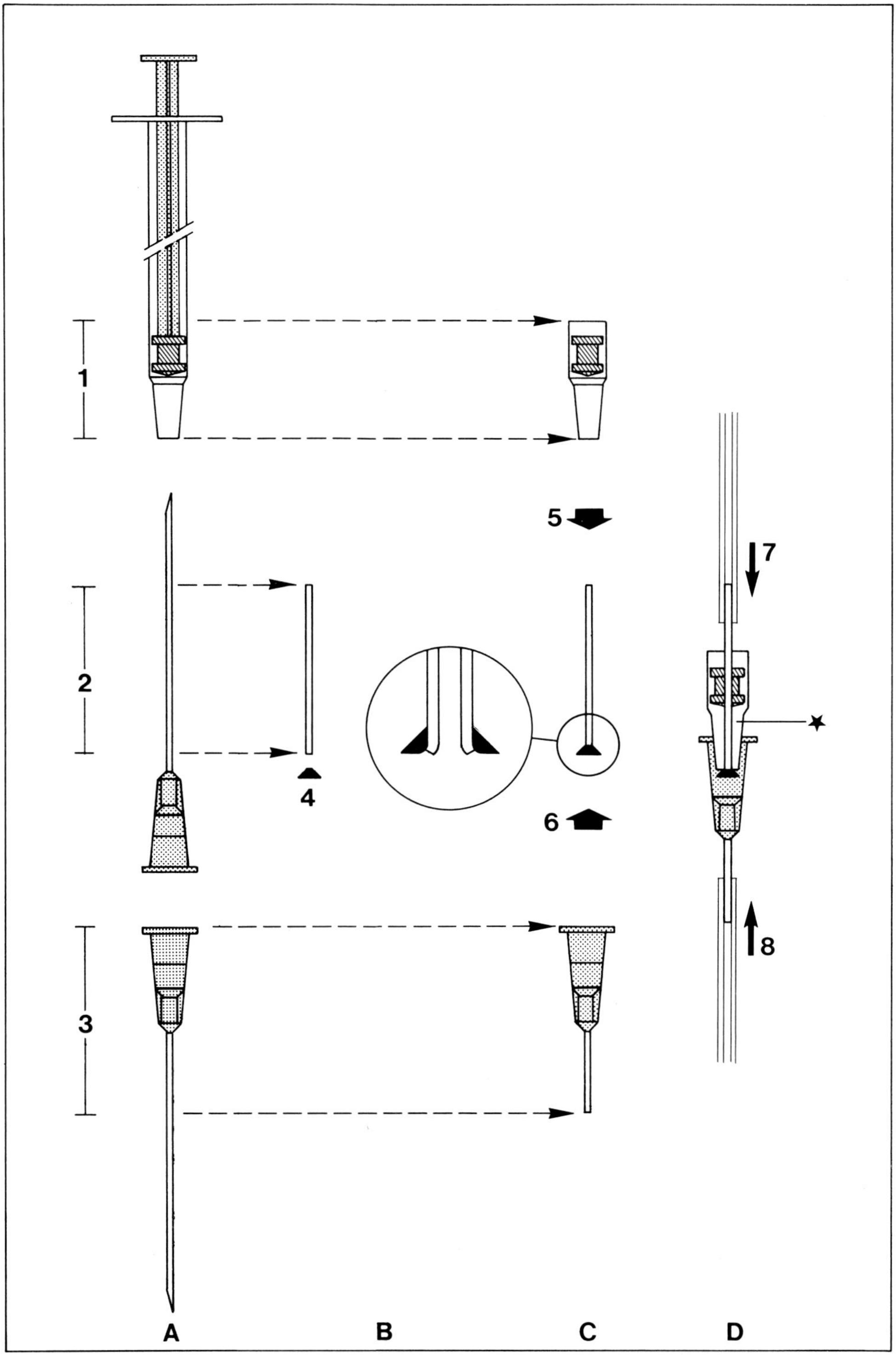
1
2
3
4
5
6
7
8
A
B
C
D

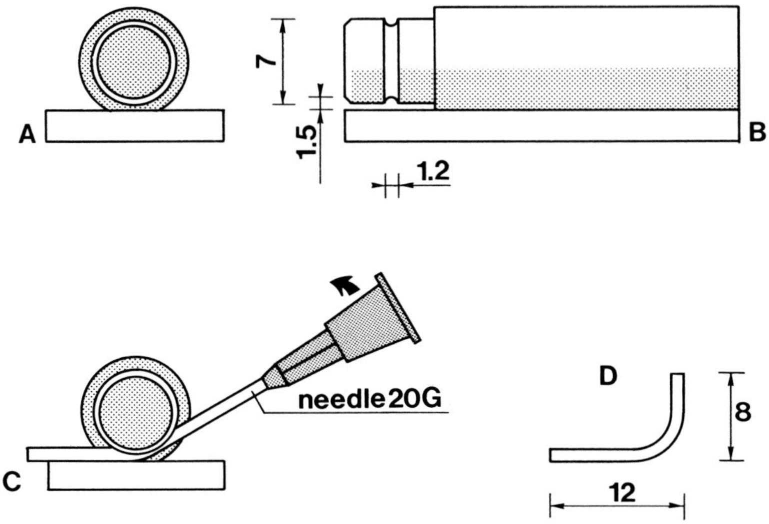

Figure 7.4.8. The mould for the preparation of the L-shaped adapter.
A. The frontal view of the mould.
B. The side view of the mould.
C. The bending of a 20G needle from which the point has already been removed.
D. The L-shaped adapter cut to its final size.
All dimensions are given in millimetres.

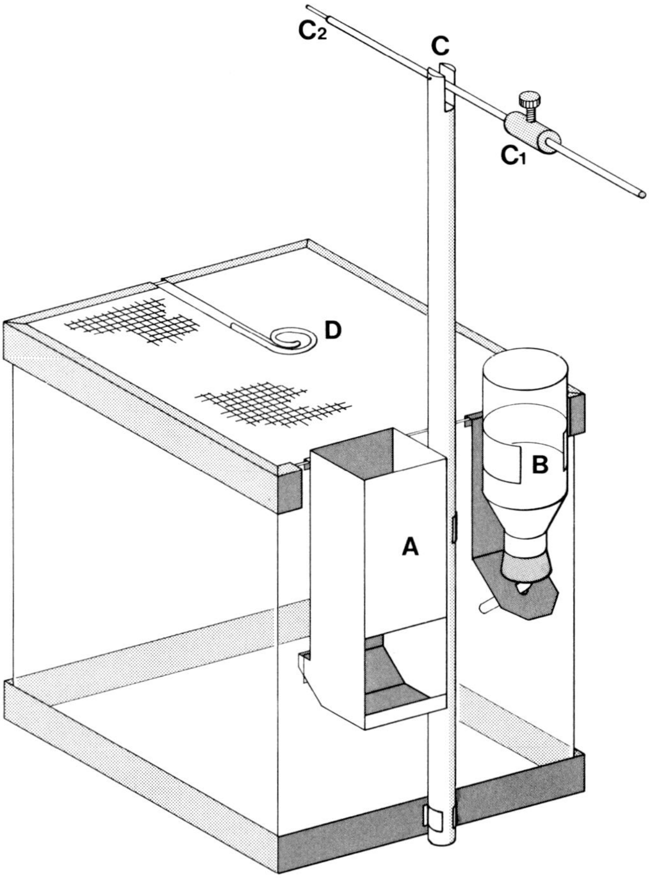

Figure 7.4.9. The experimental cage.
A. Stainless steel feeding-trough.
B. Plastic water flask in a stainless steel holder.
C. The lever with the adjustable counter-weight (c_1) and the place for the fixation of a sample cannula (C_2).
D. Stainless steel lid with an opening for the swivelled sample cannula.
A detailed plan of this experimental cage can be obtained from MD on request.

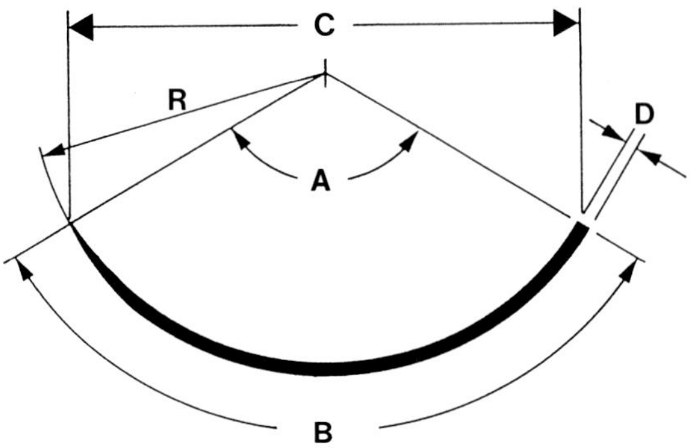

Figure 7.5.1. Description of the needle
A. Angle.
B. Arch length.
C. Chord length.
D. Diameter.
R. Radius.

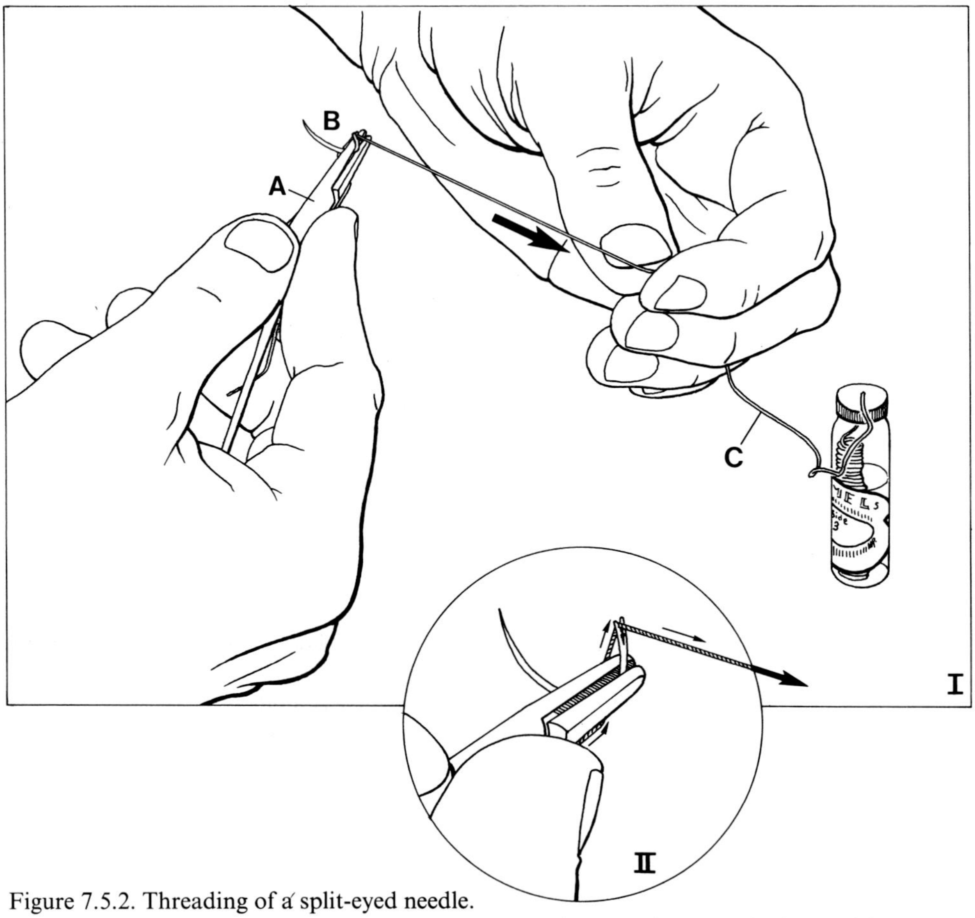

Figure 7.5.2. Threading of a split-eyed needle.
I. The thread is pulled into the split from the inside of the needle towards the outside.
II. Detail of the needle in the needle holder.
A. The needle holder.
B. The needle.
C. The thread.

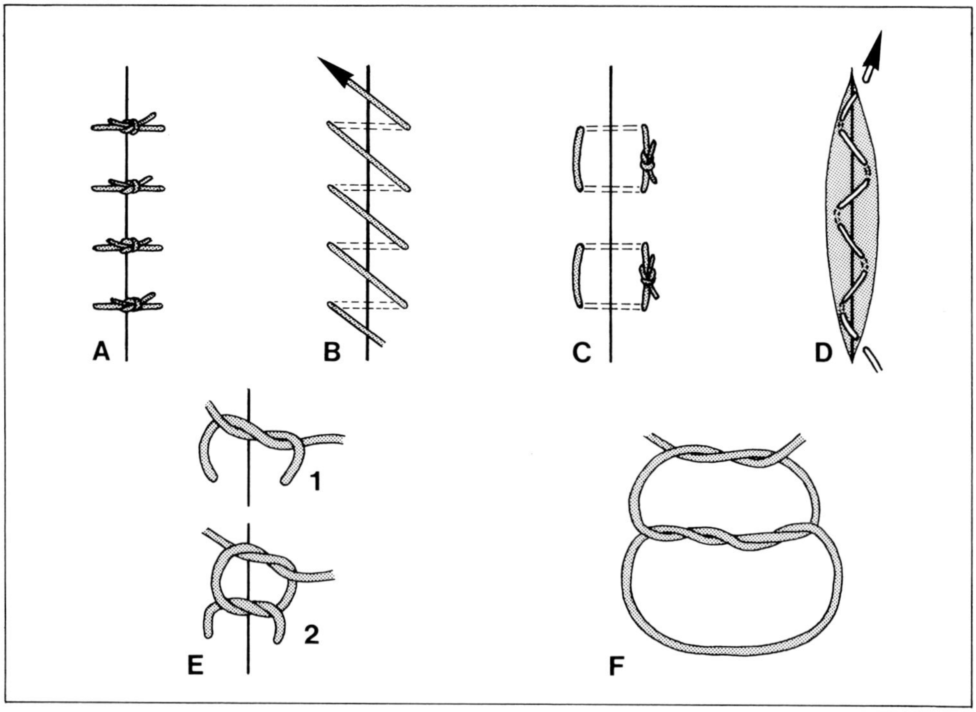

Figure 7.5.3. Most commonly used suture pattern and knots in rat surgery.
A. The interrupted suture.
B. The continuous suture.
C. The horizontal mattress suture.
D. The continuous subcuticular suture.
E. The square or reef knot:
   1. The first half of the knot
   2. The complete knot
F. The surgical knot.

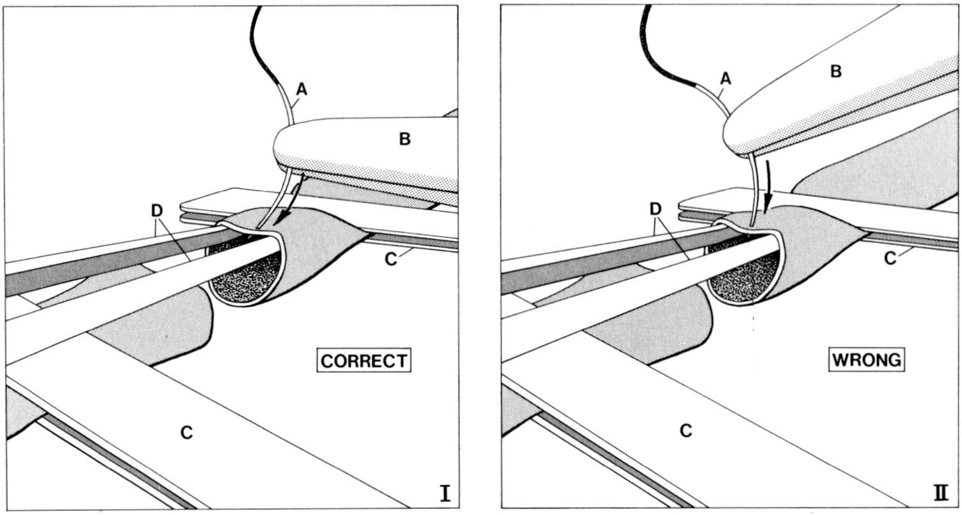

Figure 7.5.4. Correct stitch in an end-to-end anastomosis (termino-terminal anastomosis).
I. Jewellers forceps are inserted into the lumen, and slightly opened (overstretching the vessel wall must be avoided). The needle penetrates the vessel wall almost horizontally, by slight rotation of the fingers and wrist. In this way a "through-stitch" will be avoided.
II. The needle penetrates the vessel almost perpendicularly, easily leading to a fatal "through-stitch".
A. The needle.
B. The needle holder.
C. The clamps of the vessel approximator.
D. Jewellers forceps.

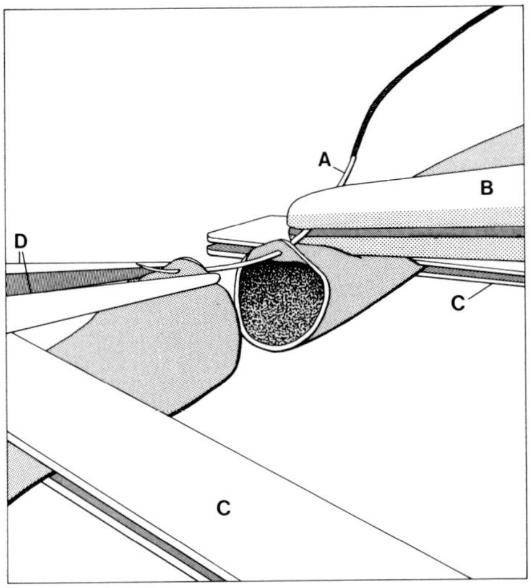

Figure 7.5.5. Completion of the first stitch in an end-to-end anastomosis.
Immediately after penetration of the first vessel wall, the opposite part of the vessel is penetrated, while the wall is supported from above by the forceps. The moment the needle holder touches the vessel, the instrument is shifted to the tip of the needle, which is pulled through the wall following its own curvature.

A. The needle.
B. The needle holder.
C. The clamps of the vessel approximator.
D. Jewellers forceps.

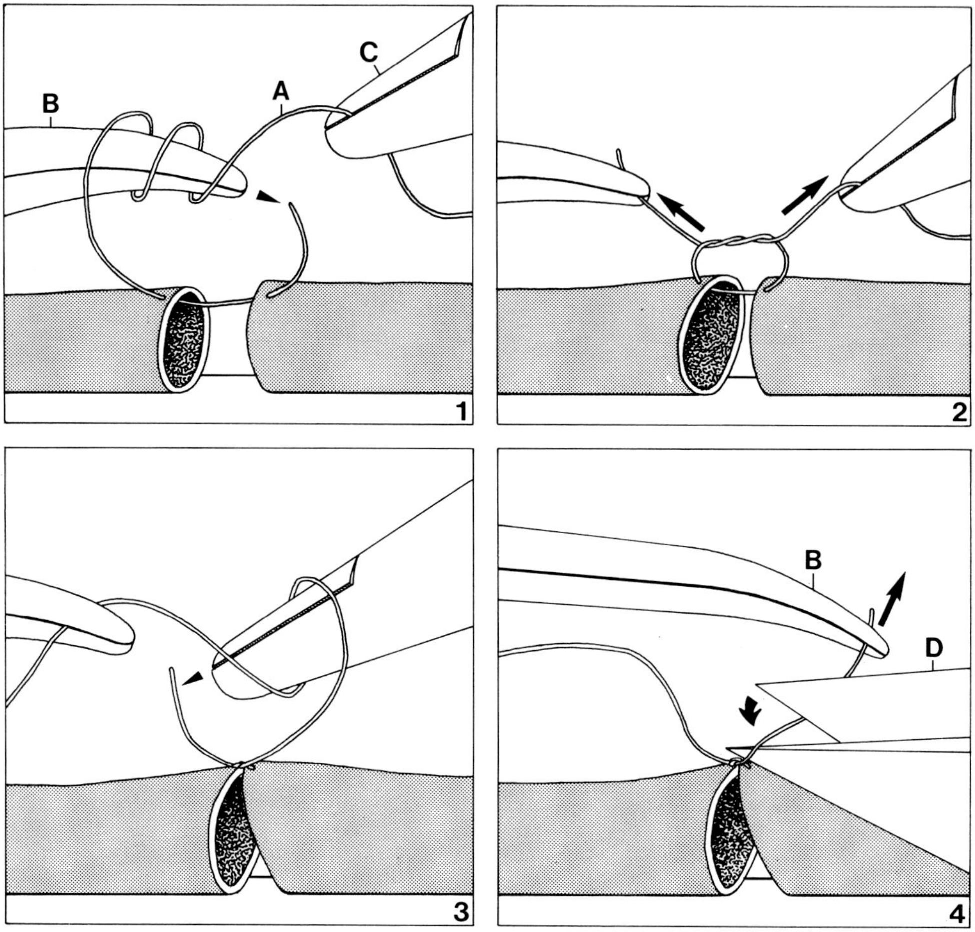

Figure 7.5.6. The surgical knot in an end-to-end anastomosis.

1. The longest thread is picked up with the needle holder, two loops are made on the tip of the left-hand forceps, and the short end is picked up with the left-hand forceps.
2. The loop is pulled off the left-hand forceps, completing the first half of the surgical knot.
3. The longest thread is picked up with the left-hand forceps, one loop is made on the tip of the needle holder, and the short end is picked up with the needle holder.
4. The loop has been pulled off, thus completing the second half of the surgical knot and the suture is cut, leaving enough length for manipulation and exposition during the application of the following stitches.

A. Suture.
B. Left-hand forceps.
C. Needle holder.
D. Scissors.

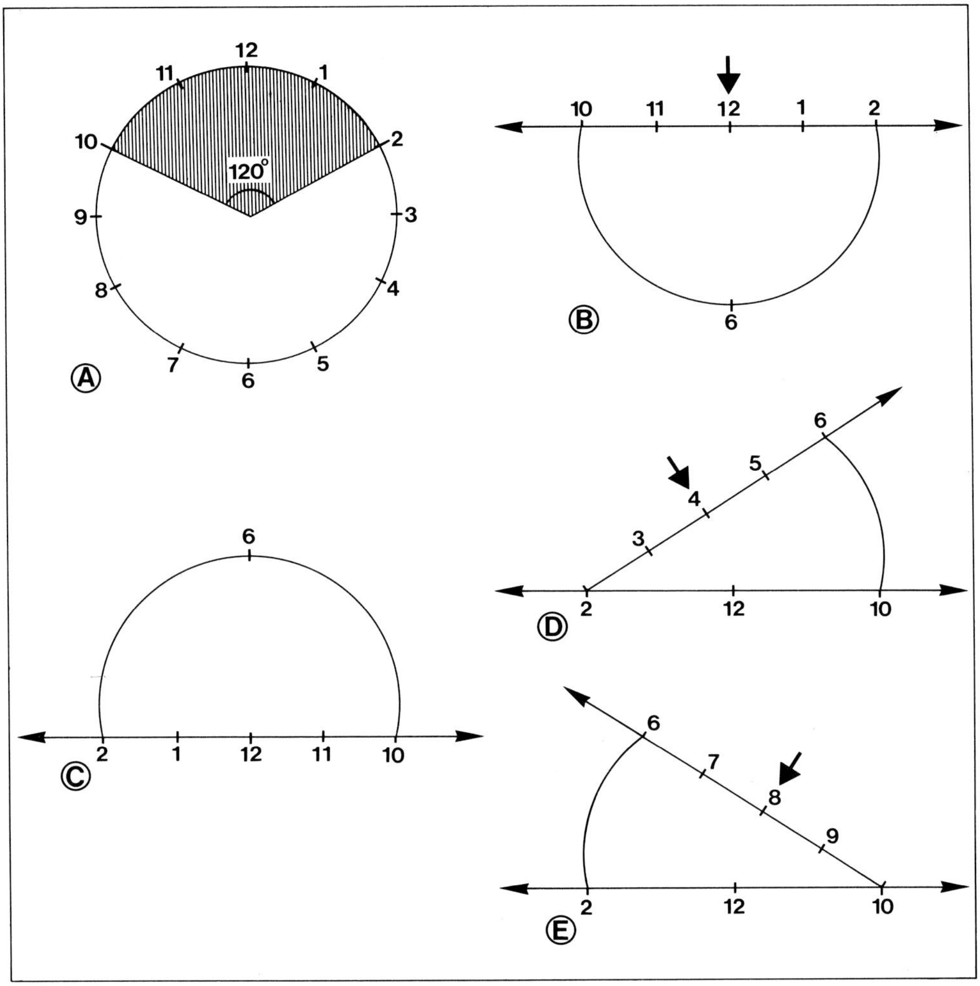

Figure 7.6.1. Schematic drawing of the steps in an end-to-end anastomosis.

A. The corner sutures are placed at 120° ("2 o'clock" and "10 o'clock").
B. Light tension is put on the corner sutures, and the next three sutures are placed. The arrow indicates the first suture to be placed.
C. The anastomosis is rotated, and the "6 o'clock" suture is placed.
D. The "6 o'clock" suture is retracted to the right, and the next three sutures are placed.
E. The "6 o'clock" suture is retracted to the left, and the anastomosis is completed.

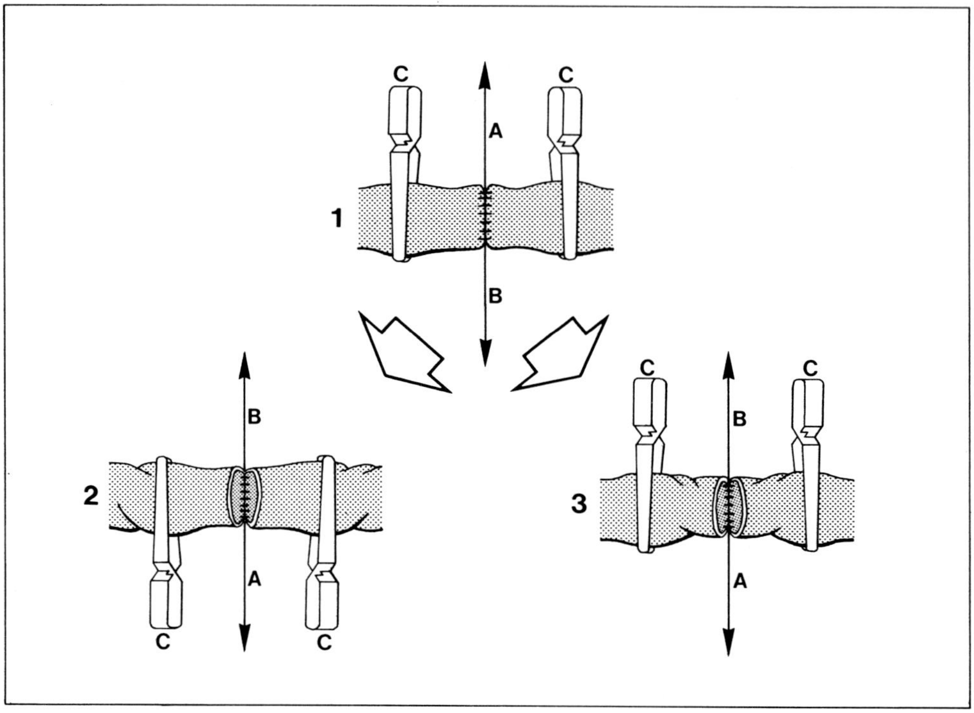

Figure 7.6.2. Rotation of the anastomosis.
1. The anterior wall has been sutured.
2. Clamp rotation: the clamps (C) are rotated and the corner sutures (A and B) are repositioned.
3. Suture rotation: the corner sutures are repositioned, while the clamps retain their position, resulting in slight torsion of the vessel.
A and B. Corner sutures. C. Clamp.

→

Figure 7.6.3. The end-to-side anastomosis (termino-lateral anastomosis) with running (continuous) suture techniques.
A. Inside suture technique.
1. Two corner sutures are placed at 180°.
2. Some tension is put on the corner sutures for purposes of exposure, and the posterior wall is sutured from the inside (see chapter 9.2.).
3. The anterior wall is sutured.
4. The anastomosis is complete.
B. Normal suture technique.
1. Two corner sutures are placed at 180°.
2. Some tension is put on the corner sutures and the anterior wall is sutured.
3. The vessel is turned over, which allows the posterior wall to become anterior, and the anterior wall is sutured.
4. The anastomosis is complete.

A

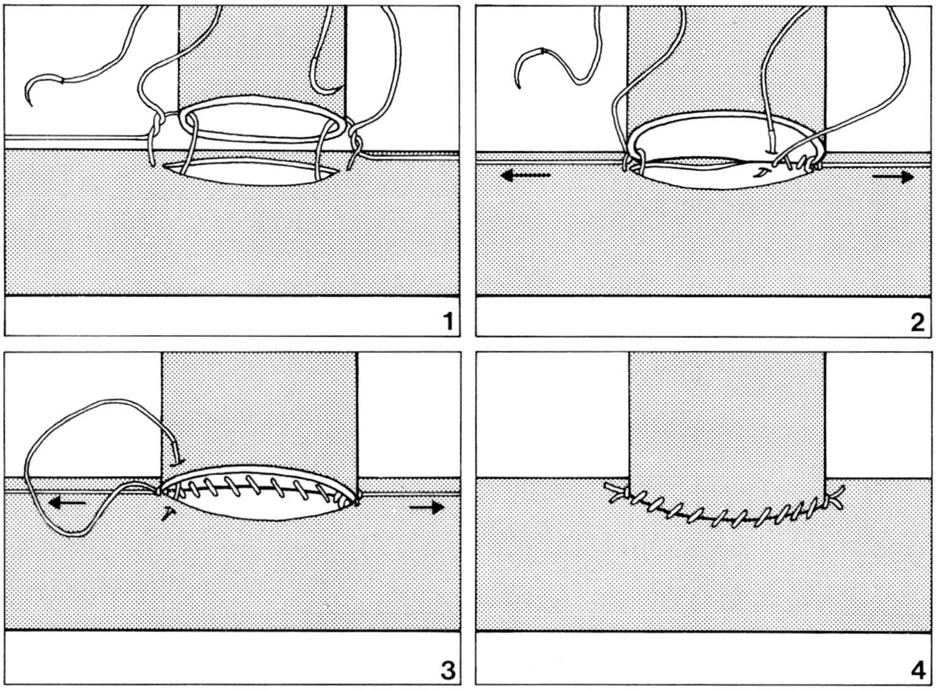

B

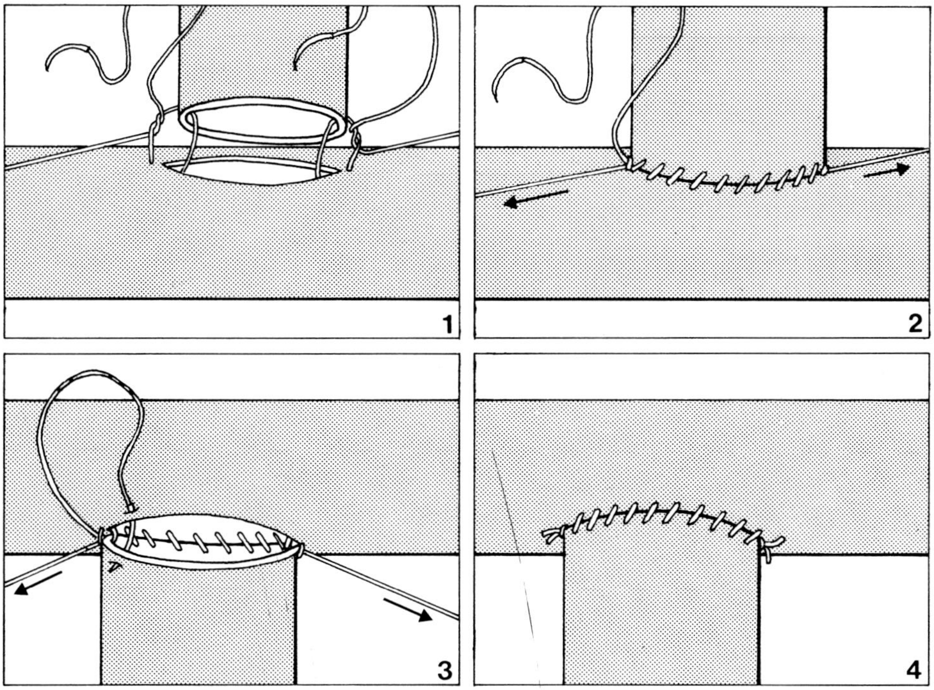

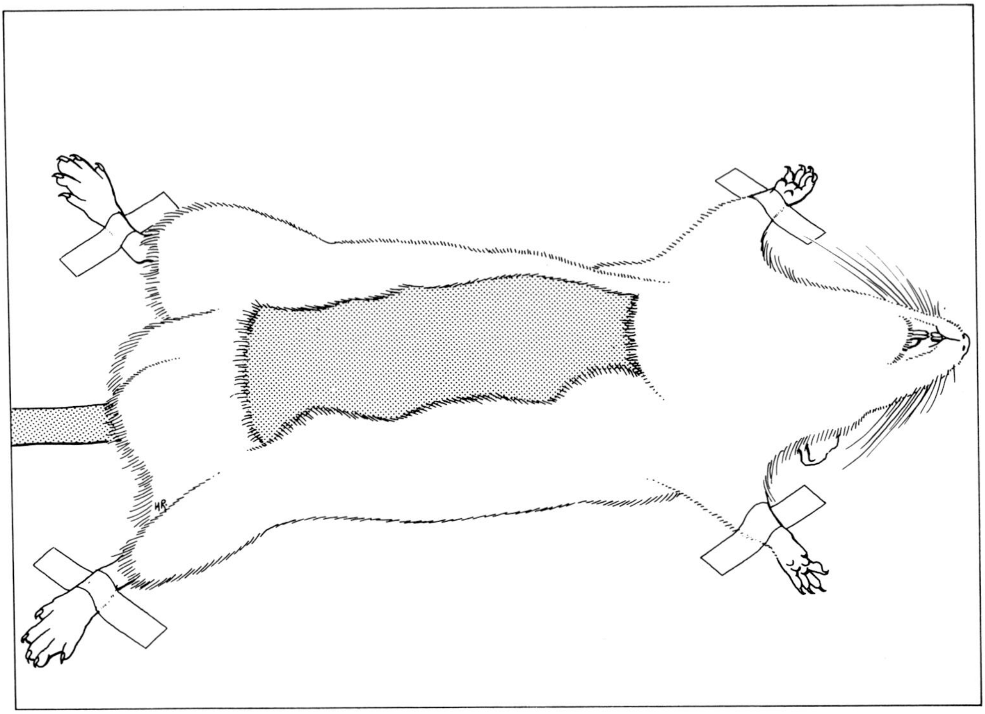

Figure 7.7.1. Opening of the abdominal wall (I).
After shaving the rat is laid on its back, and the skin is disinfected. The limbs are secured to the rat board with tape.

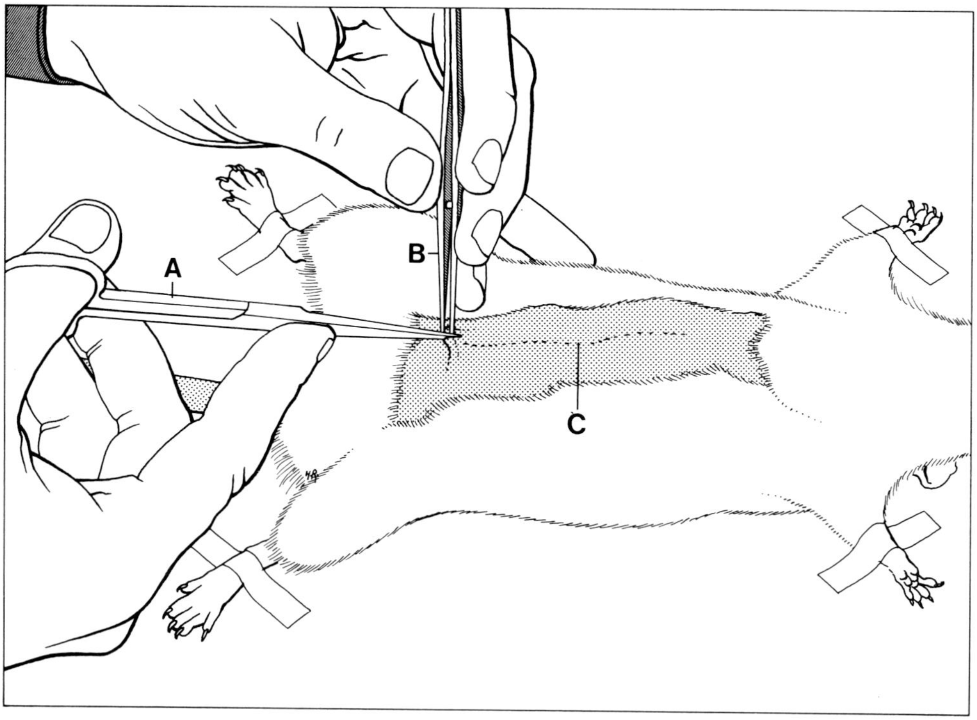

Figure 7.7.2. Opening of the abdominal wall (II).
A small incision is made in the skin using surgical forceps and a pair of ring-handled straight preparation scissors (blunt-sharp).
A. Scissors.
B. Surgical forceps.
C. Linea alba.

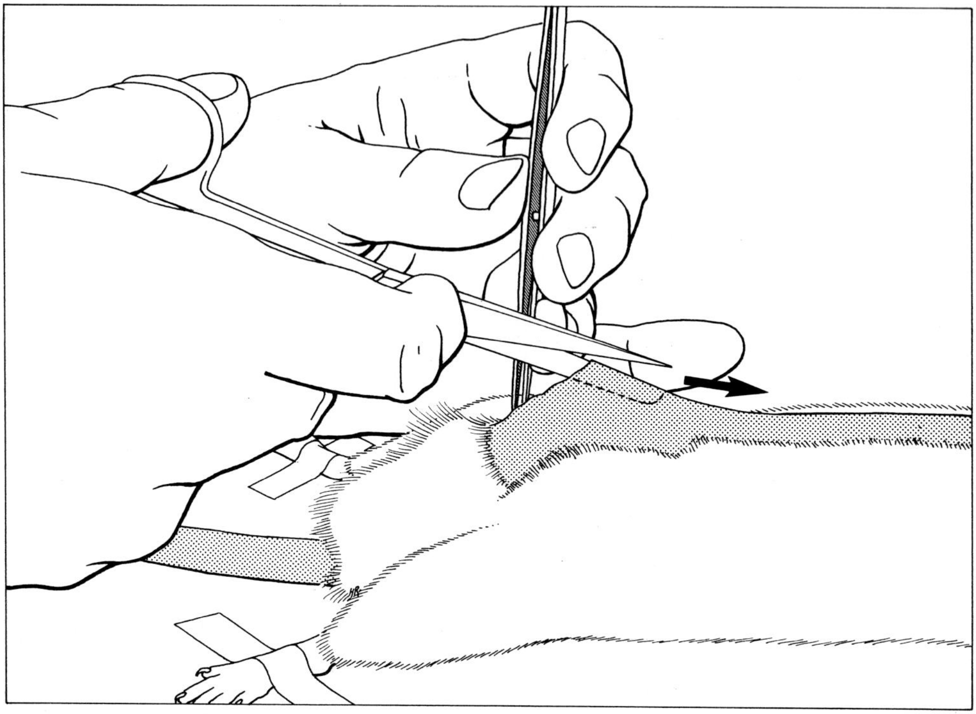

Figure 7.7.3. Opening of the abdominal wall (III).
An incision is made from the pubic bones towards the xiphoid cartilage over the linea alba by pushing the blunt part of the scissors forward under the skin.

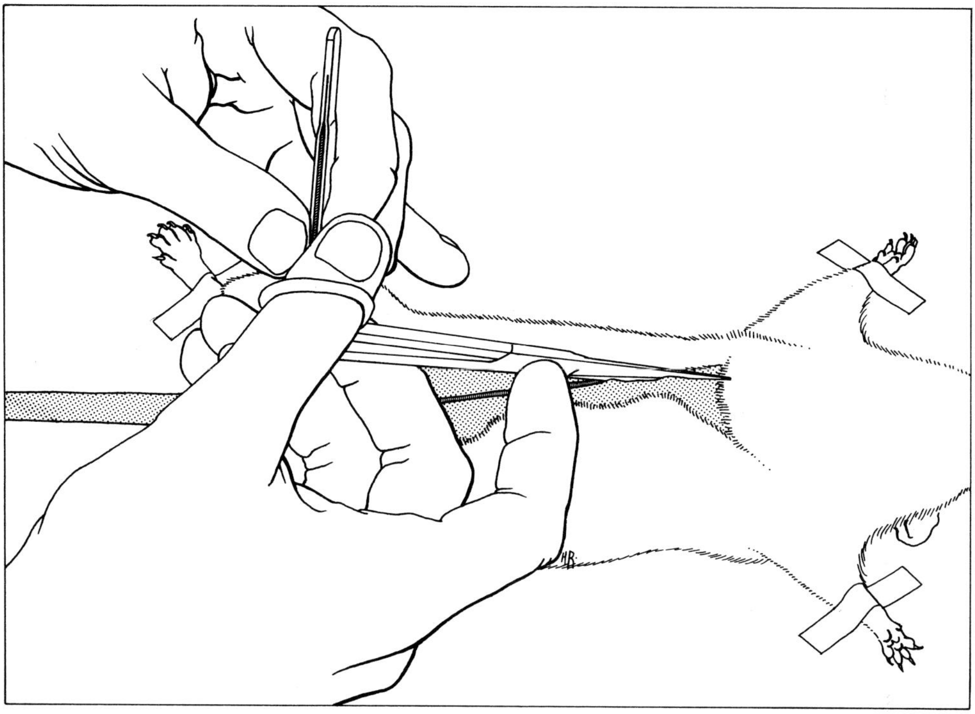

Figure 7.7.4. Opening of the abdominal wall (IV).
The incision is continued just past the xiphoid cartilage.

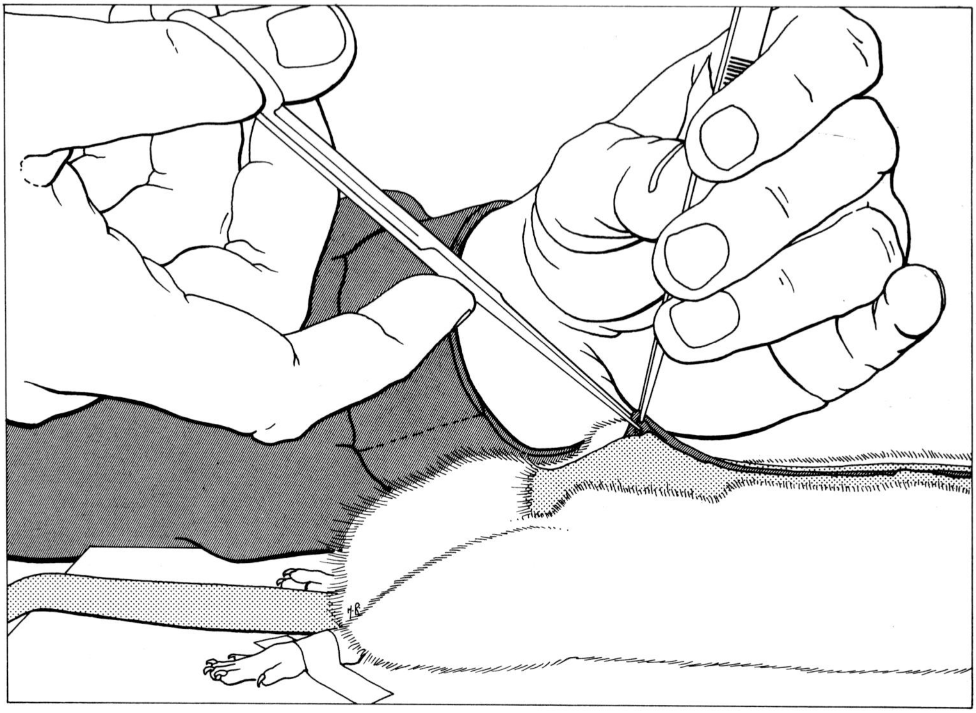

Figure 7.7.5. Opening of the abdominal wall (V).
For entry into the abdominal cavity a small transverse muscle incision is made by lifting the abdominal muscle with surgical forceps.

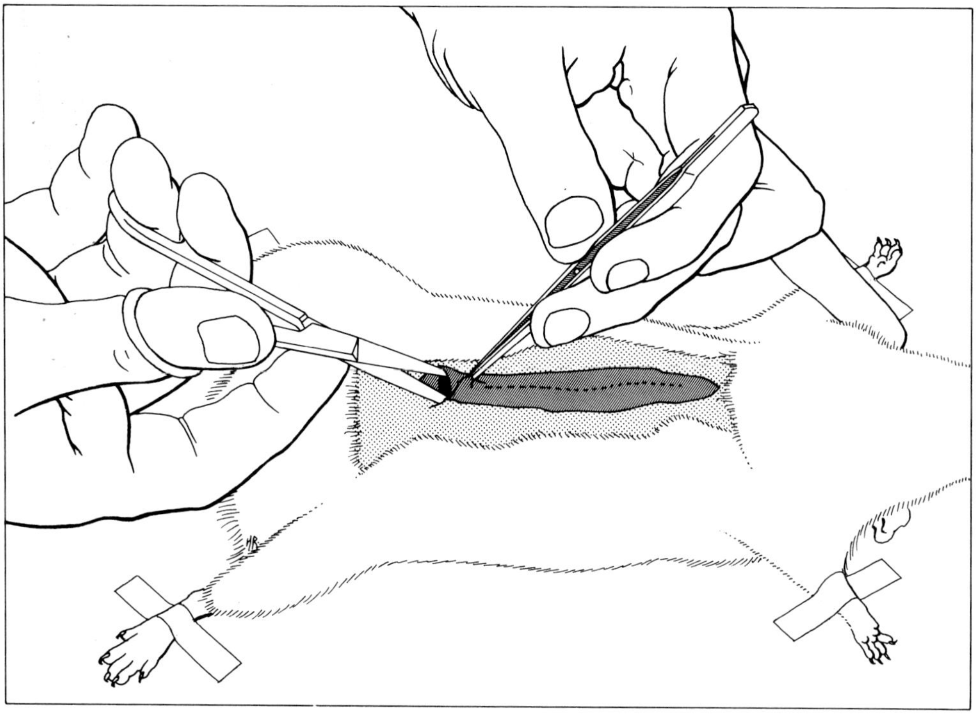

Figure 7.7.6. Opening of the abdominal wall (VI).
Both points of the closed scissors are inserted into the wound and are slightly spread transversely. Air will enter the abdominal cavity and the intestines which generally adhere to the abdominal wall, will retract and an excellent view is achieved.

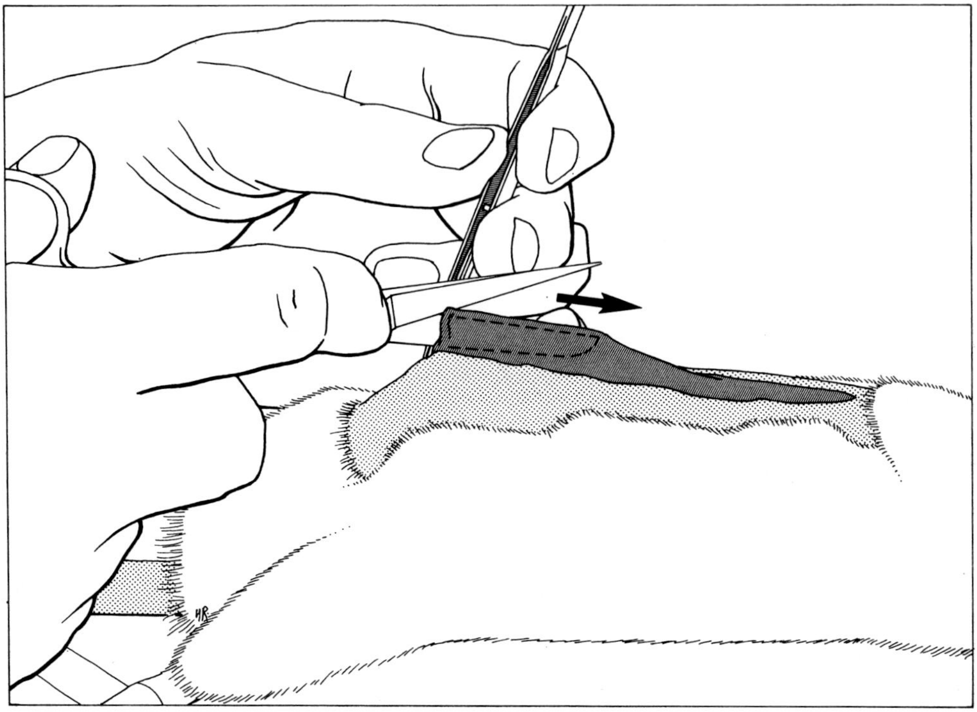

Figure 7.7.7. Opening of the abdominal wall (VII).

Again the blunt part of the scissors is inserted and a midline incision is made along the linea alba just past the xiphoid cartilage.

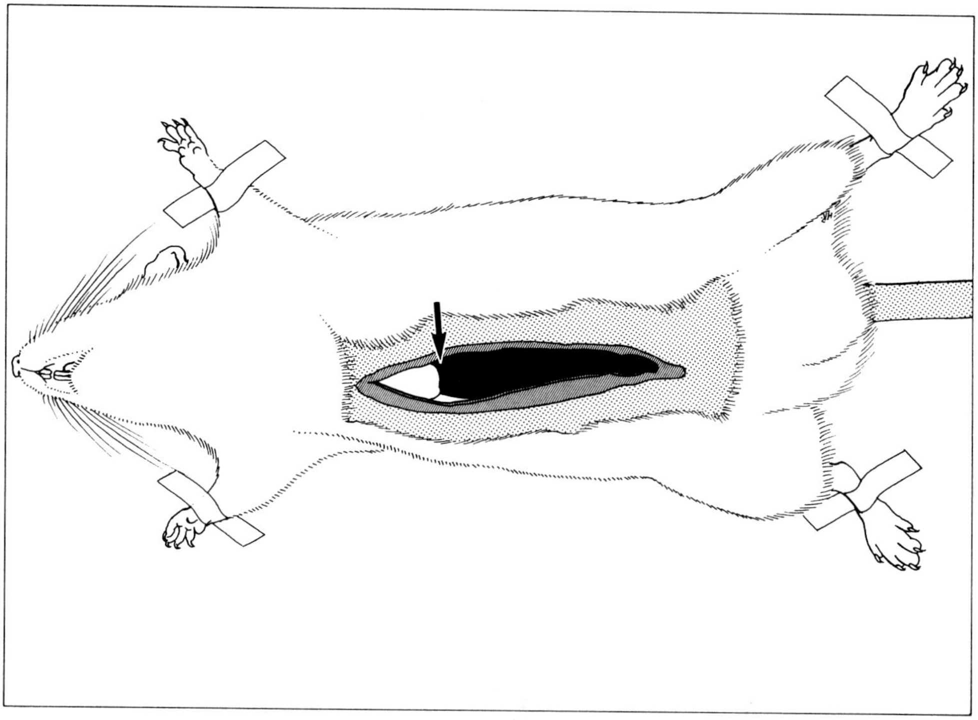

Figure 7.7.8. Opening of the abdominal wall (VIII).
Lateral to the xiphoid cartilage the ligament, indicated by the arrow, is cut.

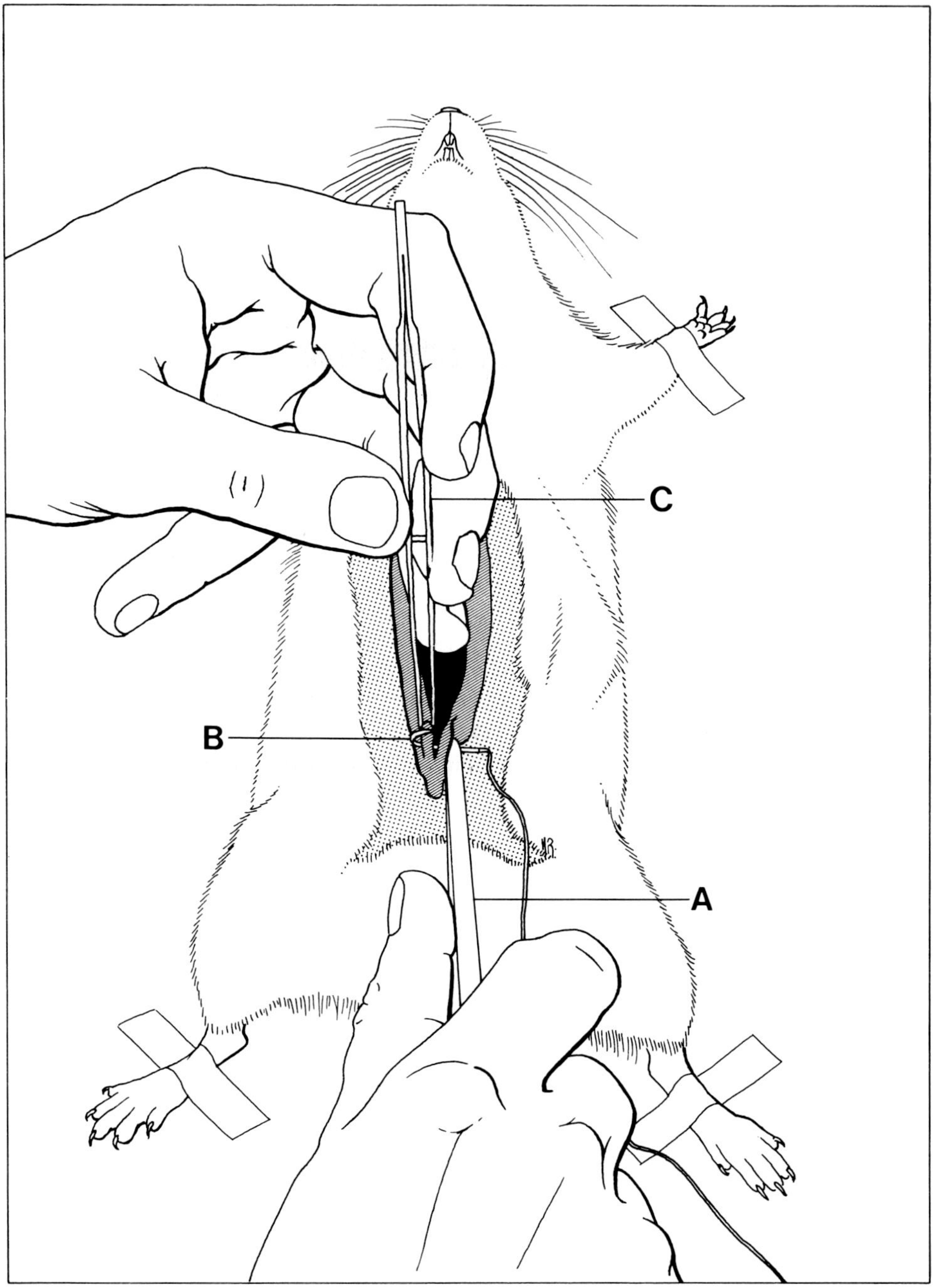

Figure 7.7.9. Closure of the abdominal wall (I).
The first stitch is placed in the rectus abdominis muscle running alongside the linea alba. The proper bit size is approximately 3–4 mm. Surgical forceps are used to support the tissue.
A. Needle holder. B. Needle. C. Surgical forceps.

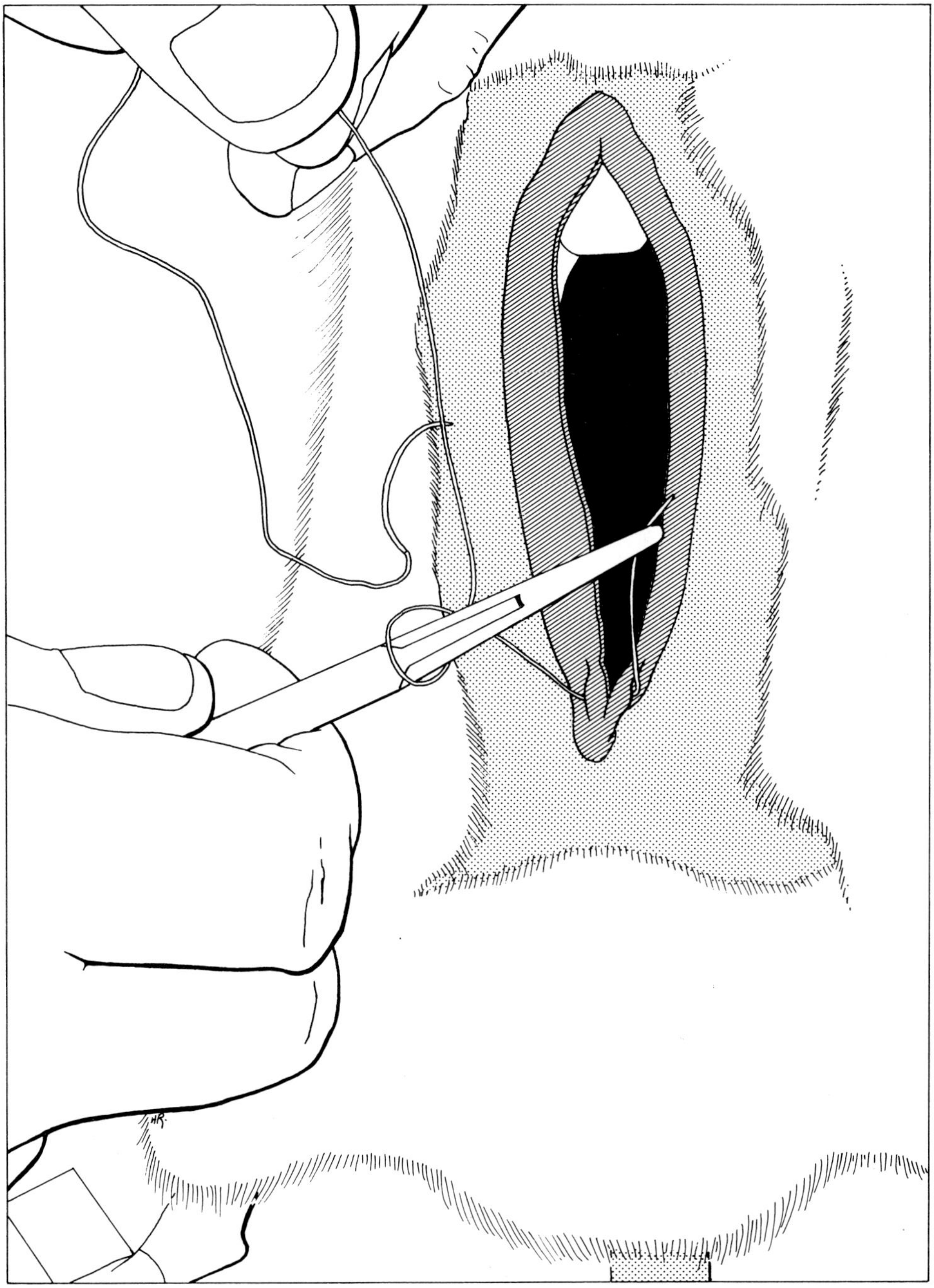

Figure 7.7.10. Closure of the abdominal wall (II).
The suture is held with the left hand, one loop is made around the needle holder, and the short end of the suture is grasped with the needle holder.

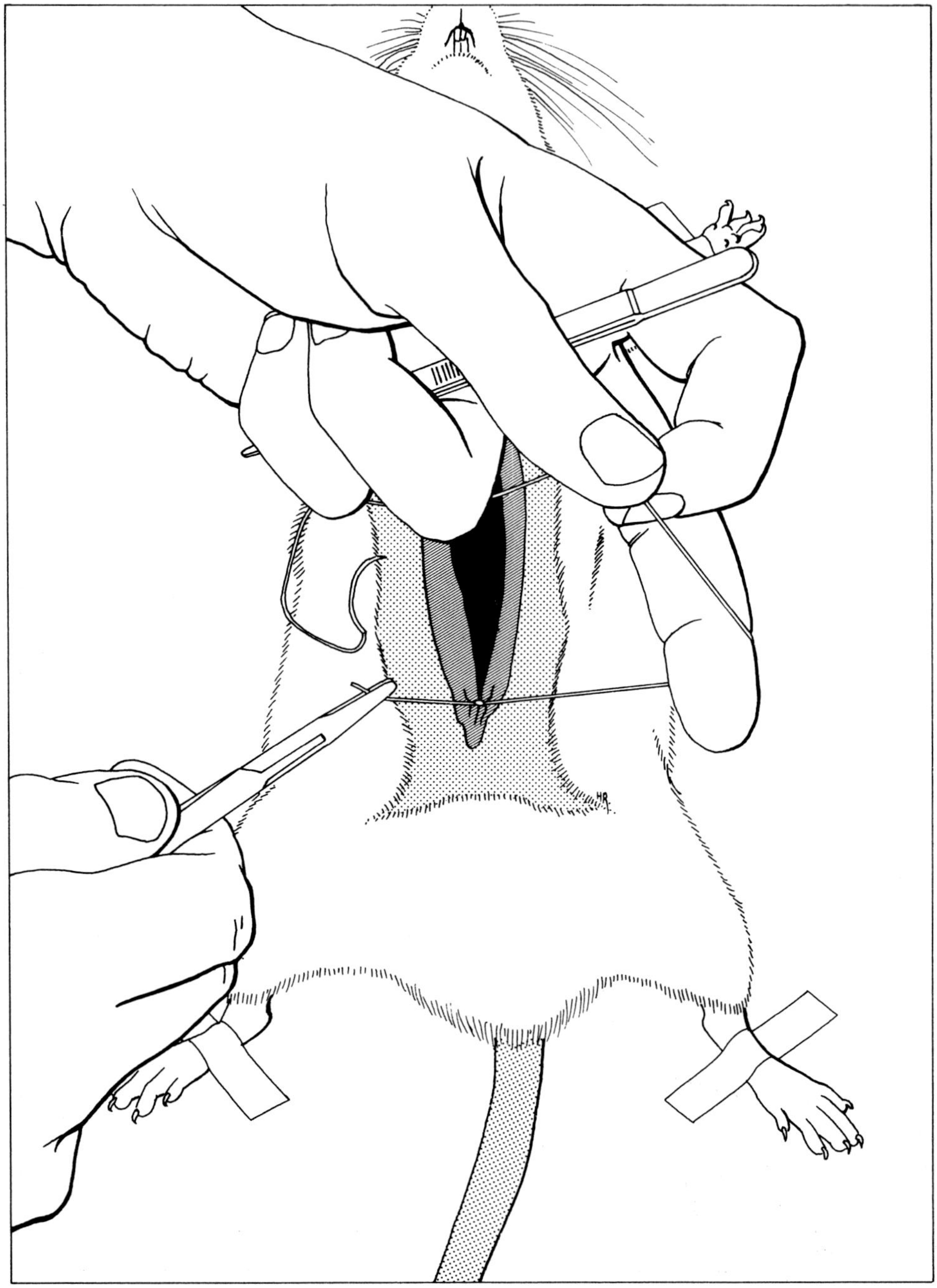

Figure 7.7.11. Closure of the abdominal wall (III).
Before the knot is tied, make sure that no underlying structures like epididymal or adipose tissue are trapped. Note that during this procedure the forceps are held in the left hand and the middle finger is used to put the appropriate tension on the suture.

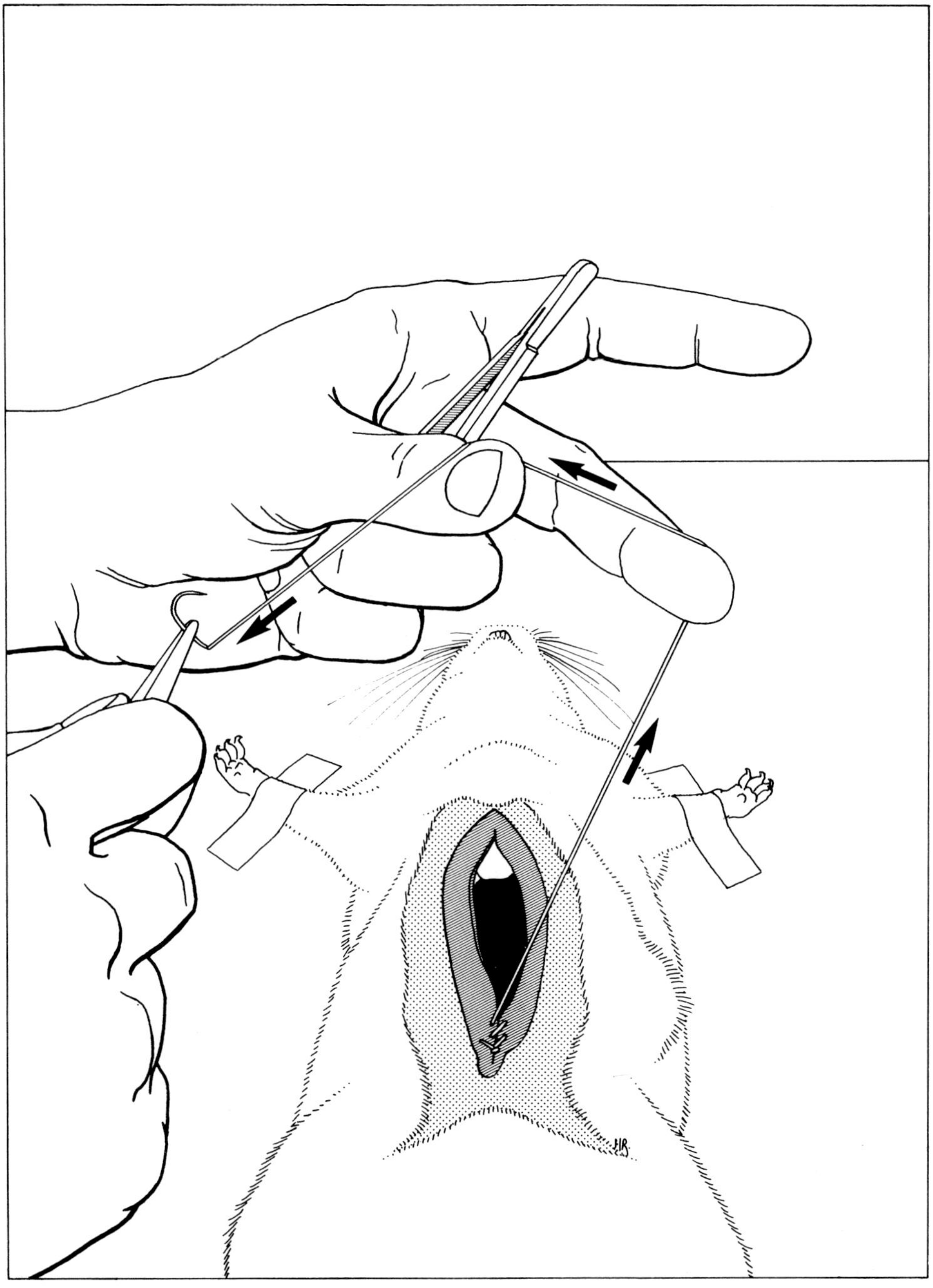

Figure 7.7.12. Closure of the abdominal wall (IV).
During the procedure the suture line should be kept under continuous tension, preventing the stitches from slipping.

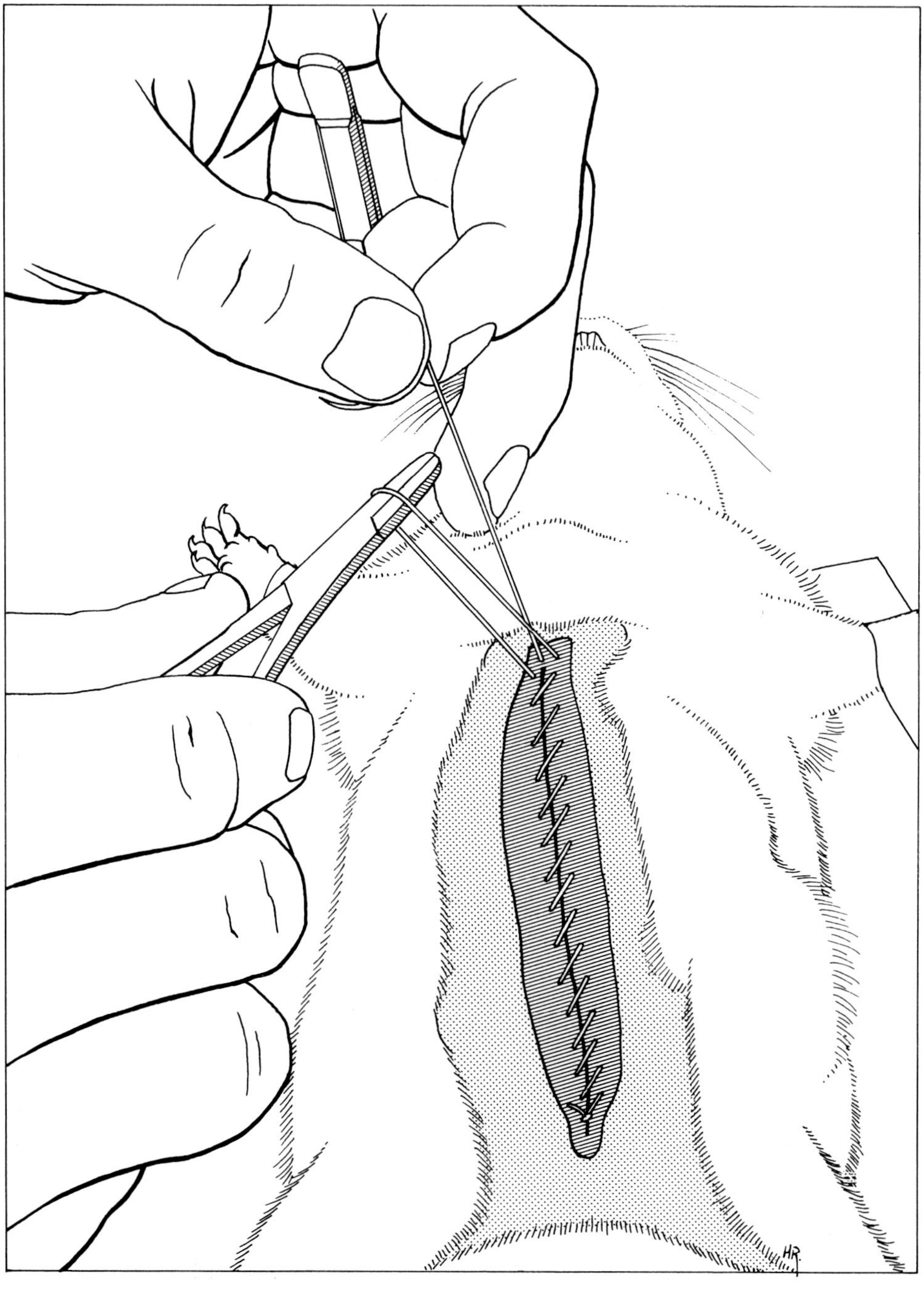

Figure 7.7.13. Closure of the abdominal wall (V).
The final knot is made. With the needle holder a loop is created holding the suture line under tension.

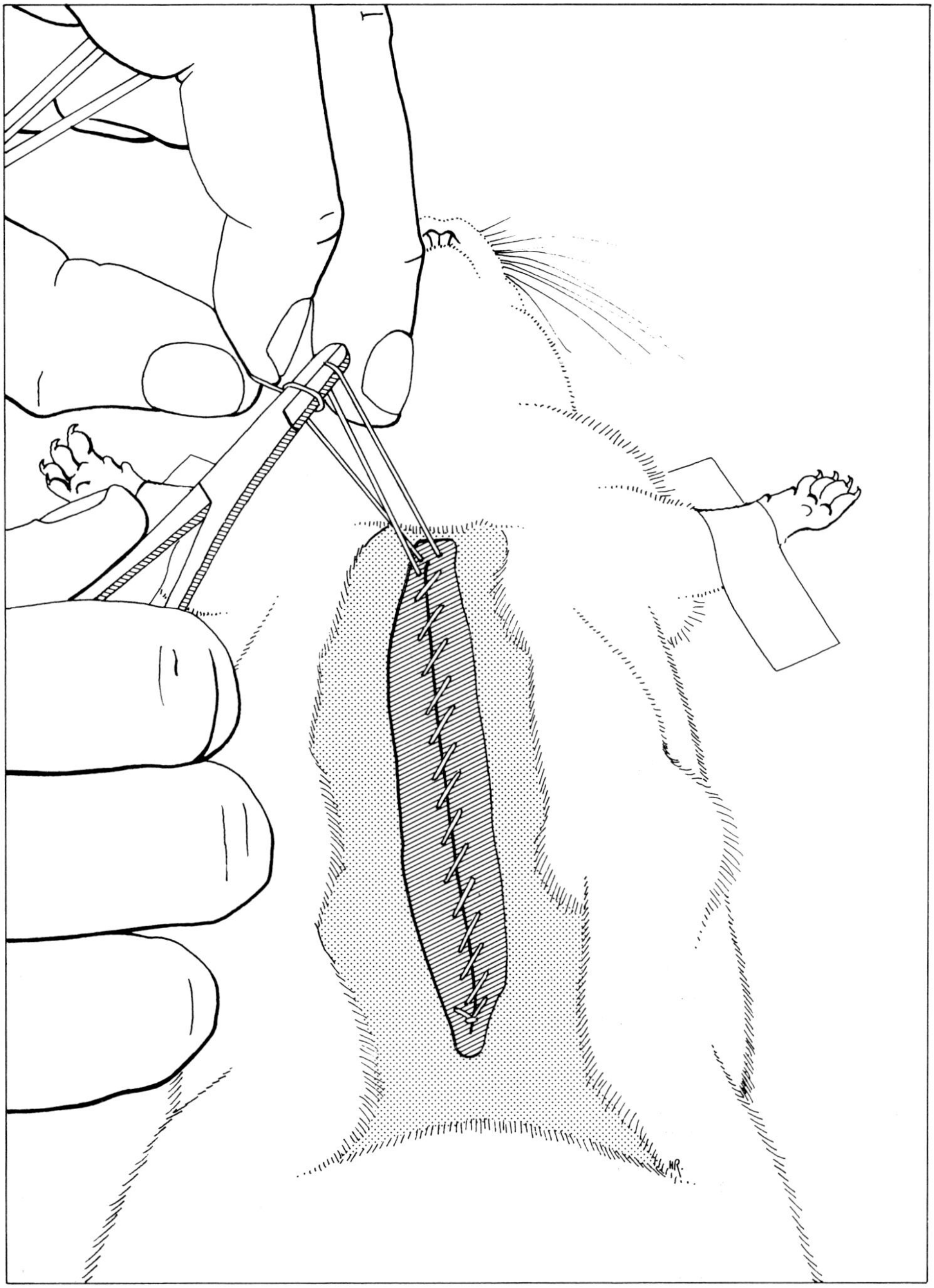

Figure 7.7.14. Closure of the abdominal wall (VI).
The thread is rotated around the needle holder, the loop is grasped while the thread is still kept under tension.

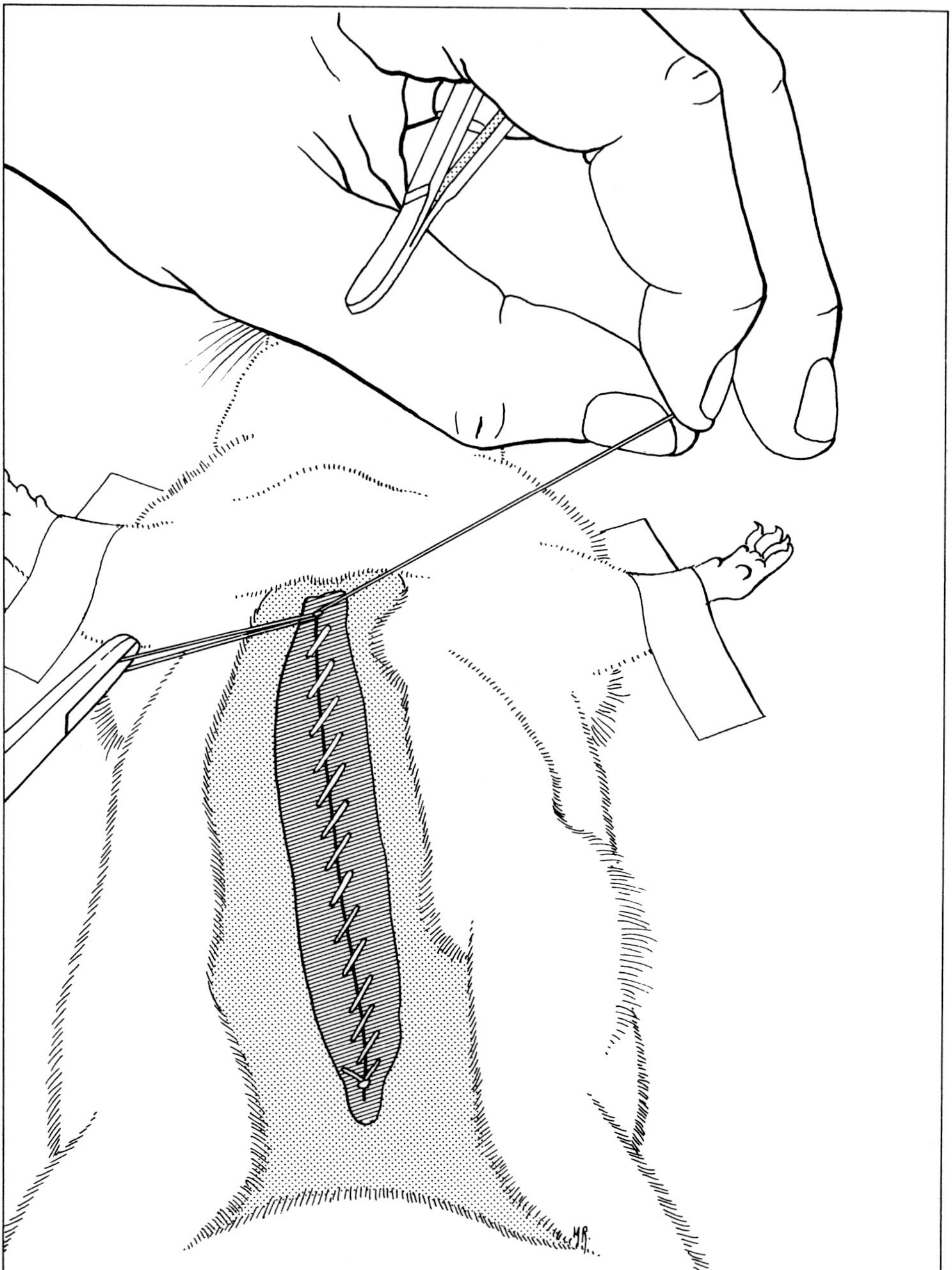

Figure 7.7.15. Closure of the abdominal wall (VII).
The loop is slipped over the needle holder and the first half knot is made. The second half knot is made using the same procedure.

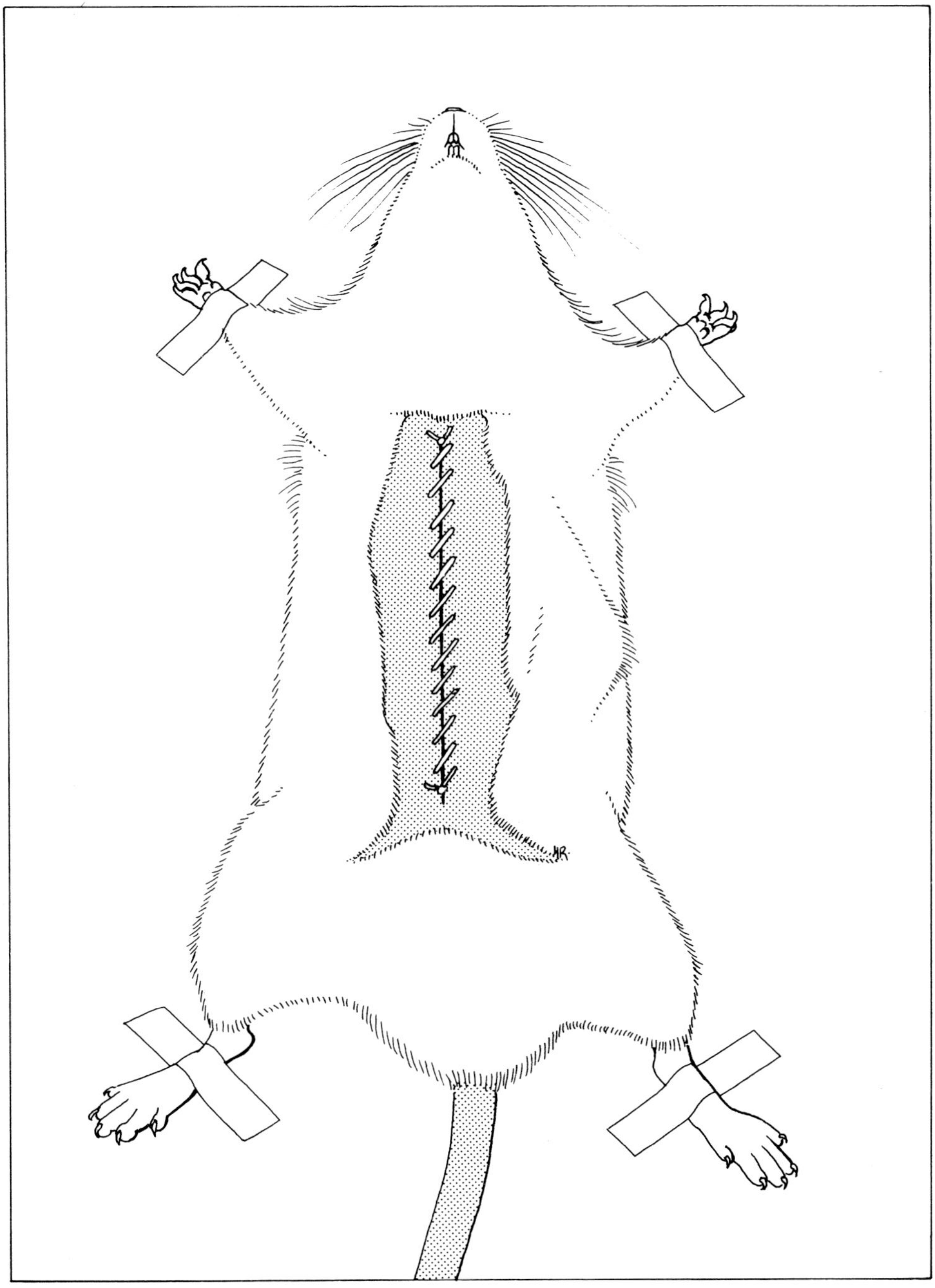

Figure 7.7.16. Closure of the abdominal wall (VIII).
The skin is closed using the same technique as described and depicted in Figures 7.7.9. to 7.7.15.

Figure 7.8.1. Subcutaneous tunnelling of cannulae (I).
The closed straight needle holder (long and slender type) is pushed into the incision on top of the head. To prevent the suture of the skin from slipping, artery forceps are used to clamp the suture.
A. Needle holder.
B. Cannulae.
C. Suture of the skin.
D. Artery forceps.

Figure 7.8.2. Subcutaneous tunnelling of cannulae (II).
While the skin of the neck is held firmly, the needle holder is pushed subcutaneously in a caudal direction for a distance of 8–10 cm, depending on the size of the animal.

Figure 7.8.3. Subcutaneous tunnelling of cannulae (III).
The needle holder is turned clockwise, as indicated by the arrow, into the direction of the aperture near the xiphoid cartilage.

Figure 7.8.4. Subcutaneous tunnelling of cannulae (IV).
The needle holder is rotated further and is pushed towards the aperture.

Figure 7.8.5. Subcutaneous tunnelling of cannulae (V).
The jaws of the needle holder are now visible. While giving some support to the abdominal skin near the aperture, the needle holder is pushed out further.

Figure 7.8.6. Subcutaneous tunnelling of cannulae (VI).
The cannulae are grasped and pulled backwards through the subcutaneous tunnel, emerging at the top of the head. Subsequently, the abdominal skin can be closed.

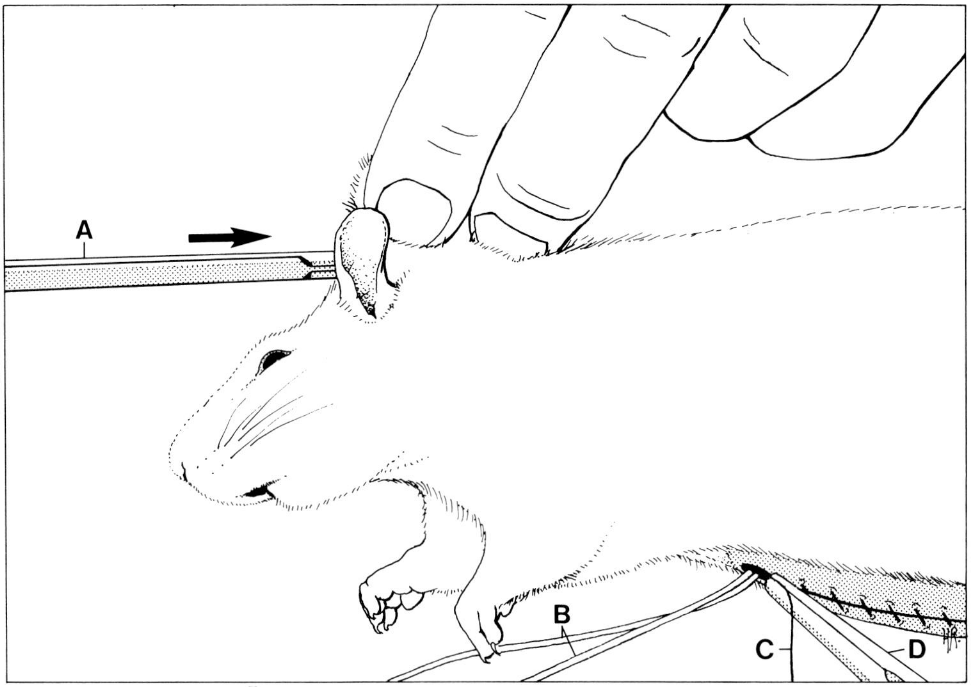

Figure 7.8.1.

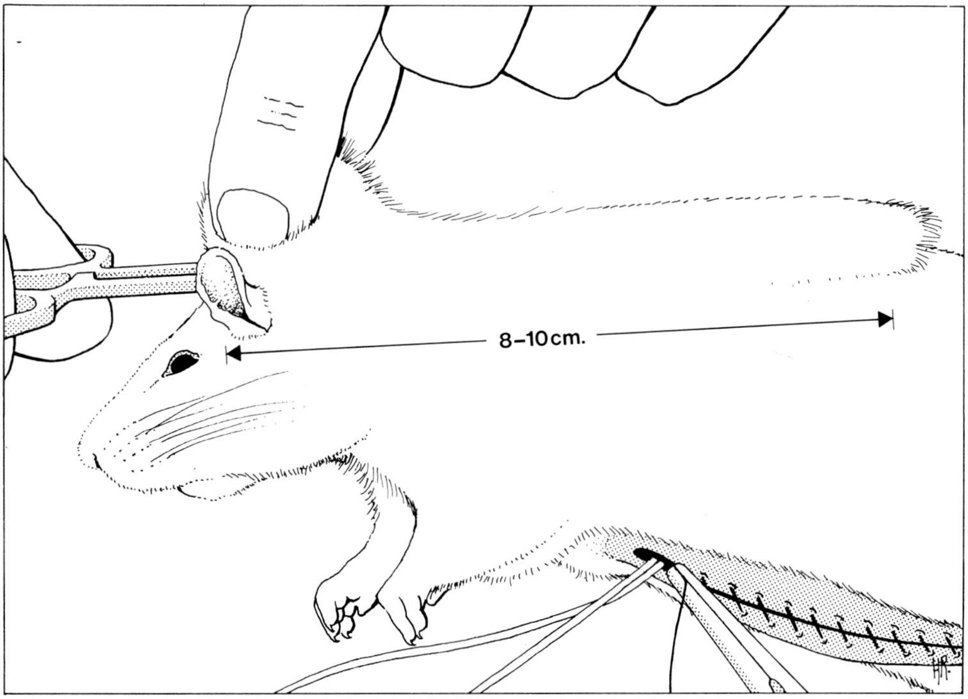

Figure 7.8.2.

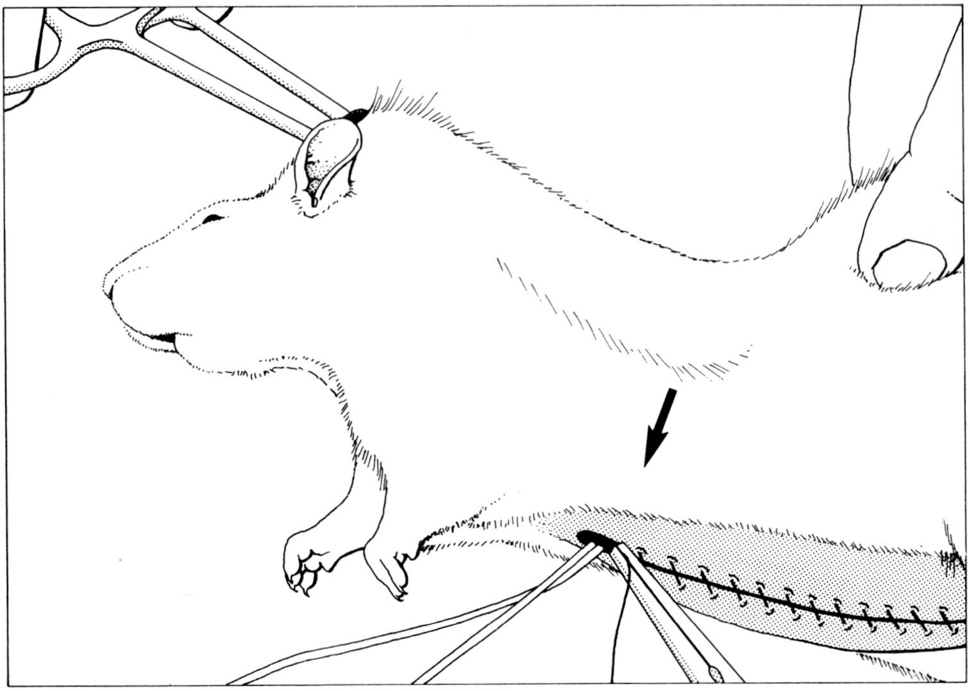

Figure 7.8.3.

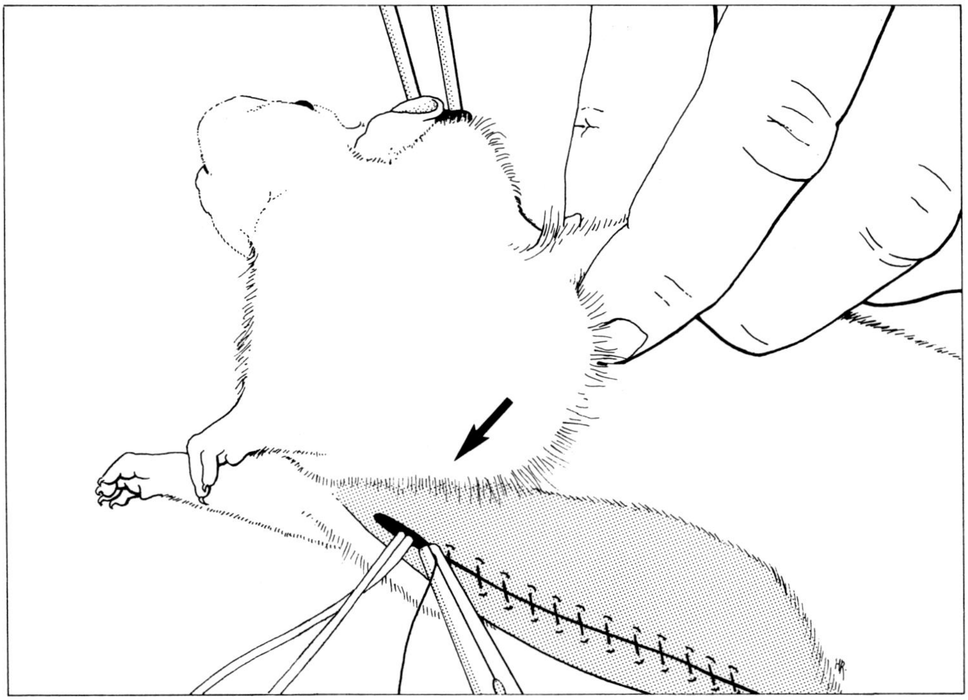

Figure 7.8.4.

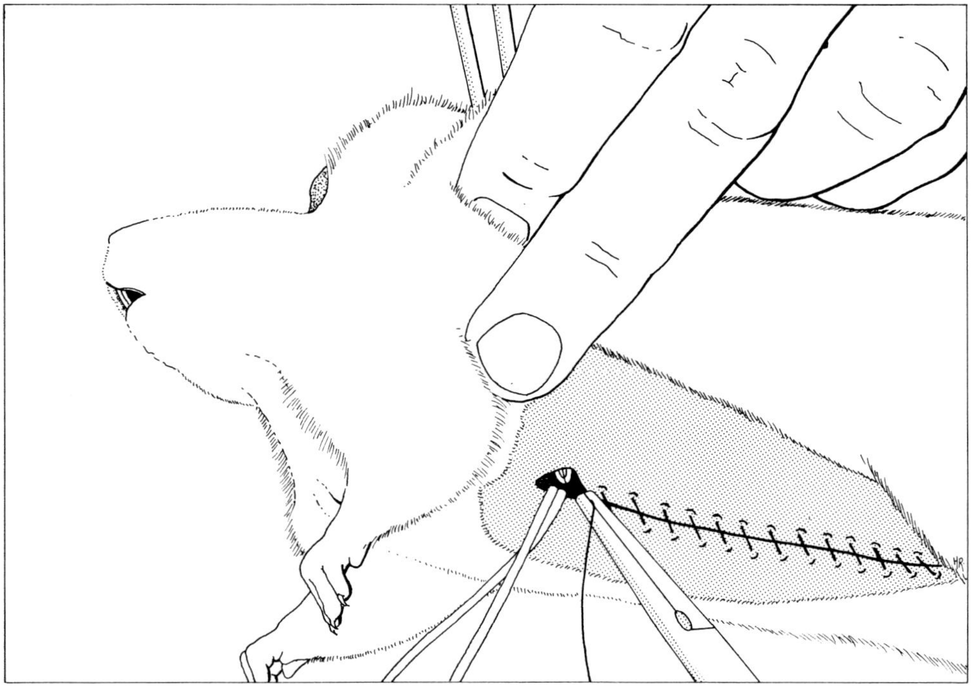

Figure 7.8.5.

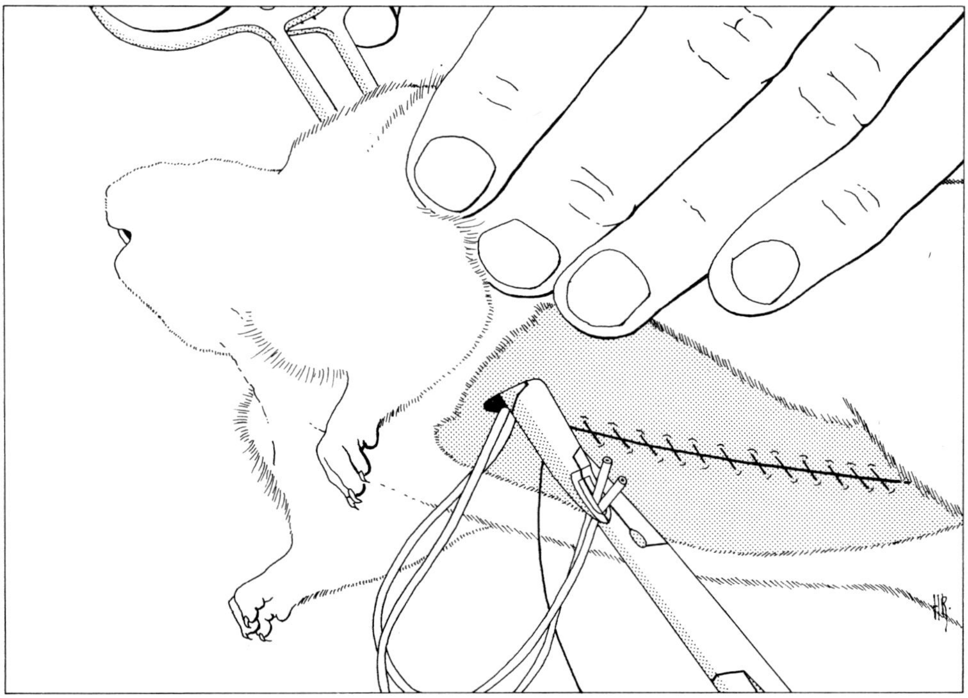

Figure 7.8.6.

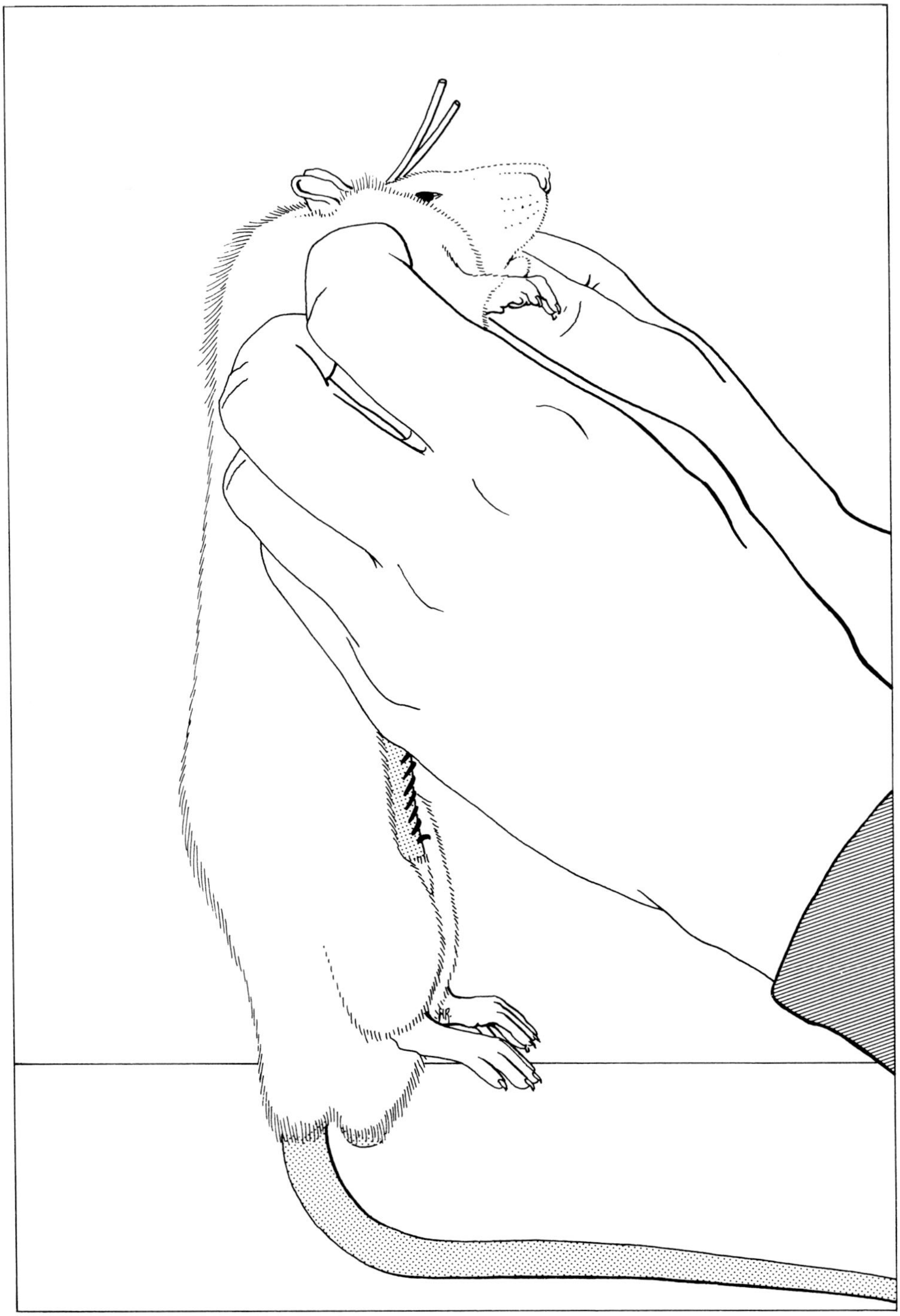

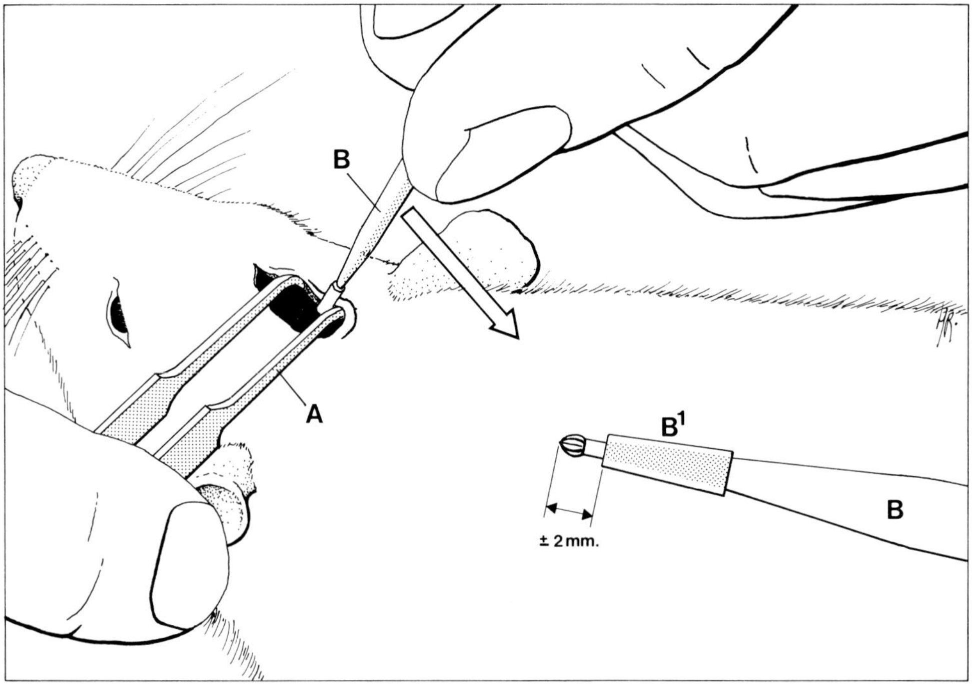

Figure 7.9.1. Preparation of the crown of the head (I).
With curved jewellers or anatomical forceps the incision on the top of the head is spread, while three holes are drilled in the skull as indicated in Figure 7.9.4., by making rotatory movements between the left hand index finger and the thumb. A piece of protective polyethylene tubing is placed over the drill bit, leaving about 2 mm of the tip uncovered. This will protect the underlying tissues from being punctured.

A. Jewellers forceps.
B. Drill bit.
B^1. Polyethylene tubing.

←

Figure 7.8.7. Subcutaneous tunnelling of cannulae (VII).
Finally the animal should be lifted by its forelegs, allowing the cannulae to set subcutaneously without being under any tension.

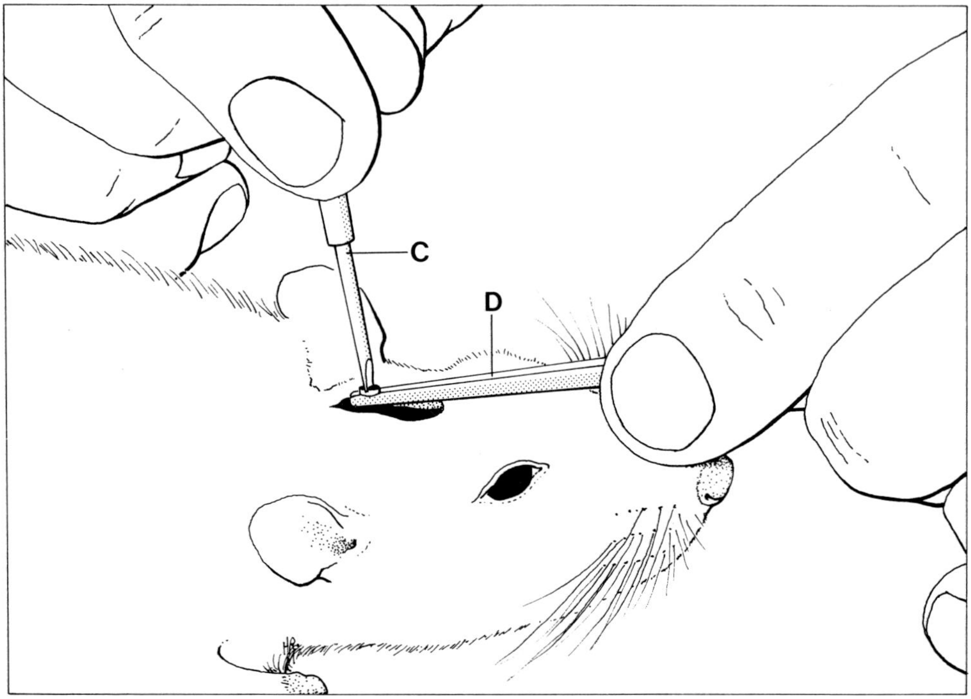

Figure 7.9.2. Preparation of the crown of the head (II).
The position of the hands and the instruments during insertion of a screw.
C. Screw driver.
D. Specially prepared surgical forceps.

→

Figure 7.9.3. Preparation of the crown of the head (III).
Detail of the head and the tip of the surgical forceps in which a 0.5 mm hole has been drilled to fixate the screws during their insertion.
C. Screw driver.
D. Tip of the specially prepared surgical forceps.

Figure 7.9.4. Preparation of the crown of the head (IV).
The situation on the crown of the skull after the screws have been placed, and the position of the screws relative to the bregma.
E. Bregma.

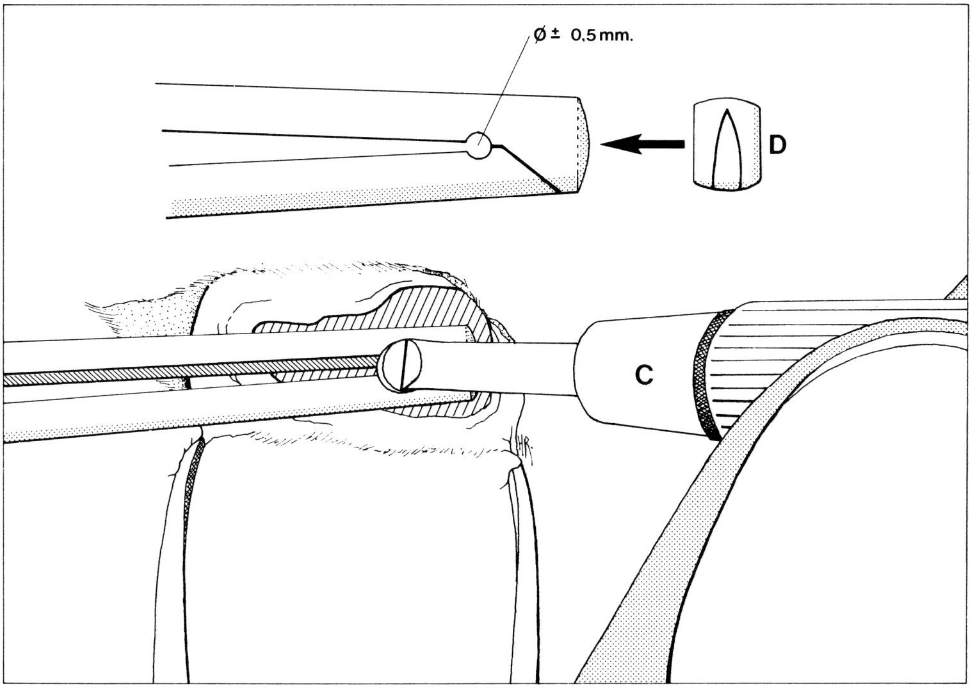

Figure 7.9.3.

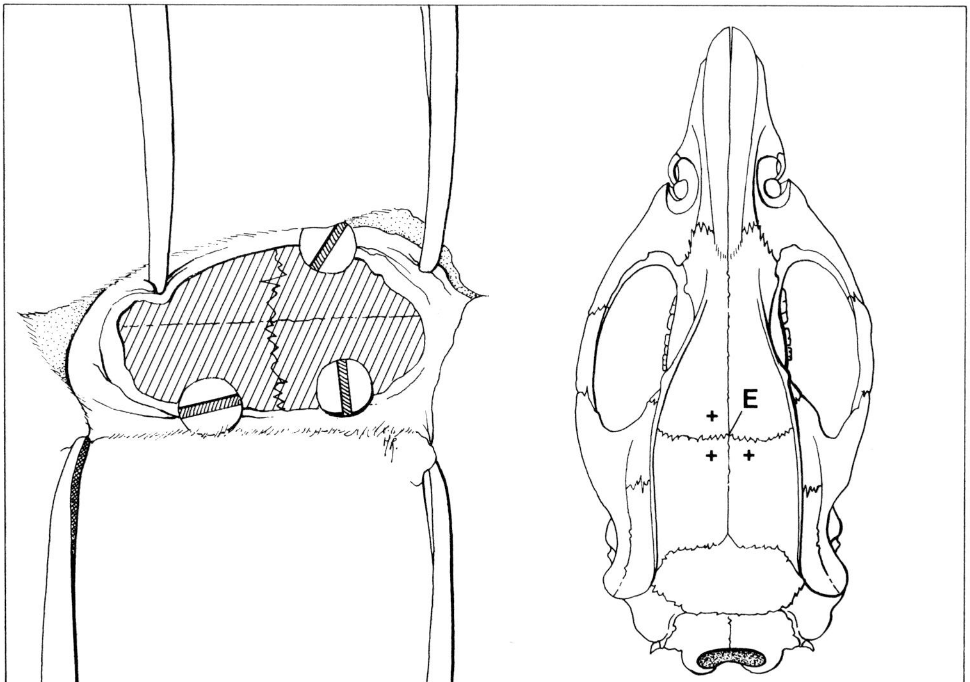

Figure 7.9.4.

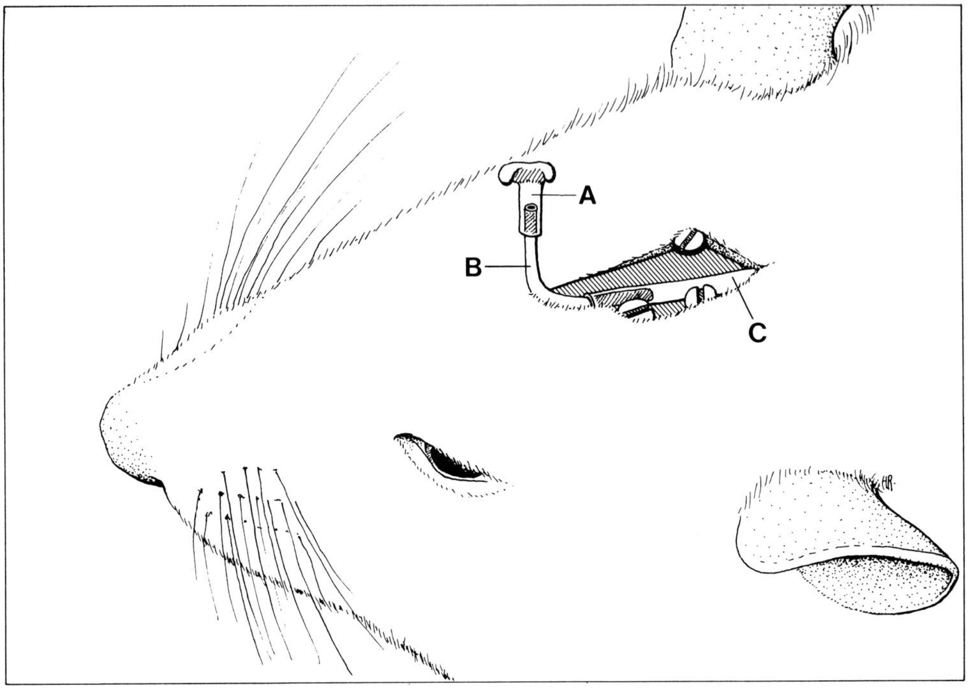

Figure 7.9.5. Fixation of cannulae (I).
The situation on the crown of the head of an animal with a permanent jugular vein cannula, after the cannula has been filled with PVP-solution, and closed with a polyethylene cap.
A. Heat sealed polyethylene cap.
B. L-shaped adapter.
C. Jugular vein cannula.

→

Figure 7.9.6. Fixation of cannulae (II).
The situation on the crown of the head of an animal with a permanent jugular vein cannula, after fixation to the skull with acrylic glue.
A. Heat sealed polyethylene cap.
B. L-shaped adapter.
D. Acrylic glue.

Figure 7.9.7. Fixation of cannulae (III).
Final situation on the crown of the head of an animal with a permanent jugular vein cannula, after closure of the skin.
A. Heat sealed polyethylene cap.
B. L-shaped adapter.
D. Acrylic glue.
E. Sutures.

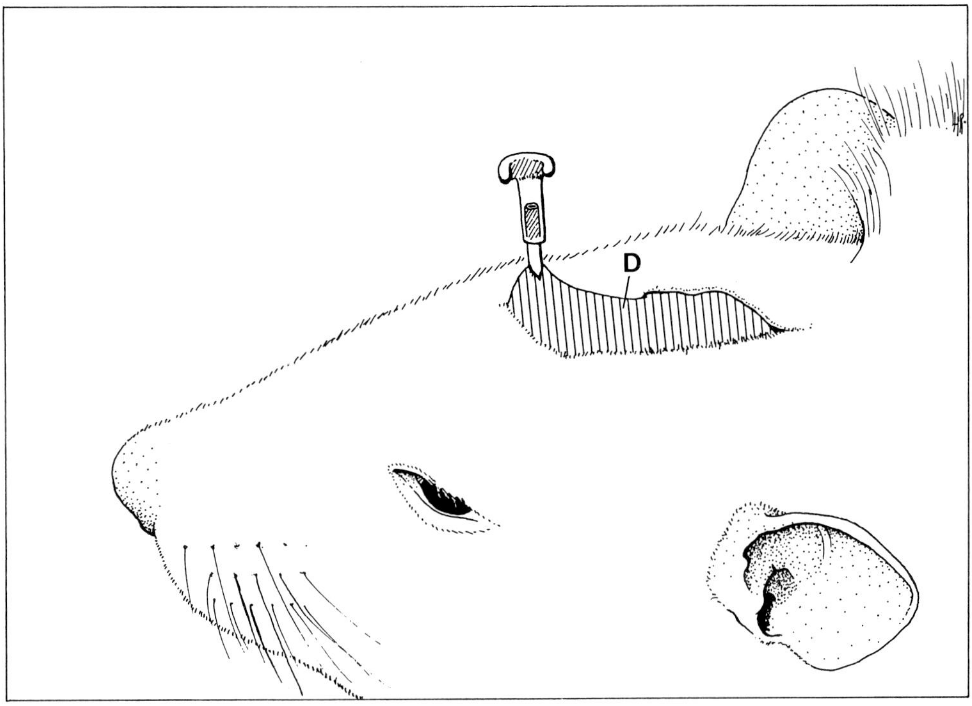

Figure 7.9.6.

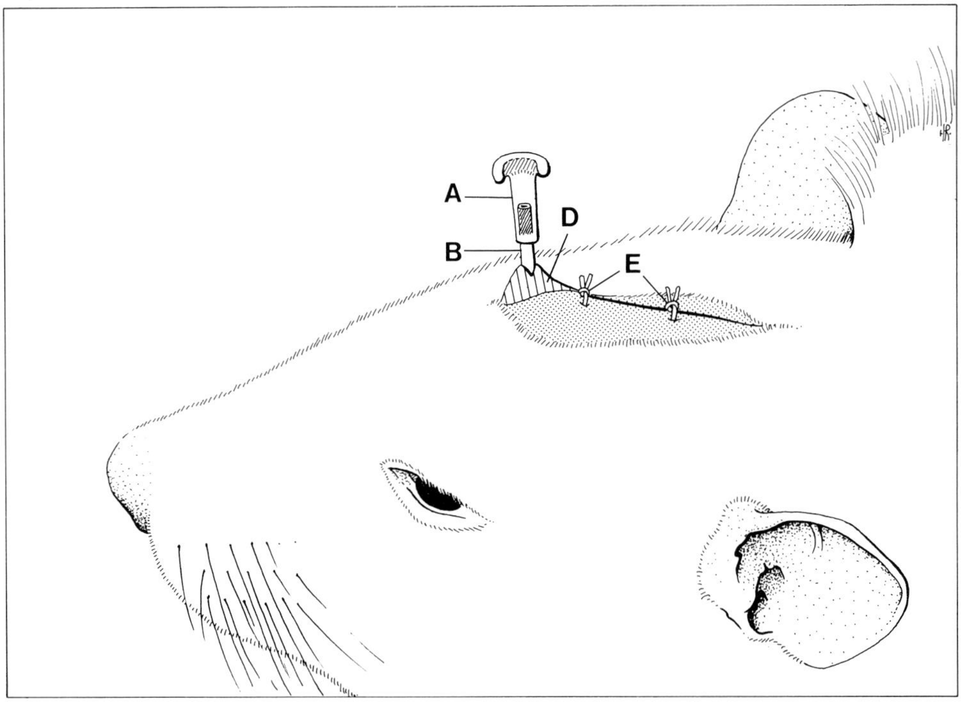

Figure 7.9.7.

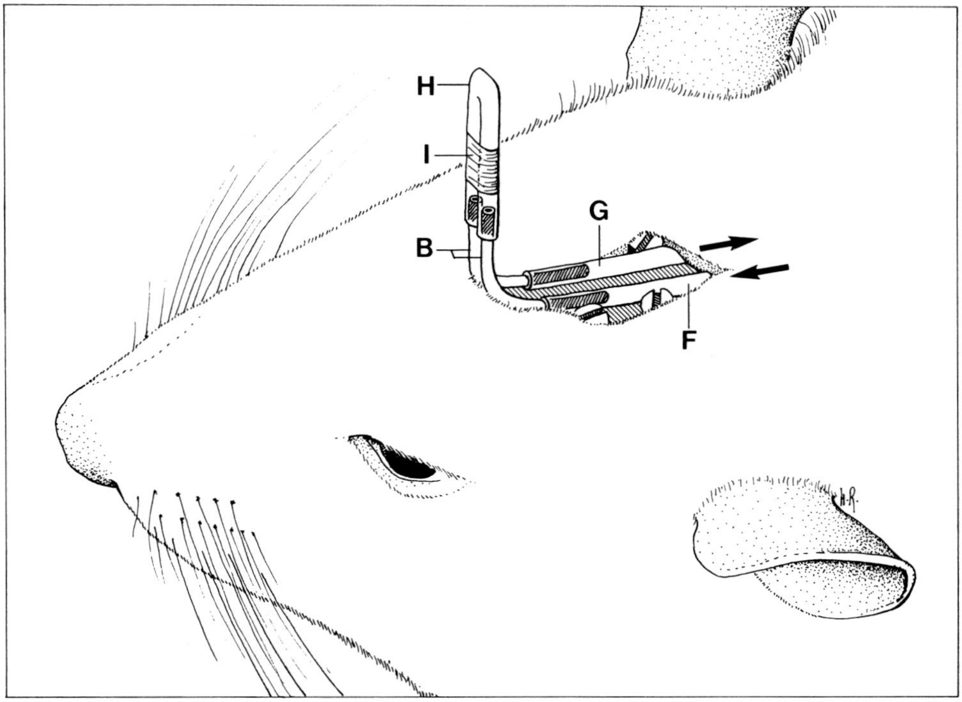

Figure 7.9.8. Fixation of cannulae (IV).
Situation on the crown of the head of an animal with a permanent double bile fistula, before the acrylic glue is applied.
B. L-shaped adapters.
F. Proximal bile cannula.
G. Distal bile cannula.
H. U-shaped piece of polyethelene tubing.
I. Adhesive tape.

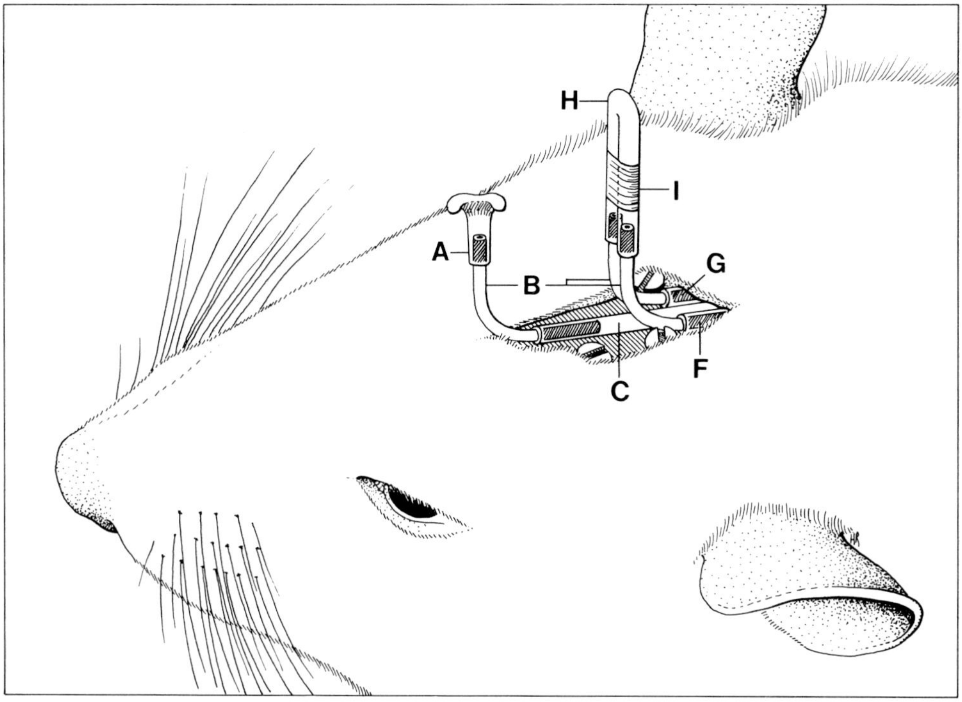

Figure 7.9.9. Fixation of cannulae (V).
Situation on the crown of the head of an animal with a permanent double bile fistula and a permanent jugular vein cannula, before the acrylic glue is applied.
A. Heat sealed polyethylene cap.
B. L-shaped adapters.
C. Jugular vein cannula.
F. Proximal bile cannula.
G. Distal bile cannula.
H. U-shaped piece of polyethelene tubing.
I. Adhesive tape.

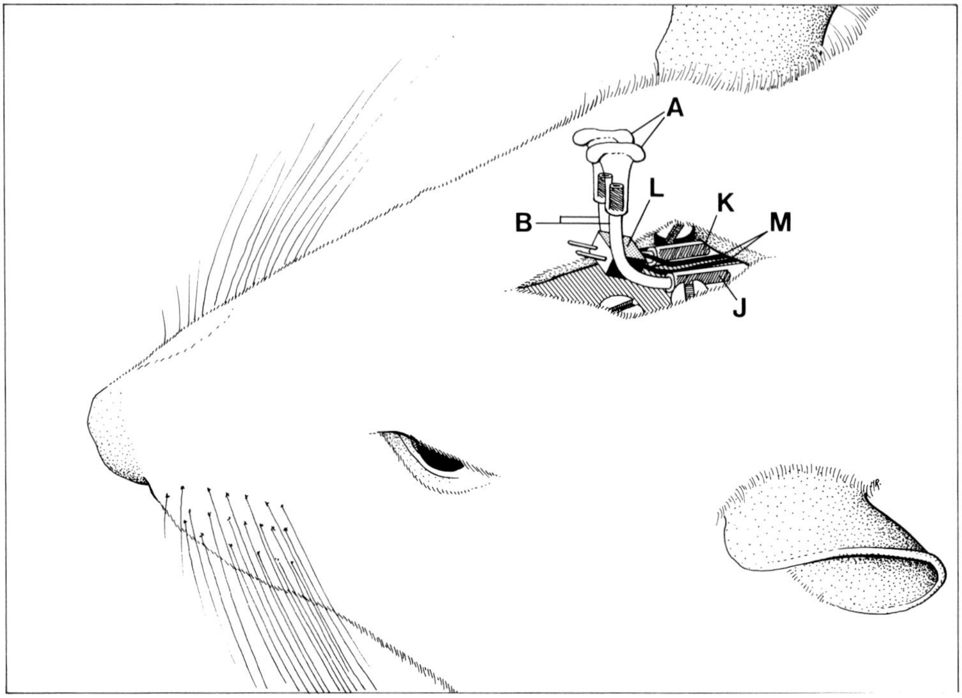

Figure 7.9.10. Fixation of cannulae (VI).
The situation on the crown of the head of an animal with a permanent portal sample and an infusion cannula, in combination with a miniature plug (modified IC-foot) attached to the stimulation electrodes, before the acrylic glue is applied.

A. Heat sealed polyethylene caps.
B. L-shaped adapters.
J. Portal sample cannula.
K. Portal infusion cannula.
L. Miniature plug.
M. Insulated silver leads.

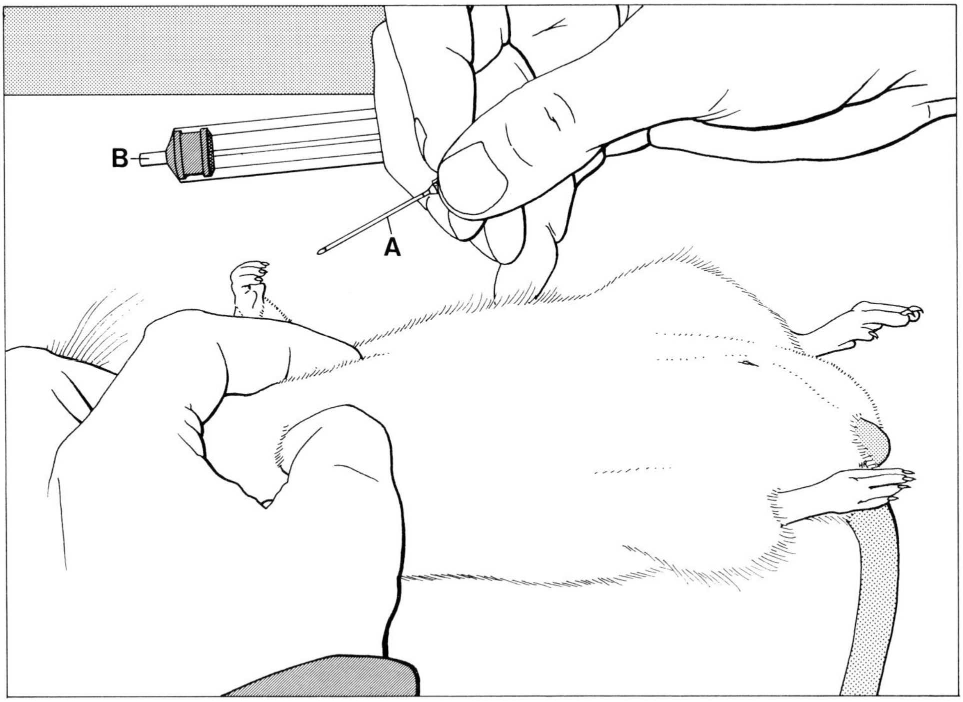

Figure 7.10.1. The heart puncture (I).
Cardiac puncture is carried out under light anaesthesia. After removal of the hair on the left part of the thorax, the skin is disinfected with iodine solution. The animal is placed in a supine position, with its head away from the surgeon. The heart is palpated during slight compression of the thorax with the index finger and the thumb of the left hand. The needle is picked up.
A. 20G needle.
B. Syringe.

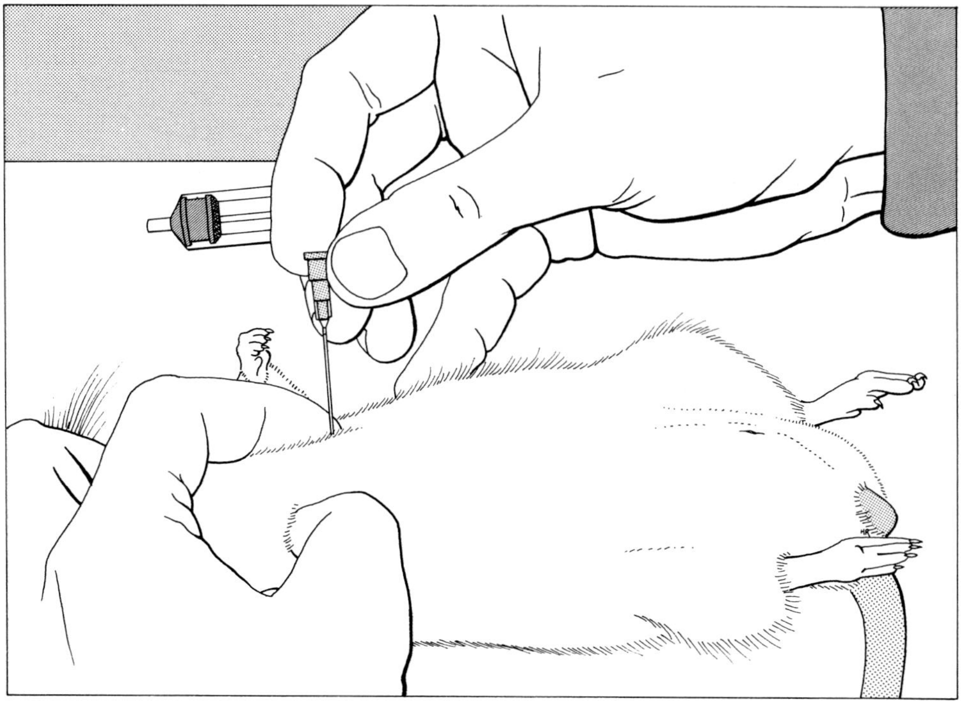

Figure 7.10.2. The heart puncture (II).
The needle is pushed through the skin into the intercostal muscles. At this moment the heart beat will be transmitted to the needle. With a short thrust the needle is pushed 3 to 4 mm into the heart, and blood will flow out of the needle.

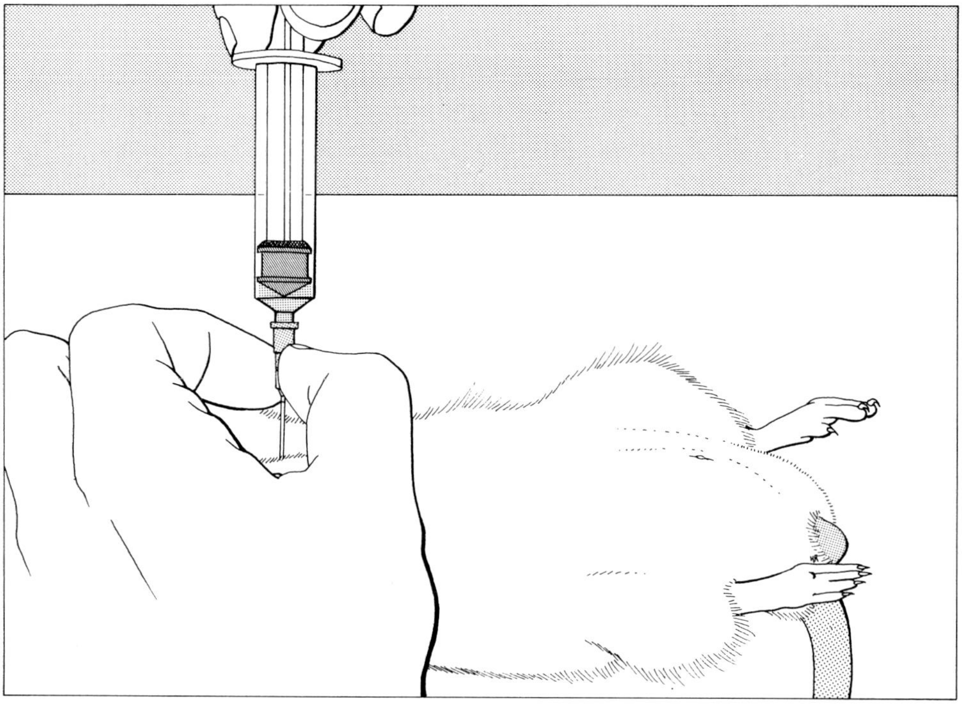

Figure 7.10.3. The heart puncture (III).
The syringe is pushed onto the needle immediately and blood is withdrawn slowly and steadily, at a rate of about 0.2 ml/sec or less.

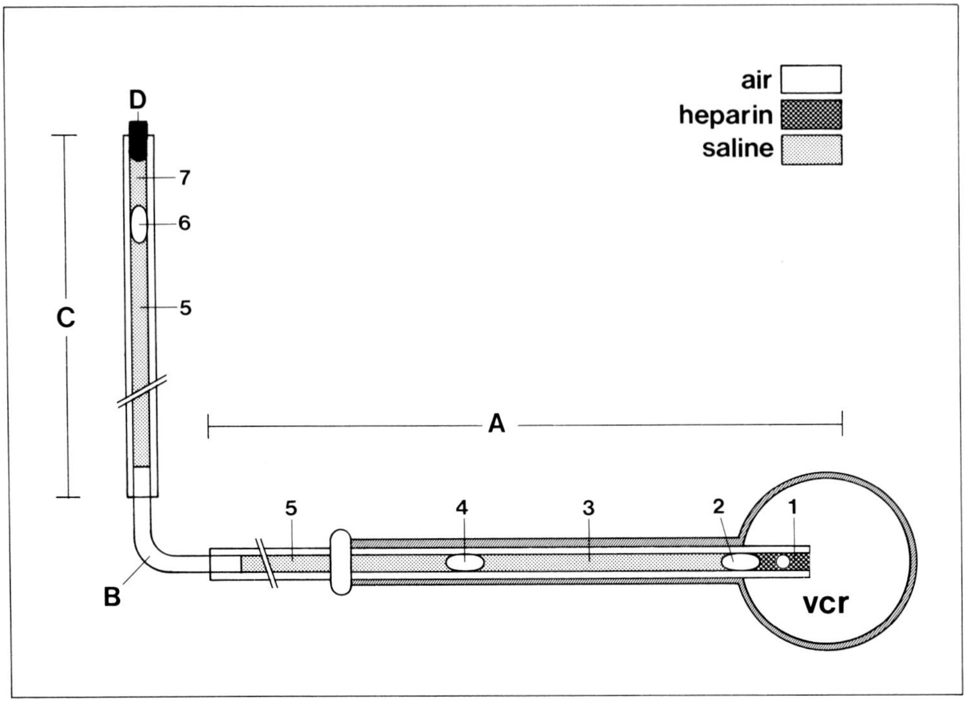

Figure 7.10.4. Schematic representation of the permanent jugular vein cannula during blood sampling.
Numbers 1 to 7 show the sequence of the procedure.
A. The cannula inside the animal.
B. The L-shaped adapter.
C. The polyethylene tubing (0.75 × 1.45 mm) attatched to the animal.
D. A copper or stainless steel nail of appropriate size.
vcr Vena cava rostralis, at the level of the right atrium.

II. EXPERIMENTAL TECHNIQUES

Manual of Microsurgery on the Laboratory Rat, Part I
Van Dongen, Remie, Rensema and Van Wunnik (eds)
© 1990 Elsevier Science Publishers B.V. (Biomedical Division)

CHAPTER 8

Permanent cannulation of the jugular vein (acc. to Steffens)

R. REMIE, J.J. VAN DONGEN and J.W. RENSEMA

8.1 Introduction

In biomedical research, blood plays a central role. Blood can be sampled from the laboratory rat in a number of ways, for example puncture of the ophthalmic venous plexus, puncture of the heart, cutting the tail or even decapitation. In all these methods, the animal is either anaesthetized or handled and restrained. This causes reactions in the animal, such as elevation of the catecholamine and corticosteroid levels, both possibly interfering with the results of the experiments. To avoid these influences it would be vastly preferable to take blood samples from the animal without causing it any disturbance. A number of techniques have been put forward. Permanent cannulation of the jugular vein in combination with a head attachment apparatus allowing easy connection of cannulae was first introduced by Steffens (1969). This technique enables continuous blood sampling from the general circulation and the infusion of fluids, in the freely moving rat. During sampling the animal remains undisturbed, which is of vital importance in experiments monitoring behaviour or where stress-factors are expected to influence results. Several modifications have been introduced amongst which the ones by Brown and Hedge (1972), who introduced the L-shaped adapter, Nicolaidis et al. (1974) who used an additional stainless steel head bolt, and Dons and Havlik (1986) who used a multilayered cannula. In our opinion, however, the technique described below is one of the most simple and reliable, and it should be regarded as one of the basic techniques in cannulation of blood vessels.

8.2 The operation

Anaesthesia

The animal should preferably be anaesthetized with N_2O_2/O_2/halothane. If this type of anaesthesia is not available, then FFM (i.p.) should be used (see Chapter 6).

The operation can be divided into four parts:

8.2.1. Preparation of the crown of the head.
8.2.2. Cannulation of the jugular vein.
8.2.3. Subcutaneous tunnelling of the cannula.
8.2.4. Fixation of the cannula to the skull.

Parts 8.2.1. and 8.2.4. are described in Chapter 7 (General techniques).

8.2.2. Cannulation of the jugular vein

The shaven neck of the animal on the right side should be disinfected with chlorhexidine solution. As depicted in Figure 8.2.1. the incision should be made just above the right clavicle. Connective and adipose tissue are pushed aside with blunt forceps and the jugular vein is exposed. The external jugular vein should be followed and the division into the maxillary vein, the facial and linguofacial vein (Figure 8.2.2.) can be identified. This bifurcation is recognizable by a small lymph node laying on the jugular vein. At this point one should decide which one of the two veins to use for cannulation. The largest vessel should be chosen and mobilized for a distance of about five millimetres.

Small artery forceps (baby-Mosquito) should be used to clamp the vessel. The vein should then be ligated rostral to the clamp with 6–0 silk, and a second ligature should be put loosely around the vessel, not tightened, as shown in Figure 8.2.3. Using iridectomy scissors (Figure 8.2.4.), a V-shaped hole (Figure 8.2.5.) should be cut in the vein 2 mm rostral from the bifurcation. Prior to its insertion into the vessel, the sterile cannula must be connected to a 1 ml syringe filled with a heparinized saline solution (50 IU/ml). There should be no air bubbles left in the cannula. See Chapter 7, for a detailed description of the cannula and its preparation.

The vessel should be dilated by means of sharp pointed jewellers forceps, the cannula slid between the legs of the forceps and gently pushed into the vessel until the silicon ring reaches the V-shaped hole (Figures 8.2.6. and 8.2.7.). At this stage there are various difficulties which may be encountered. One such example is whilst trying to push the cannula gently into the vessel, it bounces on release, then the cannula will almost certainly have entered the subclavicular vein. This can be remedied by pulling the cannula back, whilst still leaving it inside the vessel, then pushing it back in gently while lifting the animal's chest by the skin. In this way it is virtually impossible for the cannula to enter the subclavicular vein. When the silicon ring has reached the vessel, the tip of the cannula should now be at the level of the right atrium. This can be checked by removing the needle and the syringe and looking at the fluid in the free end of the cannula. During inspiration the fluid should be sucked into the cannula, while during expiration the fluid should be pushed back (intra-thoracic pressure). Moreover, the heart frequency should be superimposed on the respiratory-induced fluid movements. The catheter should be further checked by aspirating some blood, and the cannula should be flushed gently with 100 μl of the heparinized saline solution. If this can be done without problems the artery forceps should be removed, the caudal ligature gently tied, and the rostral ligature used to anchor the cannula to the vessel (Figure 8.2.8.). Subsequently, the syringe should be removed and the cannula gently clamped using a small microvascular clamp. To ensure that the cannula cannot move, one drawstring of each ligature should be tied, crossing over the silicon ring (Figure 8.2.9.).

8.2.3. Subcutaneous tunnelling of the cannula

The cannula should be tunnelled subcutaneously to emerge at the top of the head. In Figure 8.2.10. the small artery forceps are shown, just before they are pushed in longitudinally under the skin in a caudal direction to a distance of about 3 cm. Subsequently, the forceps should be turned anti-clockwise through an angle of 90 degrees, and pushed in the direction of the neck incision. The cannula should be clipped by the forceps and the forceps pulled back. Care must be taken not to twist the cannula during this procedure. The forceps should then be removed and replaced by the small microvascular clamp (Figures 8.2.11., 8.2.12., 8.2.13., 8.2.14.). The cannula should be slid over the short end of a 20G stainless steel needle bent to a 90 degree angle (the L-shaped adapter, see Chapter 7). The catheter should now be flushed with saline (0.5 ml) and filled with a 60% polyvinylpyrolidone (MW 10,000) solution in saline with 500 IU/ml heparine (PVP-solution). The long end of the L-shaped stainless steel adapter should be closed with a piece of heat sealed PE-tubing (Figure 8.2.15.). The wound in the neck of the animal should be closed with two sutures (4–0 Vicryl).

References

Brown, M.R. and Hedge, G.A. (1972) Thyroid secretion in the unanesthetized, stress-free rat and its suppression by pentobarbital. Neuroendocrinology 9: 158–174.

Dons, R.F. and Havlik, R. (1986) A multilayered cannula for long-term blood sampling of unrestrained rats. Laboratory Animal Science 36, 5: 544–547.

Nicolaidis, S., Rowland, N., Meile, M.J., Marfaing-Jallat, P. and Pesez, A. (1974) A flexible technique for long term infusion in unrestrained rats. Pharmacology Biochemistry and Behaviour 2: 131–136.

Steffens, A.B. (1969) A method for frequent sampling of blood and continuous infusion of fluids in the rat without disturbing the animal. Physiol. Behav. 4: 833–836.

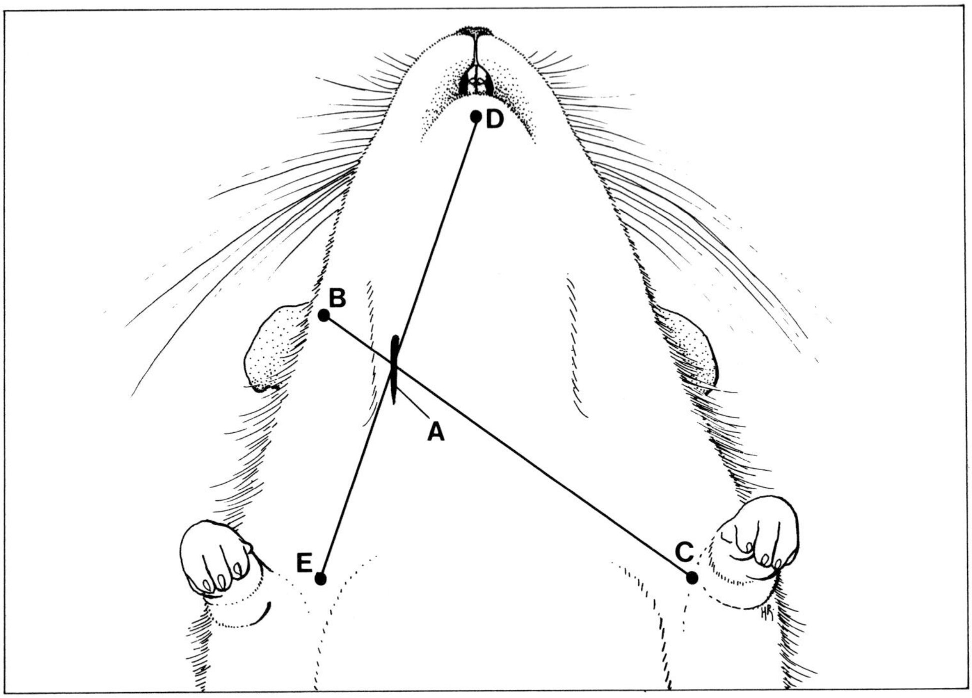

Figure 8.2.1. Place of incision.
The imaginary lines between the animal's right ear and its left armpit (B-C), and between the chin and its right armpit (D-E) are used for the determination of the incision place (A).
A. The incision.

Figure 8.2.2. Dissection of the external jugular vein.
The linguofacial vein is mobilized using blunt dissection technique.
F. Straight anatomical forceps.
lfv The linguofacial vein.

Figure 8.2.3. Clamping and ligation of the vessel.
Small artery forceps are used to clamp the vessel. The cranial ligature is tightened and the caudal ligature is put loosely around the vessel.
G. Artery forceps.
H/I. Rostral ligature.
J/K. Caudal ligature.
lfv The linguofacail vein.
mv Maxillary vein.

Figure 8.2.4. Incision of the linguofacial vein.
Position of the iridectomy scissors (L), while cutting a hole in the vein.

Figure 8.2.5. Detail of the vein with a V-shaped hole (*).

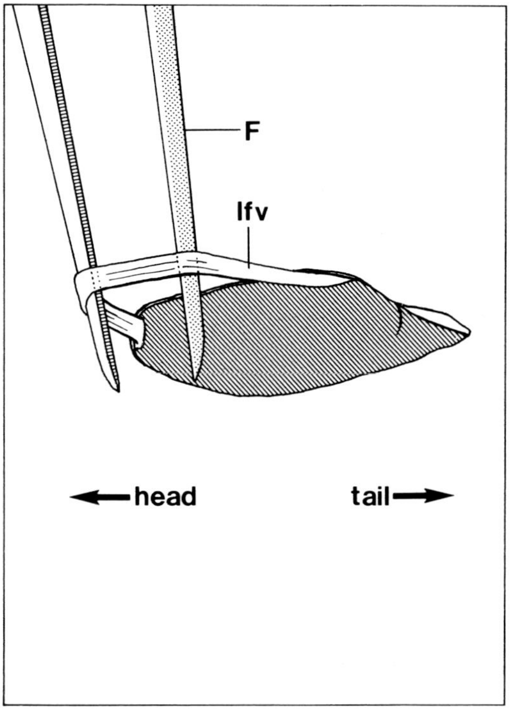

Fig. 8.2.2.

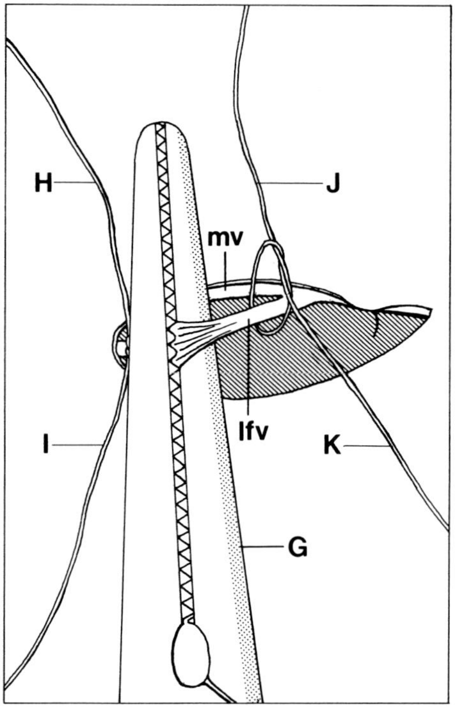

Fig. 8.2.3.

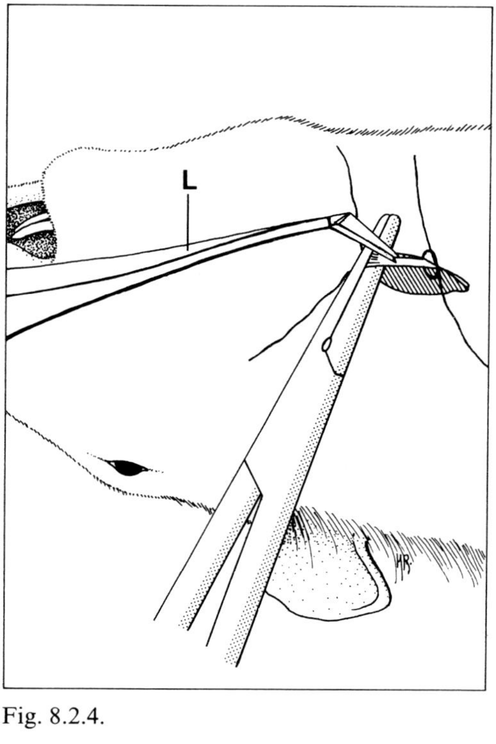

Fig. 8.2.4.

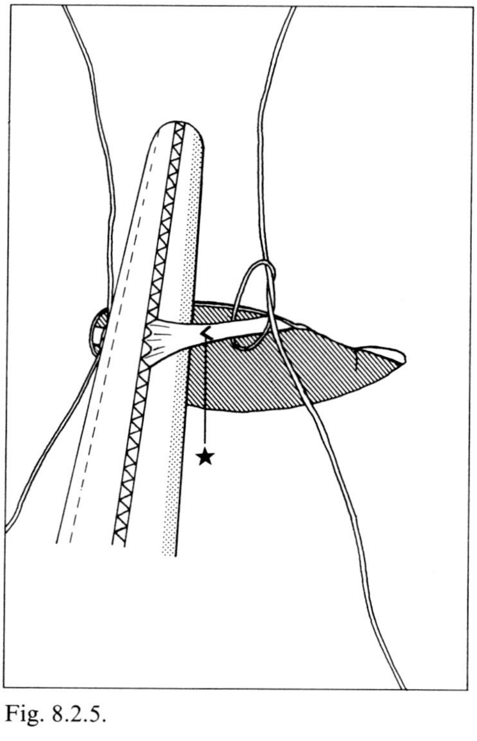

Fig. 8.2.5.

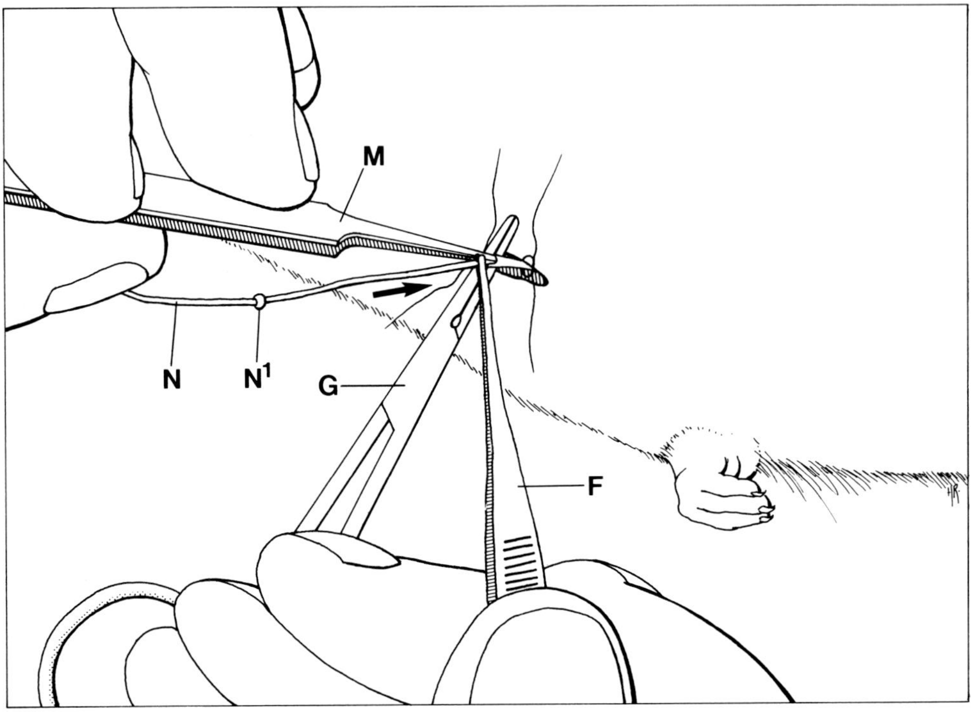

Figure 8.2.6. Insertion of the cannula.
Position of the hands and the instruments while the sterile cannula is inserted into the vein. Using jewellers forceps the vessel, held by the artery forceps, is dilated. The saline filled cannula is inserted into the vein, using anatomical forceps, and is pushed in until the silicon ring (N^1) reaches the V-shaped hole.

M. Jewellers forceps.

N. The cannula.

N^1. The silicon ring.

G. Artery forceps.

F. Anatomical forceps.

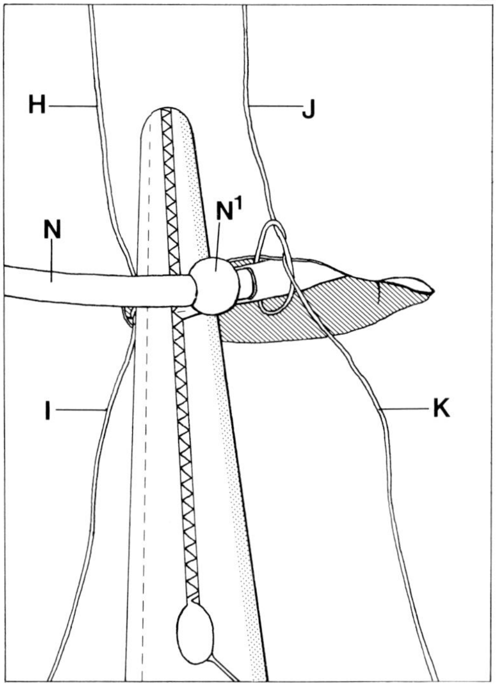

Fig. 8.2.7.

Fig. 8.2.8.

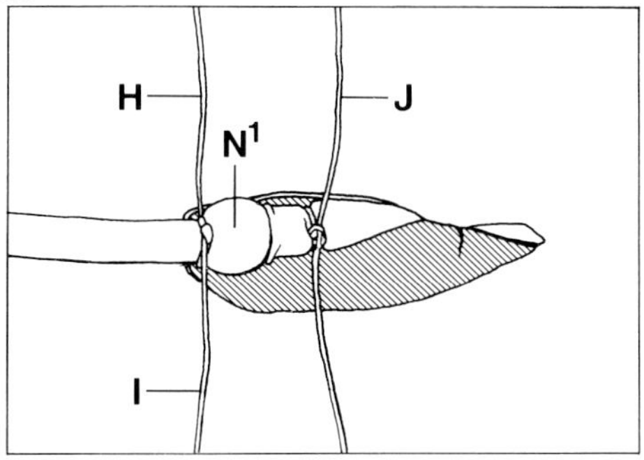

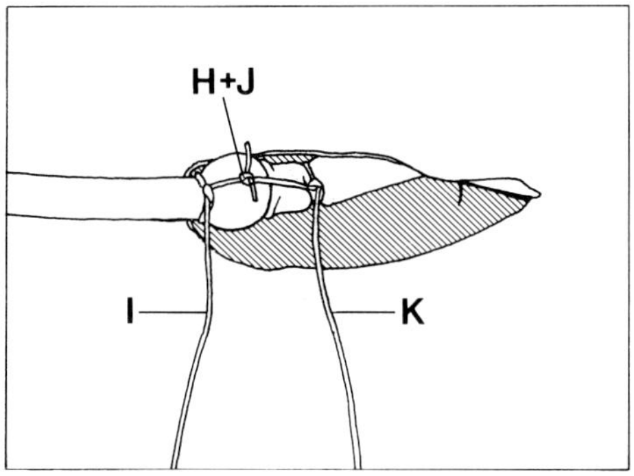

Fig. 8.2.9.

Figure 8.2.7. Fixation of the canula to the vein.
When the canula has reached the V-shaped hole, the strings J and K are tightened.

N. The canula.

N^1. The silicon ring.

H/I. Rostral ligature.

J/K. Caudal ligature.

Figure 8.2.8. Fixation of the canula to the vein.
The artery forceps are removed and the strings H and I are tightened behind the silicon ring.

Figure 8.2.9. Fixation of the canula to the vein.
The strings H and J are tightened across the silicon ring. All remaining strings are cut.

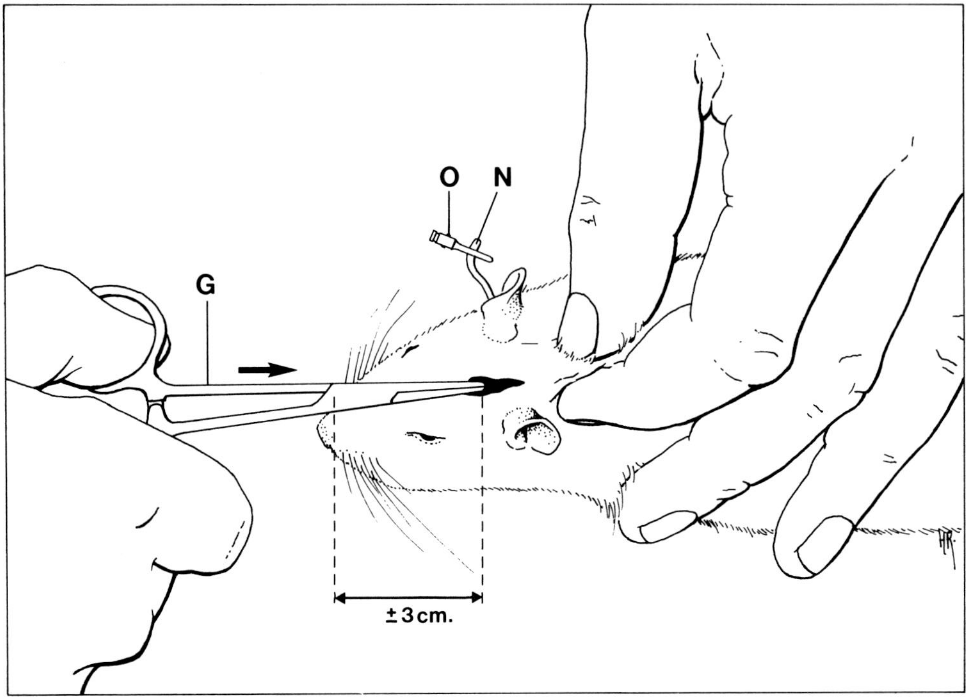

Figure 8.2.10. Subcutaneous tunnelling (I).
While the skin in the neck is held firmly, the artery forceps are inserted subcutaneously in caudal direction over a distance of about 3 cm.
O. Small vascular clip (Heifetz).
N. The cannula.
G. Artery forceps.

→

Figure 8.2.11. Subcutaneous tunnelling (II).
The artery forceps have been pushed in subcutaneously.

Figure 8.2.12. Subcutaneous tunnelling (III).
The artery forceps are turned anti-clockwise in the direction of the incision in the neck.

Figure 8.2.13. Subcutaneous tunnelling (IV).
The artery forceps emerge at the neck, the cannula is grasped and the clip removed.

Figure 8.2.14. Subcutaneous tunnelling (V).
The forceps are pulled back and the cannula emerges at the crown of the head and is reclamped with the clip.

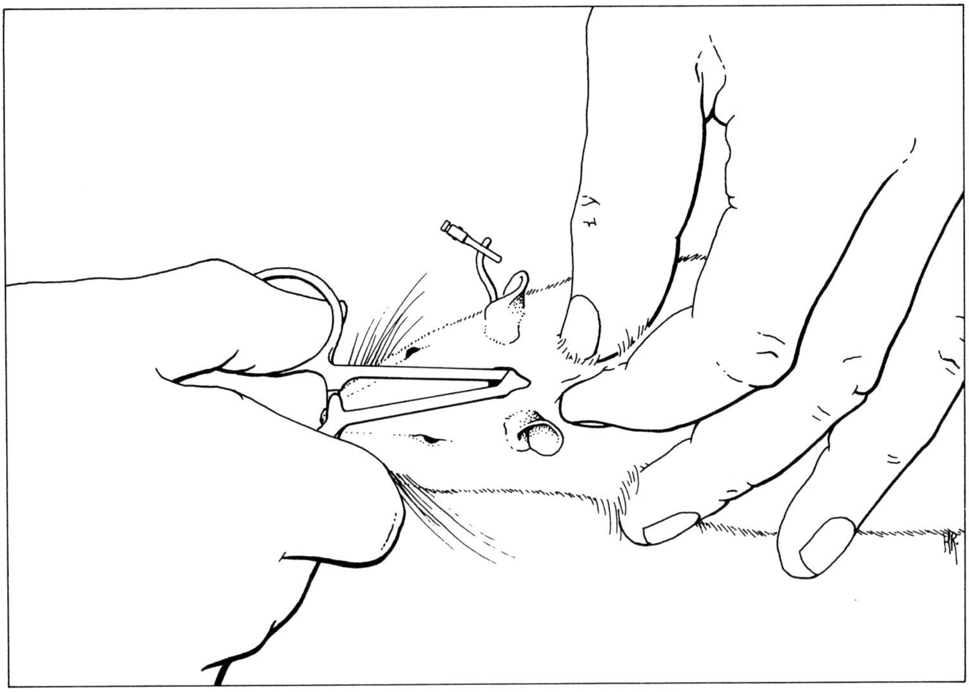

Fig. 8.2.11.

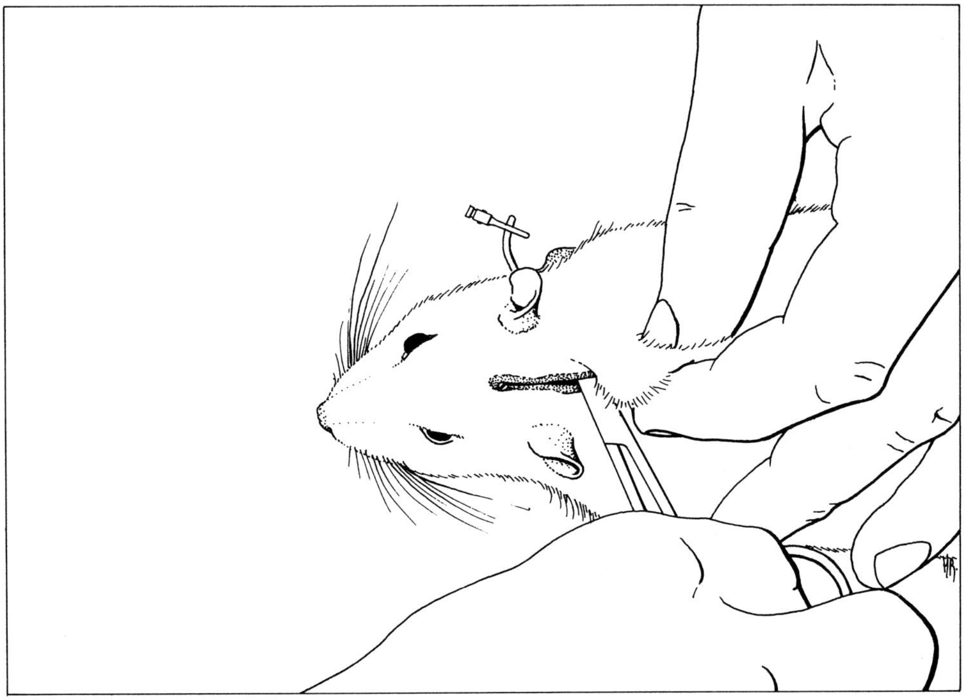

Fig. 8.2.12.

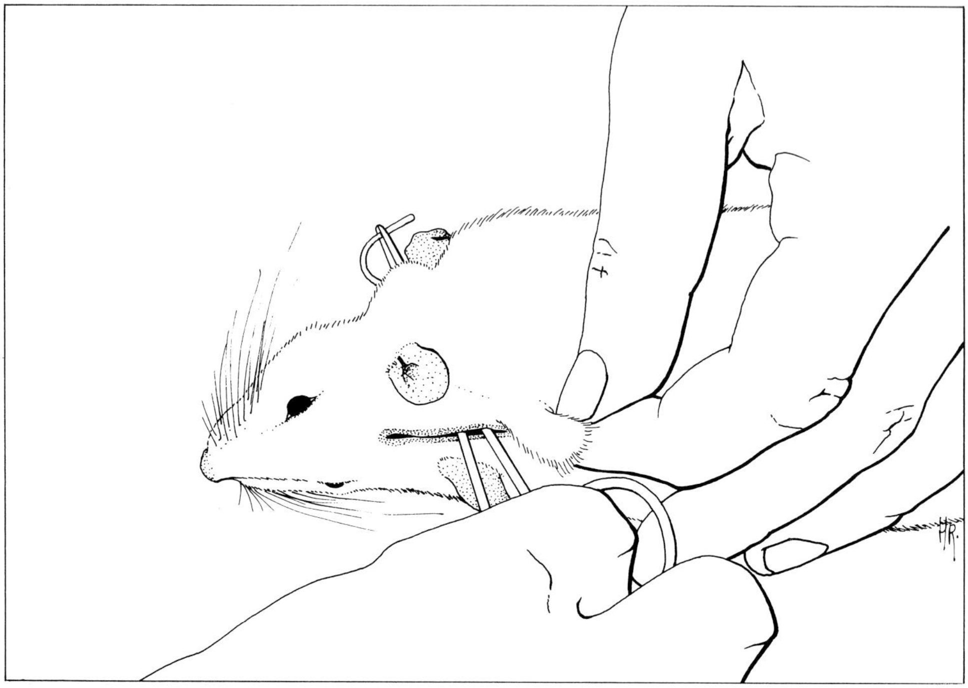

Fig. 8.2.13.

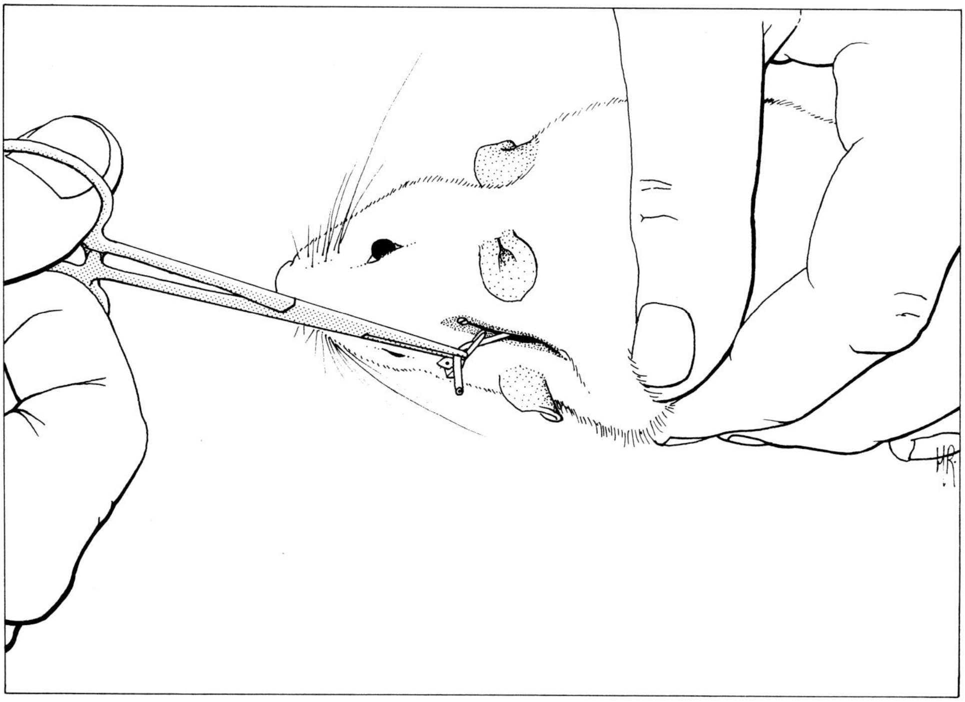

Fig. 8.2.14.

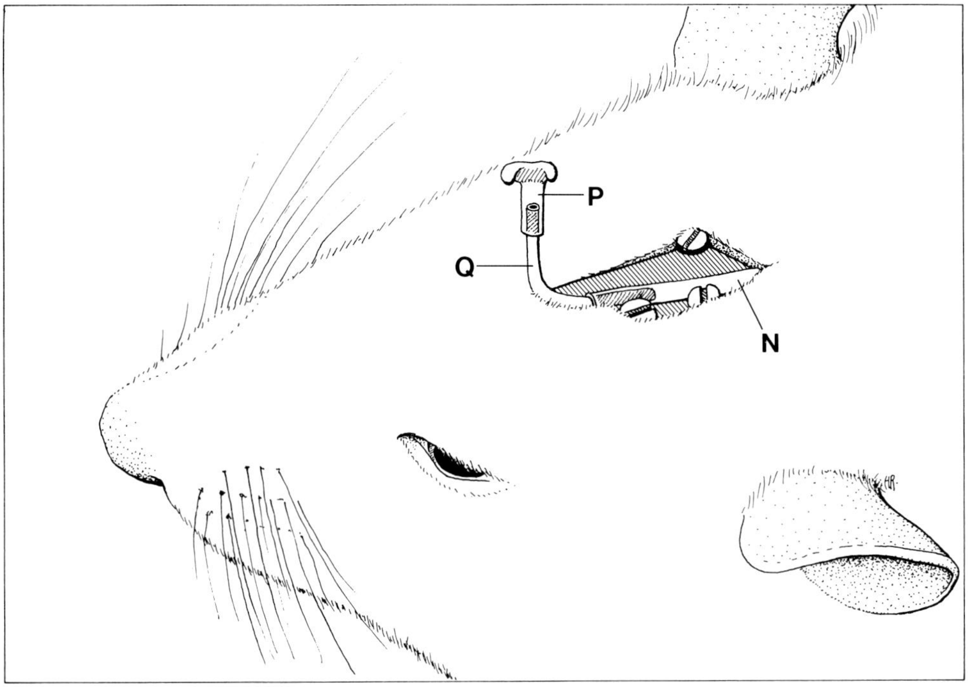

Figure 8.2.15. Fixation of the cannula.

Situation on the crown of the head of an animal with the permanent jugular vein cannula, after the cannula has been connected to the L-shaped adapter, flushed with saline solution, filled with PVP-solution, and closed with a polyethylene cap.

P. Heat sealed polyethylene cap.

Q. L-shaped adapter.

N. Jugular vein cannula.

Manual of Microsurgery on the Laboratory Rat, Part I
Van Dongen, Remie, Rensema and Van Wunnik (eds)
© 1990 Elsevier Science Publishers B.V. (Biomedical Division)

CHAPTER 9

Portacaval anastomosis

J.J. VAN DONGEN, R. REMIE, J.W. RENSEMA and
G.H.J. VAN WUNNIK

9.1 Introduction

In 1877 the Russian surgeon Nicolai Vladimirovich Eck reported the achievement of some successful portacaval shunts (PCS) in dogs. PCS are employed to study phenomena inherent to portal-systemic shunting of splanchnic blood. Since that time, many publications have discussed the haemodynamic, metabolic, and physiological consequences of such shunts. The technique to which Eck attached his name, was initially utilized and reproduced in large laboratory animals such as dogs, rabbits, swine, and monkeys. The first clinical use on a human being dates back to 1938. It was not until 1961 that Lee and Fisher succeeded in establishing a PCS in the laboratory rat. The feasibility of the PCS in a small animal like the rat gave considerable impetus to basic research on liver and brain metabolism due to the fact that a PCS induces hepatic insufficiency accompanied by encephalopathy. It appears that rats tolerate a PCS relatively well, and exhibit no or very slight encephalopathy over a period of time (de Boer et al., 1986). The usefulness of the PCS model, however, largely depends on the experience of the surgeon and the technical modification used. Both the duration of the operation, as well as the congestion of the splanchnic organs resulting from portal clamping, interfere with the results of the experiments.

One of the problems which has to be dealt with is the formation of collaterals (de Boer, 1984). During the post-operative period, collaterals sprout spontaneously from the diaphragm, the oesophagus, the stomach, the portal vein and the spleen going towards the liver. Even adipose and connective tissue can provide the liver with collaterals. These collaterals can partially restore the liver blood flow, thereby sustaining the liver function during the post-operative period. When the portal blood supply to the liver is blocked, the arterial hepatic blood supply is twice or three times its normal value, within twenty four hours after surgery.

A PCS enables us to study the interrelationship between the liver and some of the splanchnic organs. It also provides us with a model highly suited to the study of liver metabolism, regeneration of the liver, acute liver ischaemia, liver and portal blood flow, and the biochemically induced changes resulting in neurological complications.

In this chapter we will describe two variations of the PCS.
9.2.1. The button technique, based on the work of Funovics (1975).
9.2.2. The suture technique, based on the work of Lee and Fisher (1961).

9.2 The operations

Anaesthesia
The animal should be anaesthetized with N_2O/O_2 in combination with either enflurane, methoxyflurane or isoflurane. If these anaesthetics are not available then halothane should be used. Other anaesthetics will radically interfere with the results (see Chapter 6).

9.2.1. The button technique (acc. to Funovics)

The button technique can be divided into six parts:
9.2.1.1. Opening of the abdominal wall.
9.2.1.2. Exposure and dissection of the vena cava, the portal vein and the abdominal aorta.
9.2.1.3. The purse-string suture.
9.2.1.4. Placing the button on the portal vein.
9.2.1.5. Completion of the shunt.
9.2.1.6. Closure of the abdominal wall.

Parts 9.2.1.1. and 9.2.1.6. are described in Chapter 7 (General techniques) as is the preparation of the button.

9.2.1.2. Exposure of the vena cava, the portal vein and the abdominal aorta

The vena cava
After the opening of the abdominal wall, the intestines should be placed on gauze moistened with warm saline solution. They should be laid to the left of the animal (to the right as viewed by the surgeon). This provides an excellent view of the portal area (Figures 9.2.1. and 9.2.2.). Proximally and distally to the animal's right renal vein, the vena cava should then be stripped of its adipose and connective tissue, and the retroperitoneal cavity opened. Using anatomical forceps the peritoneum should be dissected from the vena cava by making small spreading movements with the for-

ceps just above the vena cava. Small pieces of adipose tissue and peritoneum can easily be removed with cotton wool sticks. Make sure that the marked area is clean.

The portal vein

Dissection of the portal vein is much more complicated, because the hepatic artery is firmly attached to it. One has to be very careful during this dissection, as the portal vein can be easily ruptured leading inevitably to massive bleeding, most probably followed by the untimely death of the animal. The portal vein should be pulled slightly to the left (and every now and than released), using straight anatomical forceps. With curved anatomical forceps, the portal vein should be freed from the hepatic artery, and the gastroduodenal artery at the points indicated (Figure 9.2.3.). Try not to damage these arteries as they easily bleed and go into spasm, causing disturbance in the liver blood flow. Therefore, time must be taken when carrying out this important part of the operation. It is vitally important to free the portal vein over a fair distance, as this will provide enough space later on for the button to be placed around the portal vein.

The abdominal aorta

Rostral to the celiac artery, the abdominal aorta which is covered with peritoneum should be freed from its lateral muscle bed, over a length of approximately 5 mm. This will provide just enough space for a small bulldog clamp to be placed on the aorta at a later stage in the operation. Clamping of the aorta is necessary in order to avoid congestion of the splanchnic organs, which would lead to small pinpoint bleedings and a drastically reduced vitality of the tissue (van Dongen et al., 1986a,b). This technique will be shown. It would, however, be preferable to clamp the celiac artery, the rostral mesenteric artery and the caudal mesenteric artery separately. In this way the normal blood flow through the kidneys and the lower extremities remains undisturbed.

9.2.1.3. The purse-string suture

Without occlusion a six fine-stitch purse-string suture should be placed in the wall of the vena cava, close to its confluence with the right renal vein. Using a Barraquer needle holder and a cotton wool stick the 7–0 silk suture, armed with a BV-1 needle, should be guided through the vessel paying special attention to the rules outlined in Chapter 7.5 and 7.6 regarding suture techniques.

Figures 9.2.4. and 9.2.5. show the position of the hands and the instruments during suturing. After each stitch, bleeding (if any) should be arrested immediately, by applying light pressure on the area, again using the cotton wool stick. After the suture has been completed a single knot should be made with the drawstrings (Figure 9.2.6.). As illustrated, the drawstrings should come together at the rostral part of the purse-string. A bulldog clamp, modified to resemble a Satinsky vascular clamp, should then be placed on the vena cava as shown in Figures 9.2.7. and 9.2.8.

9.2.1.4. Placing the button on the portal vein

Before clamping the abdominal aorta rostral to the celiac artery with a small bulldog clamp, a ligature (7–0, silk) should be placed around the portal vein as close as possible to the hilus of the liver. Subsequently, the clamp should be placed on the aorta and the ligature tightened (Figure 9.2.9.). A Heifetz clip should then be placed transversely onto the portal vein at its confluence with the gastroduodenal vein (Figure 9.2.10.). To keep the ischaemic time as short as possible, the next steps should be carried out as quickly as possible. The portal vein should be cut just distally from the ligature (Figure 9.2.11.). The button should be slipped over the arms of the left-hand straight small anatomical forceps, while the right-hand forceps are used to pass the portal vein to the left-hand anatomical forceps (Figure 9.2.12.). The vein should then be grasped and pulled through the button (Figure 9.2.13.). Subsequently, the button should be pushed as close as possible to the Heifetz clip, and clamped to the clip using a Pilling bulldog clamp (Figure 9.2.14.).

Using small straight, and curved anatomical forceps the portal vein should be reversed around the button and fixed with a previously prepared 7–0 silk suture (Figures 9.2.15. and 9.2.16.). The Pilling bulldog clamp should then be removed (Figure 9.2.17.) and replaced at the end of the Satinski clamp (Figure 9.2.18.) for reasons of stability. The vena cava is then somewhat elevated, bringing it into closer contact with the portal vein button.

9.2.1.5. Completion of the shunt

A longitudinal cut should be made in the purse-string suture using iridectomy scissors and jewellers forceps (Figures 9.2.18. and 9.2.19.). Blood clots, if present, must be removed. One drawstring of the suture should be clamped with a small haemostat and put under slight tension in a rostral direction. The button manipulated by its grip, should be pushed into the vena cava (Figure 9.2.20.). The purse-string suture is tightened with the left hand whilst the right hand still holds the button in position (Figure 9.2.21.). The button should be released, and two additional knots tied. The Satinsky clamp is removed first followed by the Heifetz clamp and the bulldog clamp on the aorta (Figures 9.2.22., 9.2.23. and 9.2.24.).

The shunt does not always work correctly instantaneously. Slight torsion of the portal vein may be the reason for the failure. If this is the case the button should be turned, while holding one suture line, letting the blood flow smoothly through the shunt. Figure 9.2.25. shows the final result.

9.2.1.6. Closure of the abdominal wall

After replacing the intestines the abdominal wall should be closed in two layers as discussed in Chapter 7.

In experienced hands the total procedure takes about 20 min, during which period the vena cava is partially occluded for 10 min and the aorta and portal vein are clamped for approximately 8 to 10 min.

9.2.2. The suture technique (acc. to Lee and Fisher)

The suture technique can be divided into six parts:

9.2.2.1. Opening of the abdominal wall.
9.2.2.2. Exposure and dissection of the vena cava, the portal vein and the abdominal aorta.
9.2.2.3. Preparations for the end-to-side anastomosis.
9.2.2.4. The corner sutures.
9.2.2.5. The anastomosis.
9.2.2.6. Closure of the abdominal wall.

Parts 9.2.2.1. and 9.2.2.6. are described in Chapter 7 (General techniques), part 9.2.2.2. is described above under 9.2.1.2.

9.2.2.3. Preparation for the end-to-side anastomosis

Having prepared the vena cava, the portal vein and the aorta, curved atraumatic artery forceps should be placed on the vena cava. A small oval aperture should be cut in the clamped segment (Figure 9.2.26.) using iridectomy scissors and jewellers forceps. To avoid congestion of the splanchnic organs, the aorta should be occluded prior to the clamping of the portal vein and the gastroduodenal vein.

After ligation of the portal vein, as close as possible to the hilus of the liver, the vessel should be divided between the ligature and the clip as close to the ligature as possible (Figure 9.2.26.). The portal vein should then be brought next to the aperture in the vena cava to compare dimensions. If necessary the hole in the vena cava should be adapted. When the diameters of the vessels correspond well, the anastomosis is made much easier.

9.2.2.4. The corner sutures

The anastomosis of a vein requires less stitches compared with an artery of equal diameter. It is not possible to stipulate a minimum or maximum number of stitches. More information about the end-to-side anastomosis can be found in Chapter 7 (Anastomosis).

The needle can be used as a tool to expose the aperture of the vessel in such a way that the adventitia of the wound edges can be grasped easily with the forceps. After the wound edge of the portal vein is visible, the first stitch should be placed on the rostral side of the portal vein wall, working from the outside to the inside. Subsequently, the aperture cut into the wall of the vena cava should be exposed using forceps in the left hand and a needle holder with a needle in the right. The adventitia of the vena cava wall should be picked up near the wound edge, and the lumen exposed by using the tip of the needle. The tip of the needle enters the lumen on the rostral side and penetrates the vena cava from the inside to the outside. A surgical knot should be made and the edges must be lined up although the knot is not tightened as yet. The second stay suture should then be applied at 180° to the first suture in the same way as described above, and the edges lined up by tightening the knots (Figure 9.2.27.). The animal should be rotated through 180°. Light tension should be put on the stay sutures by applying a small bulldog clamp just behind the needle on the left suture line. This clamp can be positioned just outside the abdominal cavity. The second clamp should be fixed on the needleless end of the right suture, and laid aside on the thorax of the animal.

9.2.2.5. The anastomosis

As the portal vein cannot be turned over allowing suturing of the posterior wall, one has to start suturing the posterior wall from the right to the left. The running suture should be made by over and over stitches about one millimetre apart varying from radial to perpendicular thereby providing a sealing effect. The lumen of the portal vein should then be exposed, and the needle should penetrate the portal wall from the outside to the inside, close to the stay suture on the rostral side (Figure 9.2.28.). The posterior wall of the vena cava and the portal vein are penetrated from the inside to the outside, and from the outside to the inside respectively, as close to the stay suture as possible. In this way, any possibility of leakage which can occur near the stay sutures of the anastomosis will be diminished. The next stitch should be made from the inside to the outside of the vena cava and from the outside to the inside of the portal vein wall. The posterior suture line should be completed in this way (Figure 9.2.29.). Special attention must be paid when making the last stitch as this one has to penetrate the vena cava wall just behind the stay suture going from the inside to the outside. Using a surgical knot, the needleless drawstring of the stay suture should be tied.

The animal should be turned through 180°, and the anterior wall sutured using standard technique (Figure 9.2.30.). The clamp on the vena cava should be released first, followed by the one on the portal vein. Any bleeding which occurs should be stopped by applying mild pressure on the anastomosis with cotton wool sticks. Figure 9.2.31. shows the final result.

9.2.2.6. Closure of the abdominal wall

After replacing the intestines the abdominal wall should be closed in two layers as discussed in Chapter 7.

In experienced hands the total procedure should take about 25 min, during which time the vena cava is occluded for 10 min and the aorta and the portal vein are clamped for approximately 10 min.

References

Boer, J.E.G. de (1984) Branched chain amino acid metabolism in portal-systemic shunting. Experimental studies in the rat. Thesis, University of Limburg, Maastricht, the Netherlands.

Boer, J.E.G. de, Janssen, M.A., van Dongen, J.J., Blitz, W., Oostenbroek, R.J., Wesdorp, R.I.C. and Soeters P.B. (1986) Sequential metabolic characteristics following portacaval shunt in rats. Eur. Soc. Surg. Res. 18: 96–106.

Dongen, J.J. van, de Boer, J.E.G., Rensema, J.W., van Dijk, P.J., van Eijk, H. and Soeters, P.B. (1986a) Improvement of portacaval shunting techniques in rats. Proceedings of the 27th Dutch Fed. Meeting, Groningen, nr. 96.

Dongen, J.J. van, de Boer, J.E.G., Rensema, J.W., van Dijk, P.J., Ruers, T.J.M. and Soeters, P.B. (1986b) Improvement of heterotopic auxiliary heart transplantation with pulmo-portal outlet and of orthotopic total small bowel transplantation in rats. Proceedings of the 27th Dutch Fed. Meeting, Groningen, nr. 97.

Eck, N.V. (1877) On the question of ligature of the portal vein. Voen. med. J., St. Petersburg, Med. J. 130,(2): 1–2. Translation by Child, C.G., III, (1953) Surg. Gynecol. Obstet., 96: 375–376.

Funovics, J.M., Cummings, M.G., Shuman, L., James, J.H. and Fischer, J.E. (1975) An improved non suture method for portacaval anastomosis in the rat. Surgery 77: 661–664.

Lee S.H. and Fischer B. (1961) Portacaval shunt in the rat. Surgery 50: 668–672.

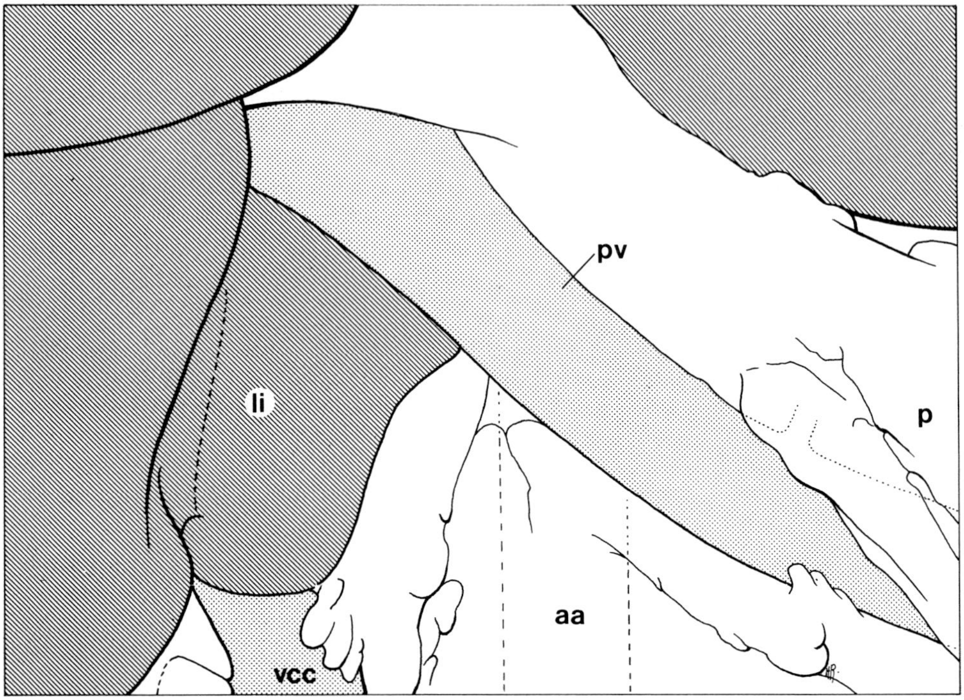

Fig. 9.2.1.

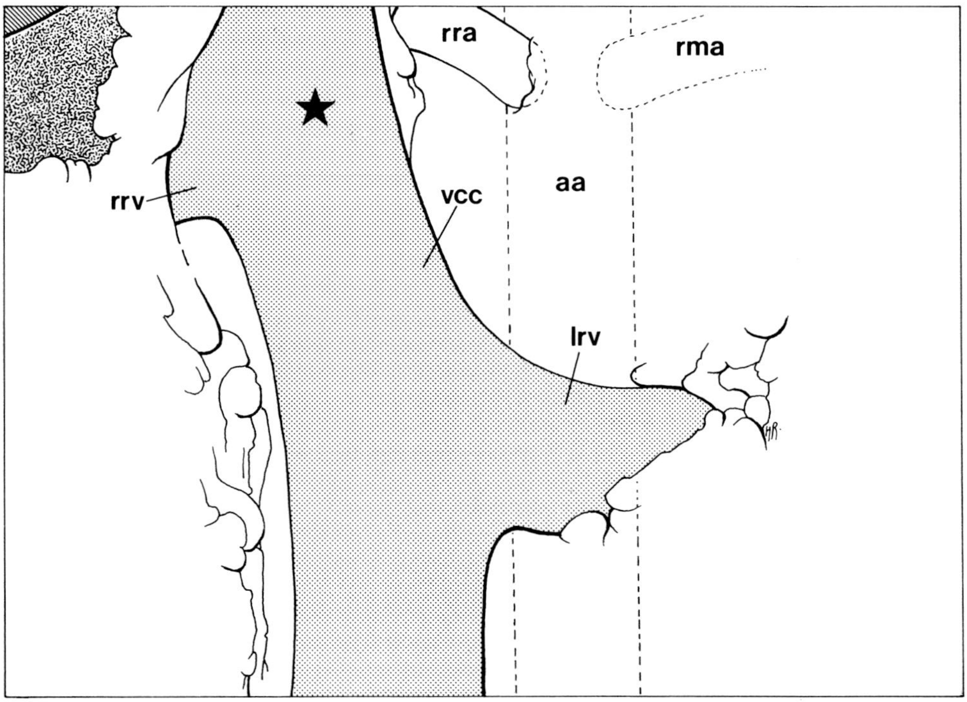

Fig. 9.2.2.

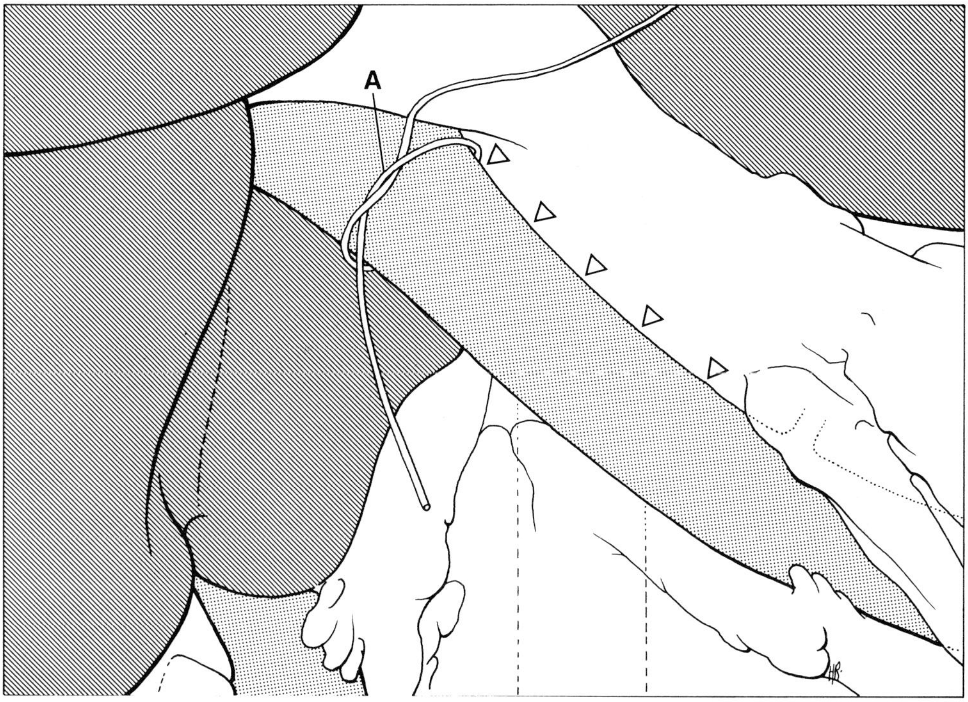

Figure 9.2.3. Preparation of the portal vein.
After freeing the portal vein of its surrounding tissue (△ △ △), a ligature is placed around it and not tightened as yet.
A. Ligature.

←
Figure 9.2.1. Anatomy of the portal area (I).
View on the portal area.

aa Abdominal aorta.
vcc Vena cava caudalis.
pv Portal vein.
p Pancreas.
li Liver.

Figure 9.2.2. Anatomy of the portal area (II).
Marked spot (*) indicates the place of the purse-string suture near the entrance of the right renal vein. Retroperitoneal, adipose and connective tissue within this region should be removed.

rra Right renal artery.
rma Rostral mesenteric artery.
rrv Right renal vein.
vcc Vena cava caudalis.
lrv Left renal vein.
aa Abdominal aorta.

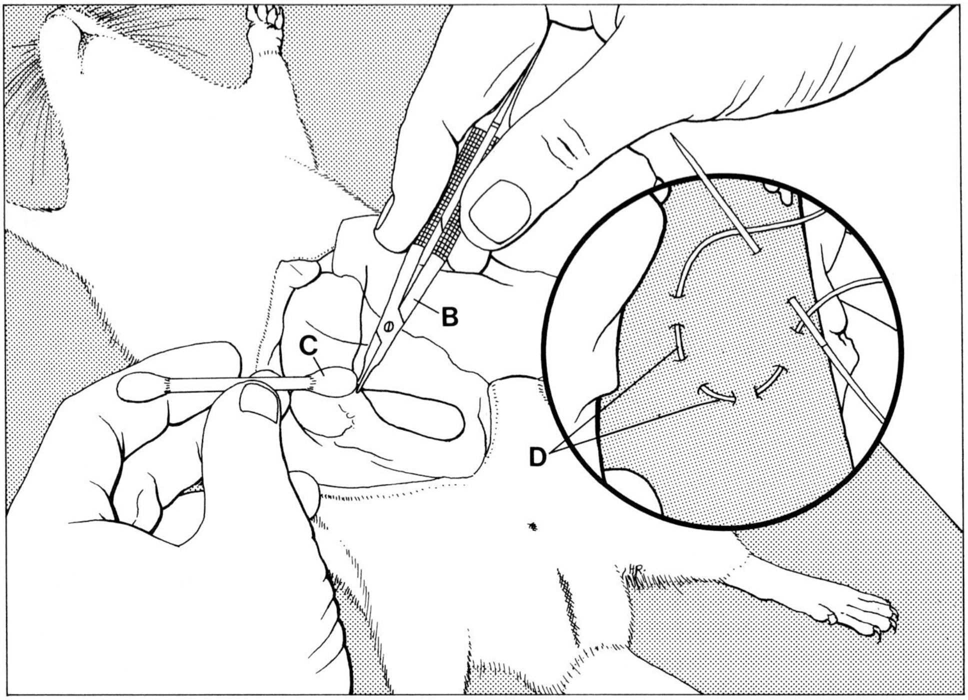

Figure 9.2.4. The purse-string suture (I).
The final stitches of the purse-string suture placed in the wall of the vena cava. The vessel wall is supported with a cotton wool stick.
B. Needle holder.
C. Cotton wool stick.
D. Stitches of the purse-string suture.

→

Figure 9.2.5. The purse-string suture (II).
The thread is pulled through in the entrance-exit direction, while the cotton wool stick is supporting the tissue.

Figure 9.2.6. The purse-string suture (III).
The suture is finished.

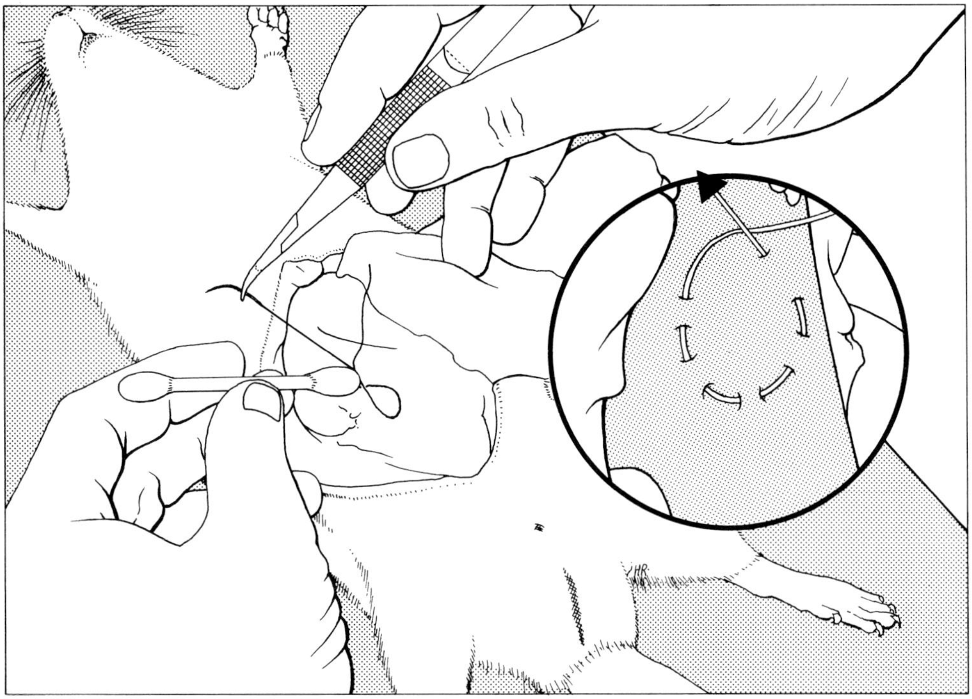

Fig. 9.2.5.

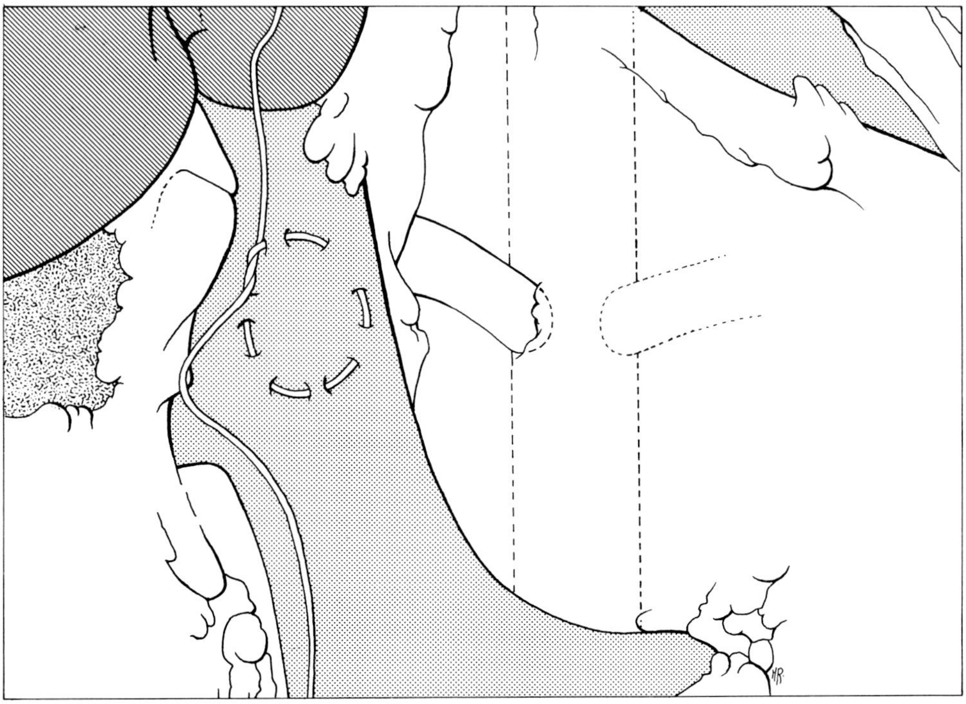

Fig. 9.2.6.

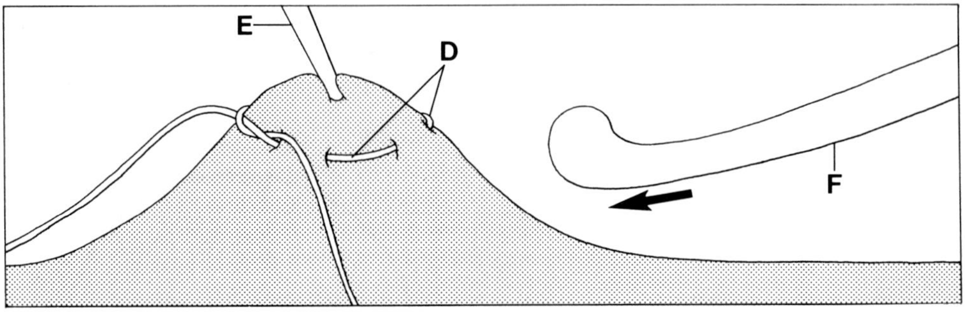

Figure 9.2.7. Clamping of the vena cava (I).
The vena cava is lifted by picking up the vessel wall within the purse-string suture. A modified bulldog clamp is about to be placed on the vena cava and approaches from the caudal direction.

D. Purse-string suture.
E. Anatomical forceps.
F. Modified bulldog clamp.

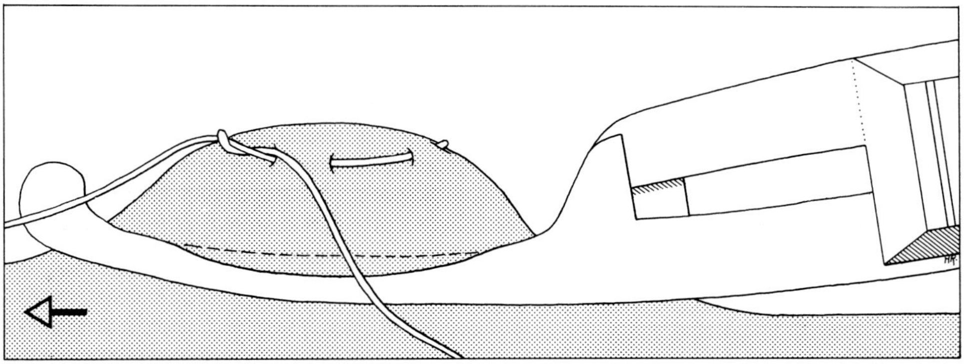

Figure 9.2.8. Clamping of the vena cava (II).
Vena cava is clamped just beneath the purse-string suture. The open arrow indicates the blood stream towards the heart.

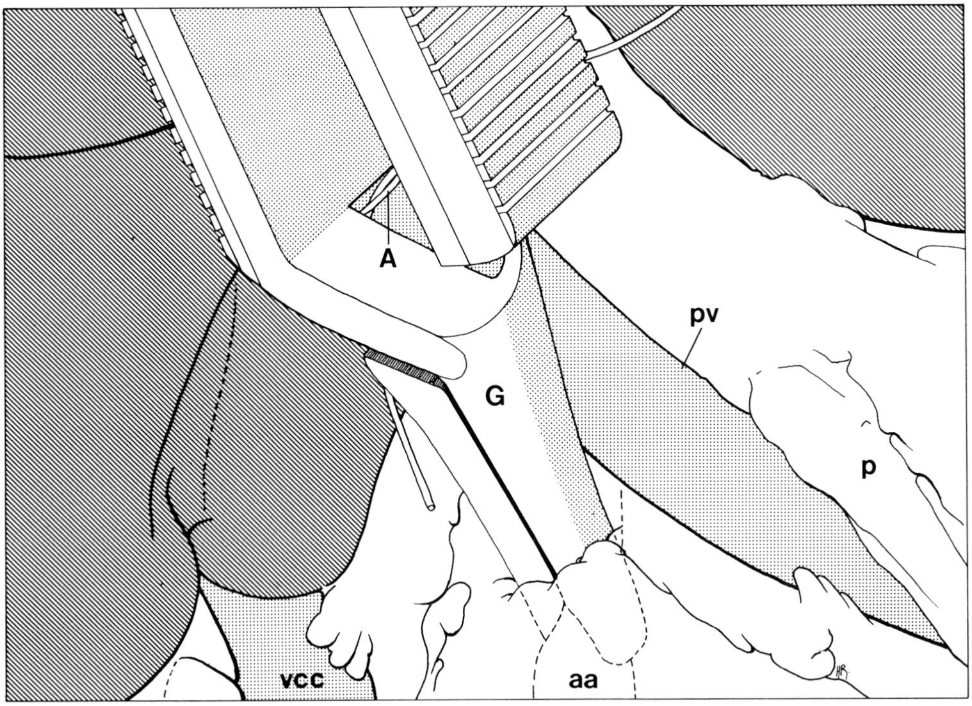

Figure 9.2.9. Clamping of the aorta.
A small clamp is placed on the aorta proximal to the celiac artery avoiding entering of blood into the splanchnic organs. Before application of the clamp a ligature is placed around the portal vein, but is not tightened yet.
G. Bulldog clamp.
A. Ligature around the portal vein (not tightened).
vcc Vena cava caudalis.
pv Portal vein.
aa Abdominal aorta.
p Pancreas.

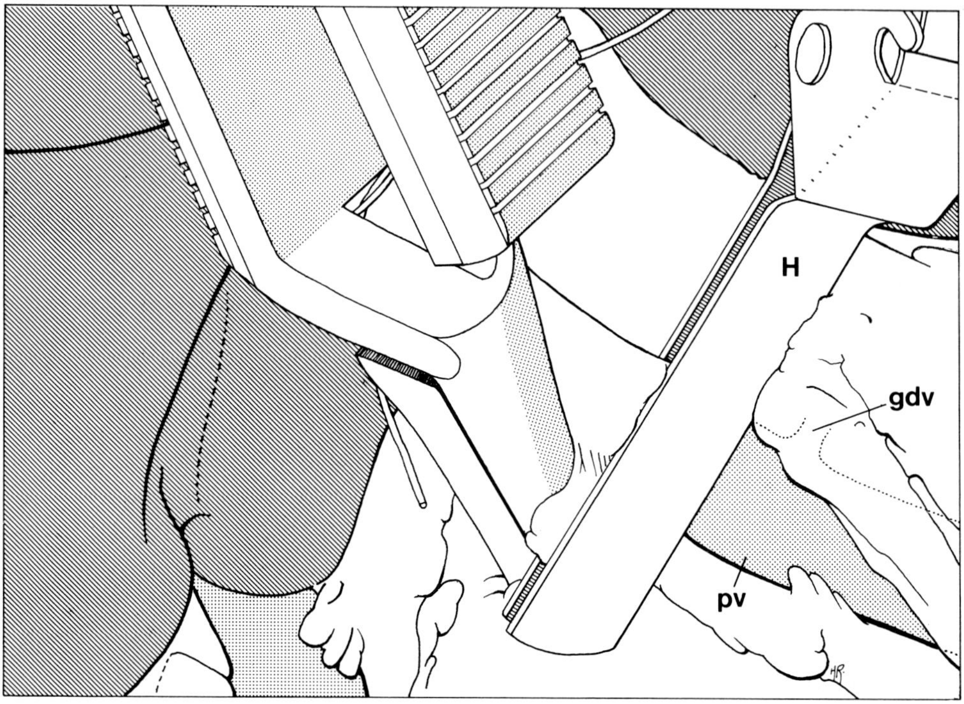

Figure 9.2.10. Clamping of the portal vein.
A Heifetz clip is placed on the portal vein as close as possible to the gastroduodenal vein, thus obtaining sufficient length to place the button and to reverse the vessel.
H. Heifetz clip.
pv Portal vein.
gdv Gastroduodenal vein.

→

Figure 9.2.11. Cutting of the portal vein.
The ligature is tightened (1), and the portal vein is cut just distal to the ligature (2-2).

Figure 9.2.12. Placement of the button (I).
The button is slipped over the tips of the left-hand forceps, while the portal vein is loosely helt by the right-hand forceps.
D. Bulldog clamp.
H. Heifetz clip.
I. Right-hand forceps.
J. Button.
K. Left-hand forceps.

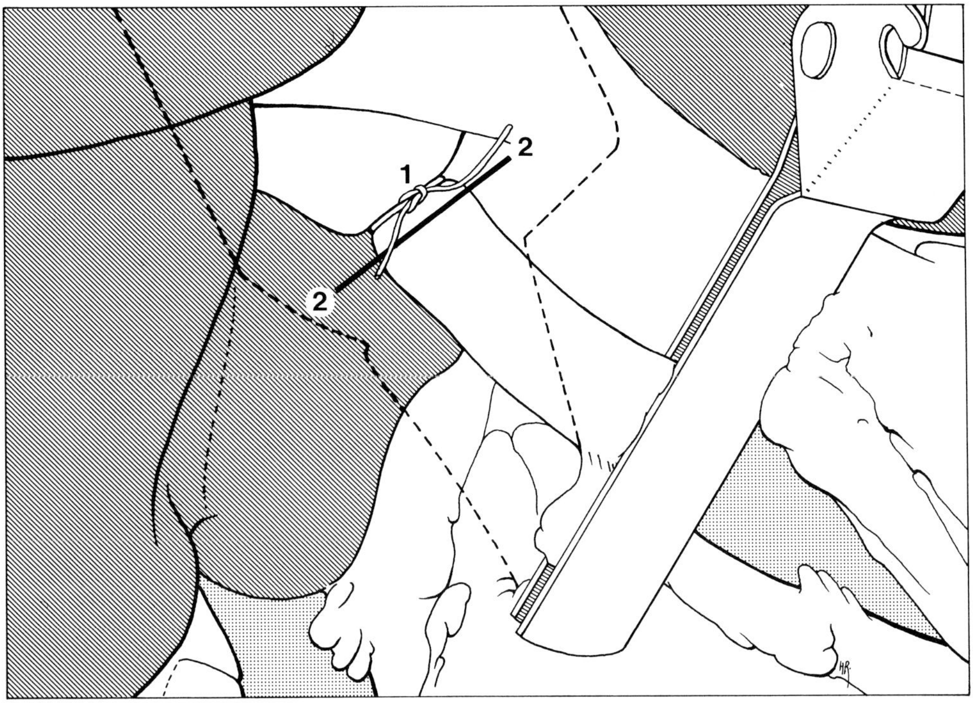

Fig. 9.2.11.

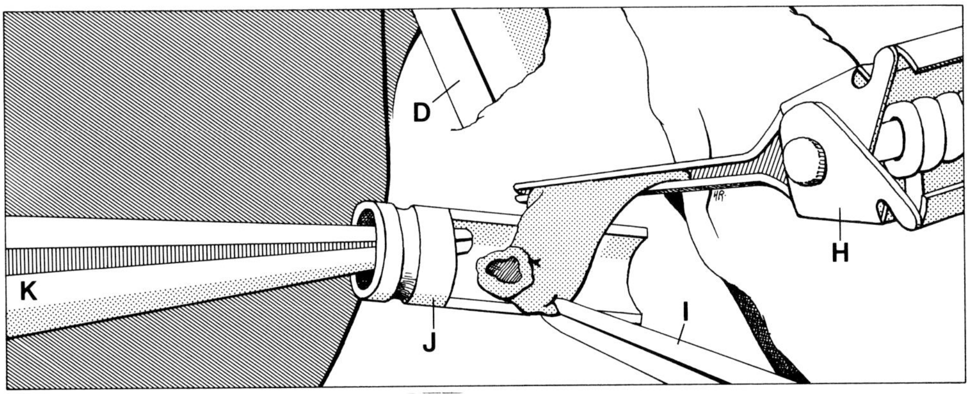

Fig. 9.2.12.

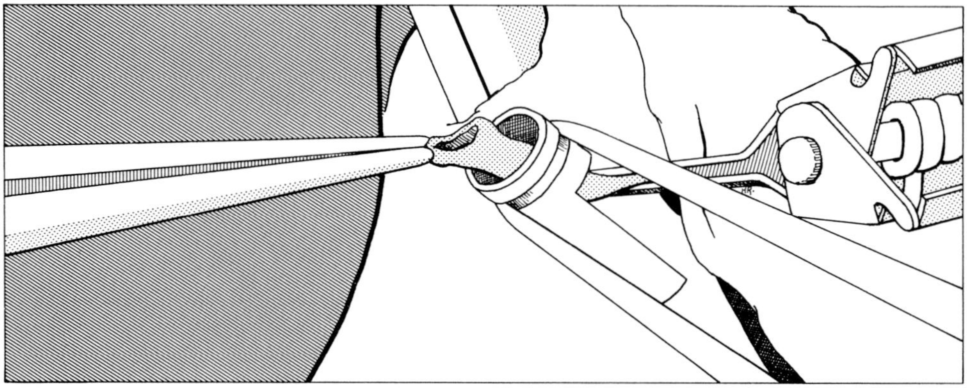

Figure 9.2.13. Placement of the button (II).
The vessel is pulled through the button by the left-hand forceps, and the button is pushed towards the clip.

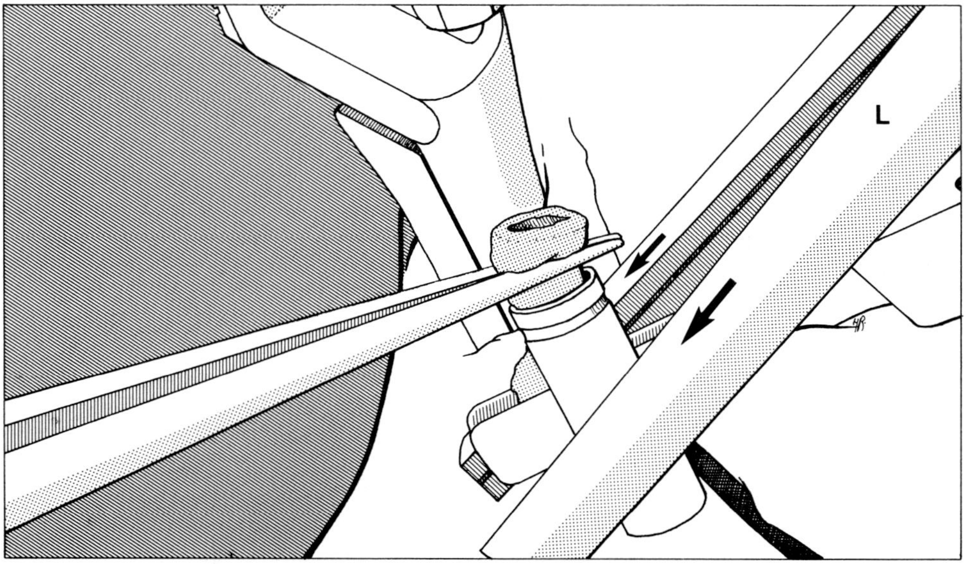

Figure 9.2.14. Placement of the button (III).
The vessel is taken over into the right-hand forceps, and is regrasped with the left-hand forceps. A large Pilling clamp is used to fixate the button against the clamped portal vein.
L. Large (5 cm) Pilling clamp.

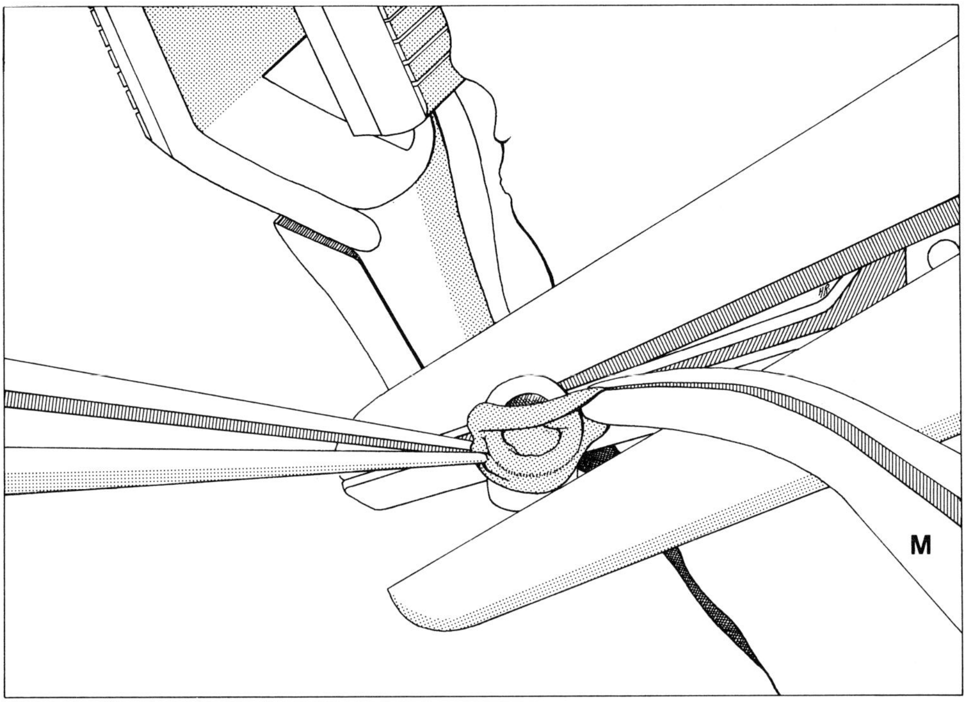

Figure 9.2.15. Reversion of the portal vein.
The portal vein is reversed around the button using straight and curved anatomical forceps.
M. Curved forceps.

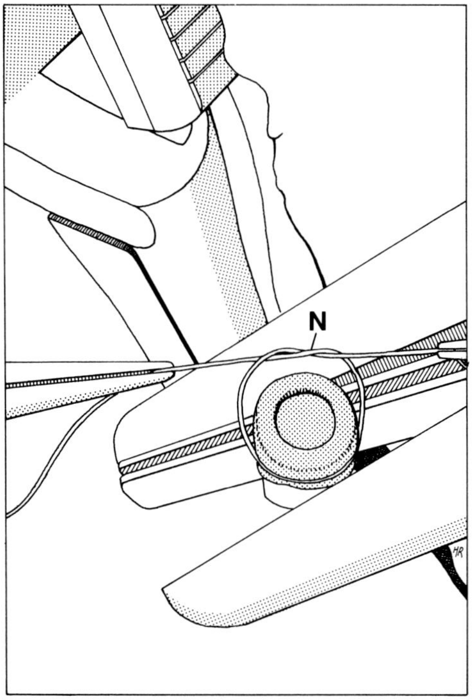

Fig. 9.2.16.

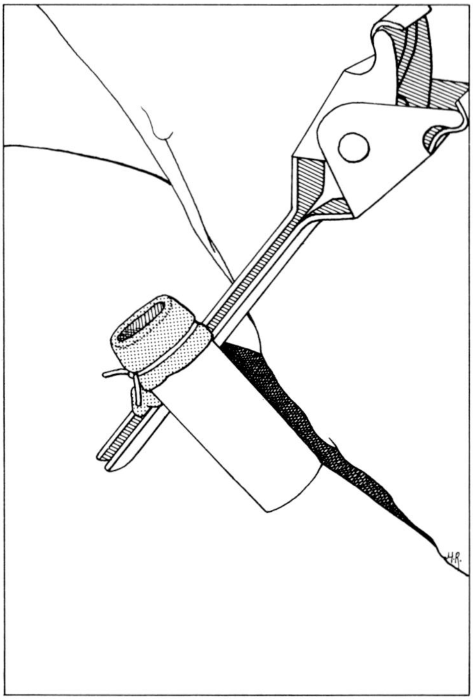

Fig. 9.2.17.

Figure 9.2.16. Fixation of the portal vein to the button (I).
The reversed portal vein is fixed to the button with a ligature, which is pulled into the groove of the button.
N. Ligature.

Figure 9.2.17. Fixation of the portal vein to the button (II).
The portal vein seen from the side.

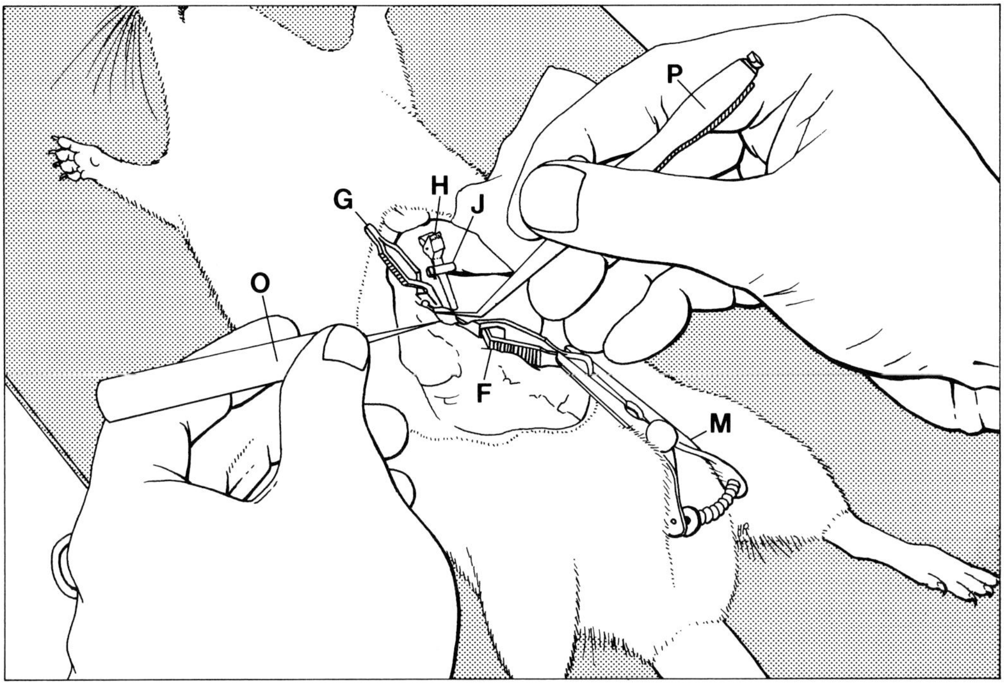

Figure 9.2.18. Cutting the purse-string suture (I).
The large Pilling bulldog clamp is replaced to stabilize the clamp on the vena cava, and an aperture will be cut in the purse-string suture.

F. Modified bulldog clamp.
G. Bulldog clamp.
H. Heifetz clip.
J. Button.
M. Pilling clamp.
O. Jewellers forceps.
P. Iridectomy scissors.

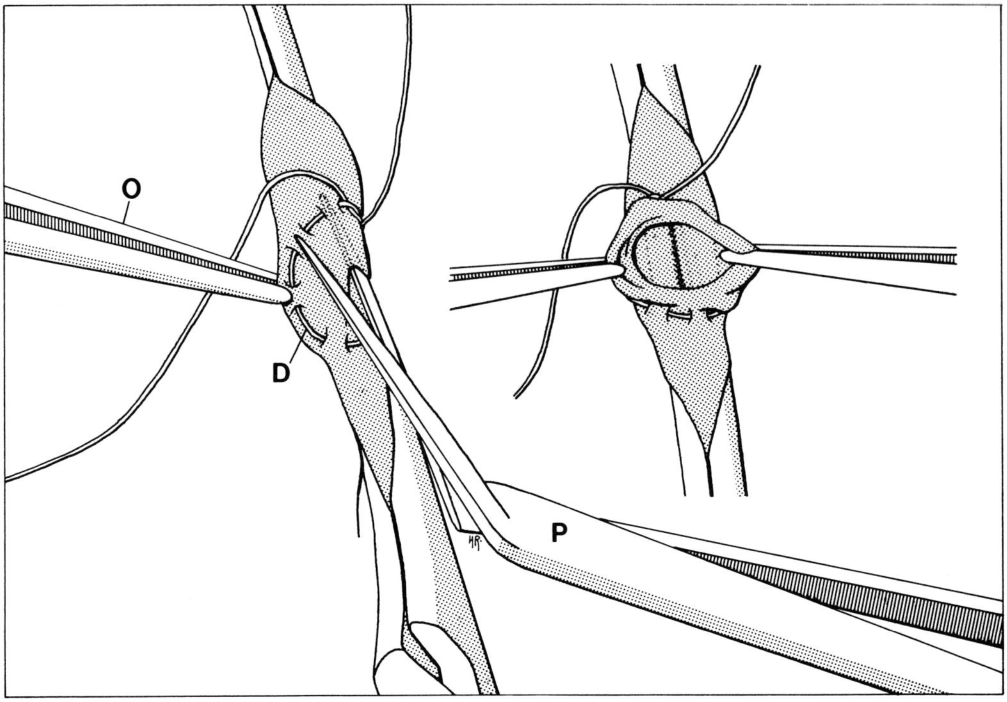

Figure 9.2.19. Cutting the purse-string suture (II).
Left: An aperture is cut into the vena cava. Right: The aperture is spread and dilated using jewellers forceps, to ensure easy insertion of the button.
D. Purse-string suture.
O. Jewellers forceps.
P. Iridectomy scissors.

→

Figure 9.2.20. Insertion of the button (I).
The proximal suture line is clamped and fixated to the rat board under minimal tension, the button is handled by its grip and inserted into the vena cava. For reasons of clarity the bulldog clamp on the aorta has not been drawn.
F. Modified bulldog clamp.
H. Heifetz clip.
J. Button.

Figure 9.2.21. Insertion of the button (II).
The purse-string suture is tied and pulled into the groove of the button. Because the proximal suture is fixated the right hand can keep the button positioned, while the left hand ties the purse-string.

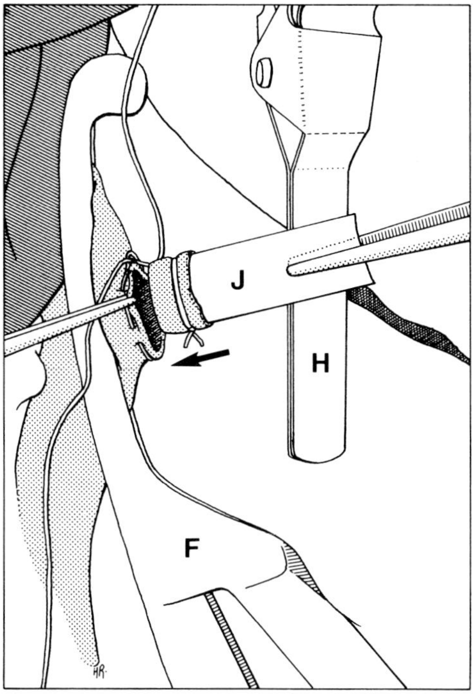

Fig. 9.2.20.

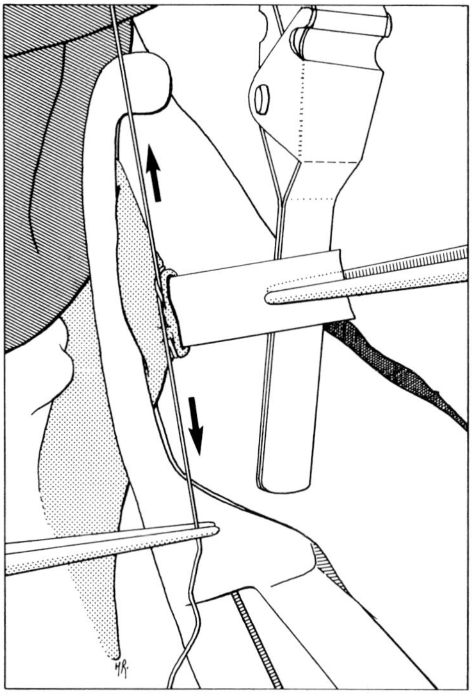

Fig. 9.2.21.

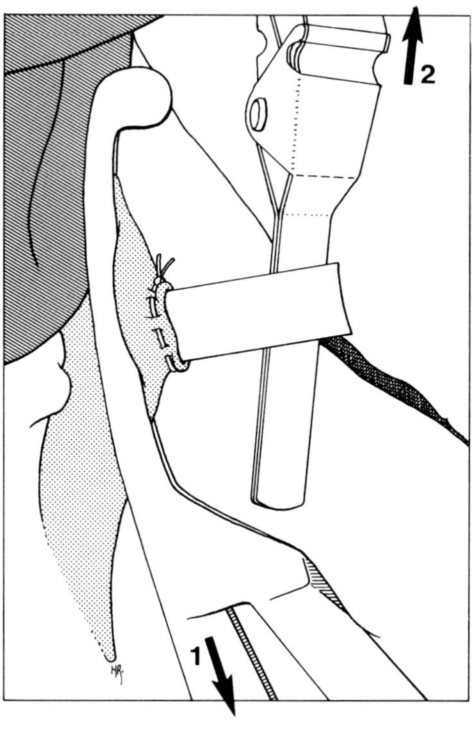

Figure 9.2.22. Removal of the clamps (I).
First the modified bulldog clamp is removed (1).
Since the aorta and portal vein are still occluded there will be no pressure on the shunt.
Next, the Heifetz clip will be removed (2).

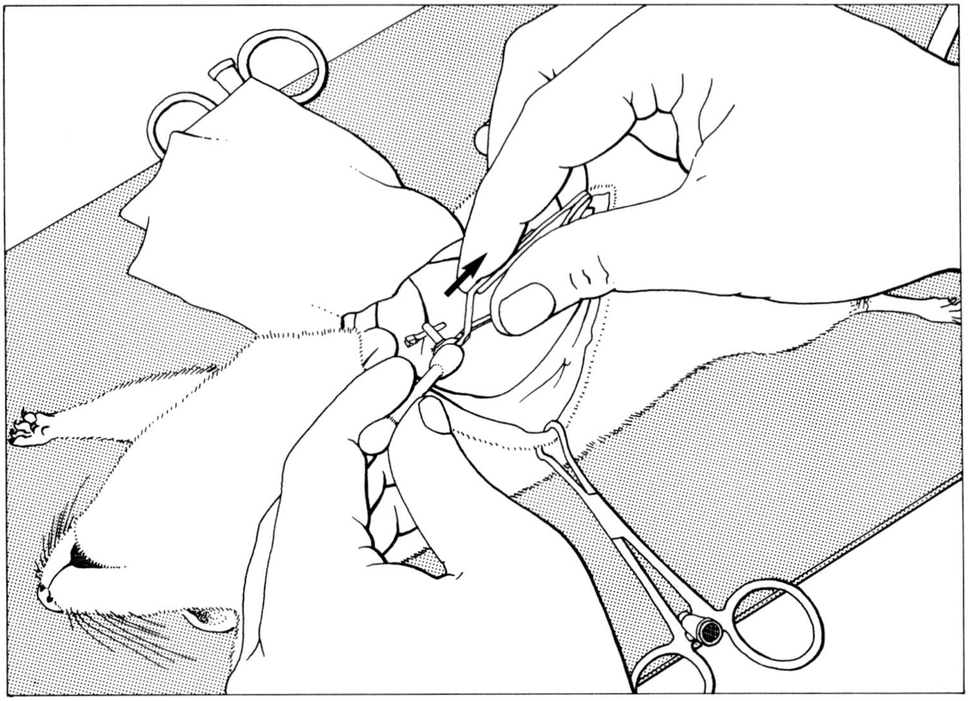

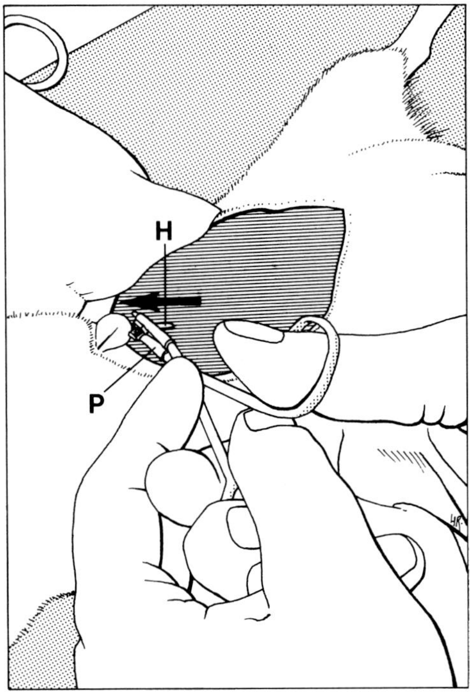

Figure 9.2.23. Removal of the clamps (II). The bulldog clamp is removed in the direction of the arrow, while the shunt is supported with a cotton-wool stick.

Figure 9.2.24. Removal of the clamps (III). The Heifetz clip is removed in rostral direction (see the arrow) using artery forceps.
H. Heifetz clip.
P. Artery forceps.

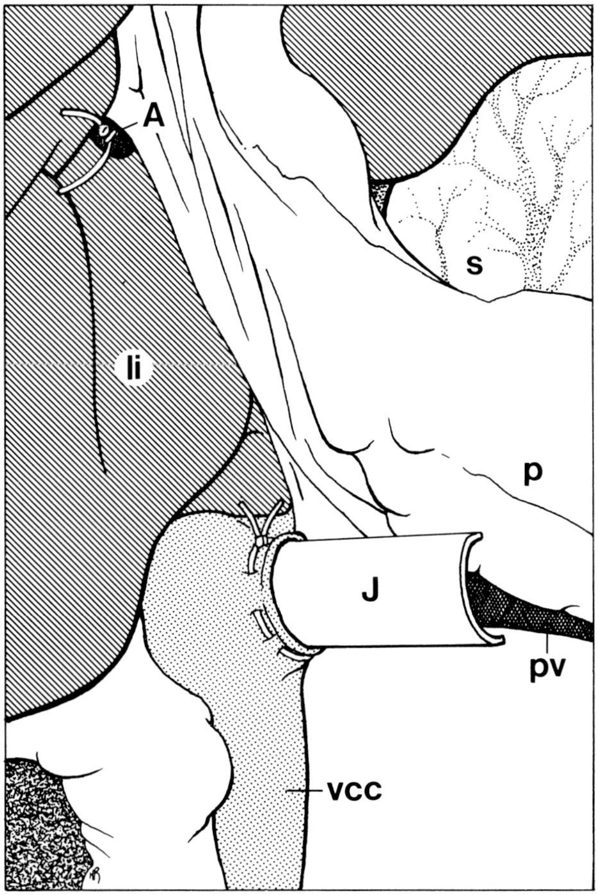

Figure 9.2.25. Final result.
A functioning portacaval shunt by means of a button, according to the technique of Funovics.
J. Button.
A. Ligature on the portal vein.
li Liver.
pv Portal vein.
vcc Vena cava caudalis.
p Pancreas.
s Stomach.

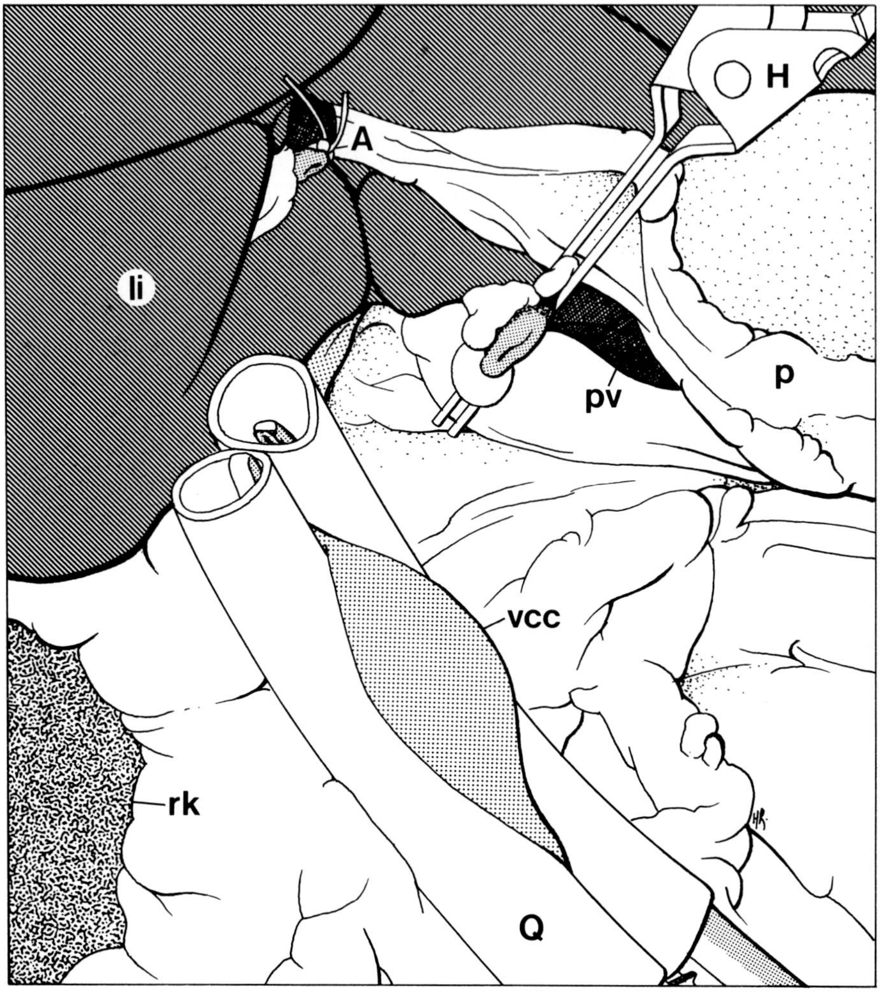

Figure 9.2.26. Clamping of the vena cava.
The vena cava is clamped with curved atraumatic artery forceps, which are for safety's sake covered with Silastic tubing.

A. Ligature on the portal vein.
H. Heifetz clip.
Q. Atraumatic artery forceps.

rk	Right kidney.
vcc	Vena cava caudalis.
pv	Portal vein.
p	Pancreas.
li	Liver.

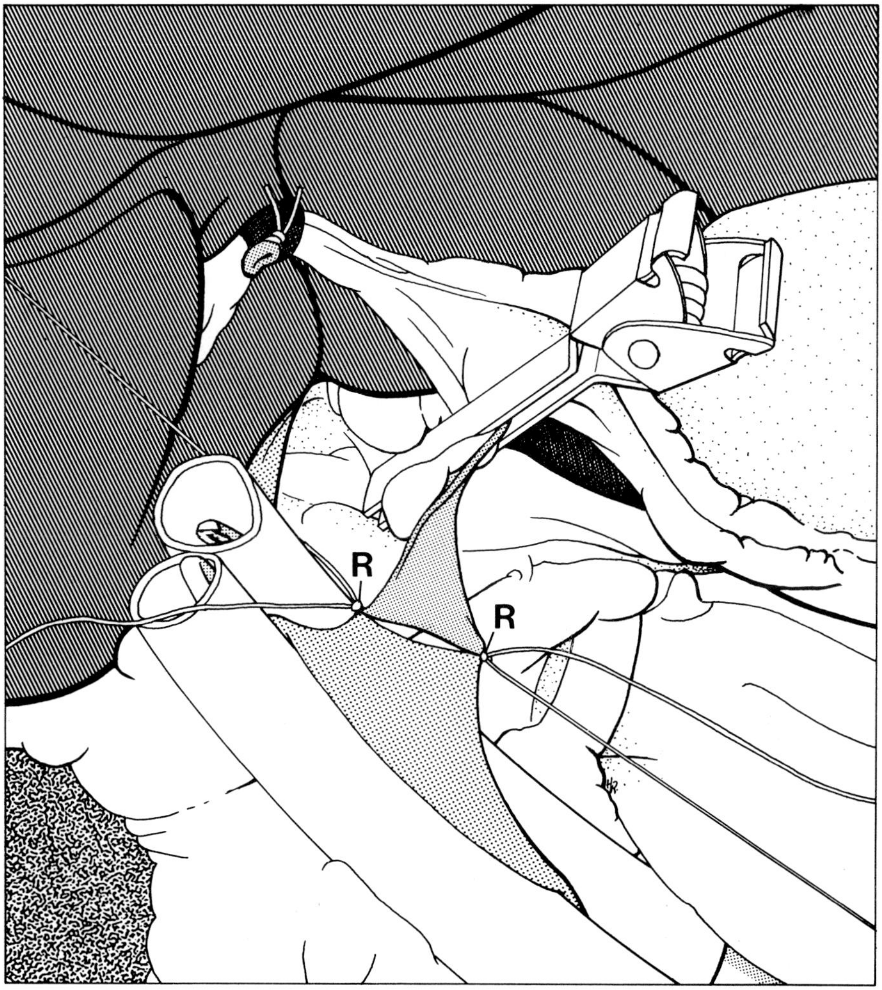

Figure 9.2.27. The corner sutures.
The two corner sutures (R) are placed and the anastomosis is slightly distended.

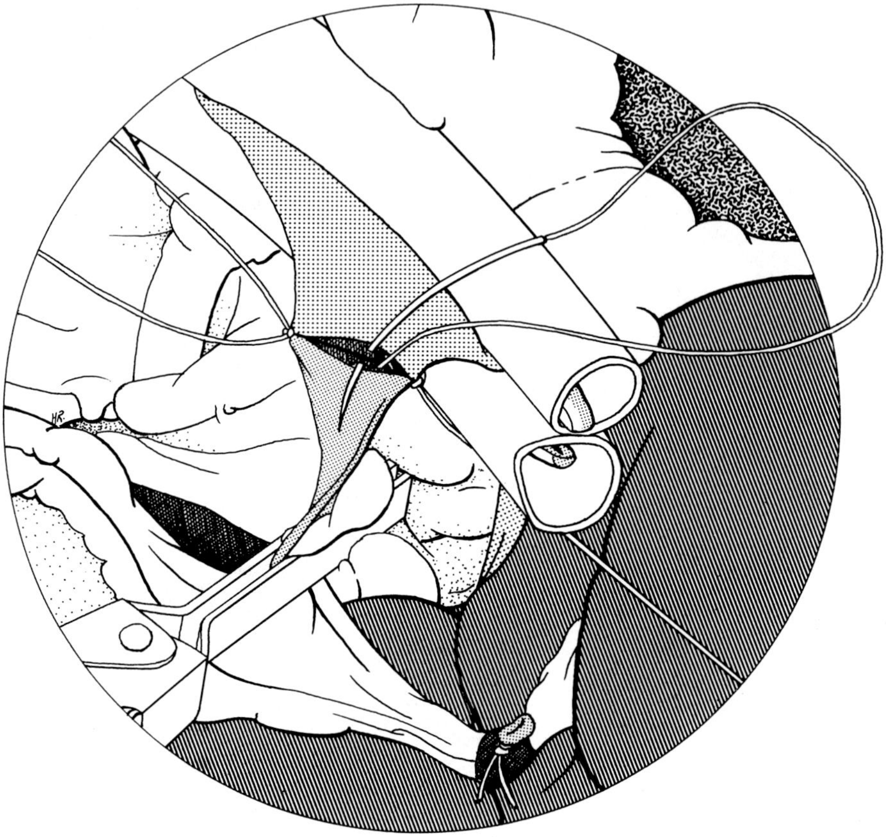

Figure 9.2.28. The first stitches in the posterior wall.
The animal has been turned through 180°. The needle is introduced into the lumen of the vessels via the portal vein wall, as near to the corner suture as possible. With running suture technique the posterior wall is closed.

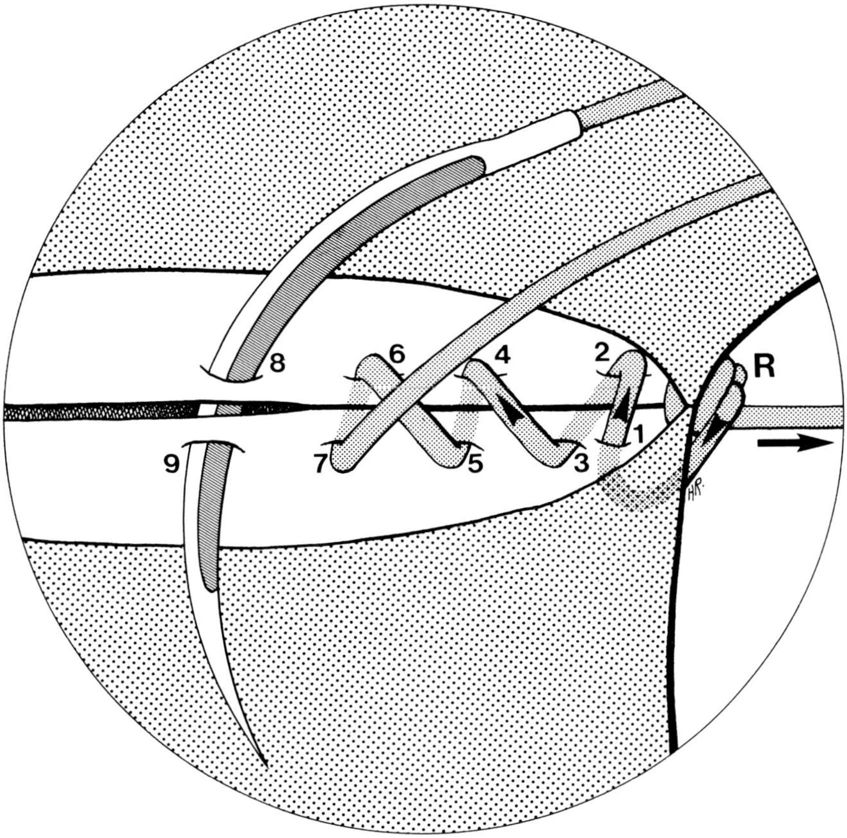

Figure 9.2.29. Detail of the first stitches in the posterior wall. R. Corner suture.

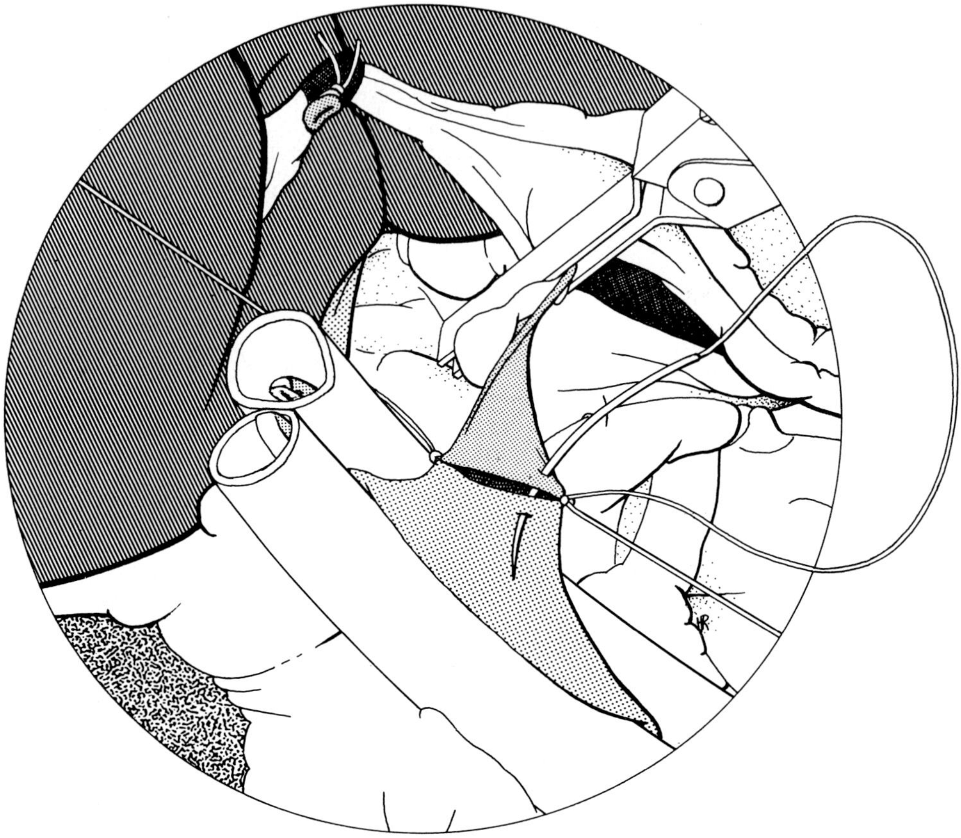

Figure 9.2.30. The anterior wall suture. Continuous suture of the anterior wall by over and over stitches.

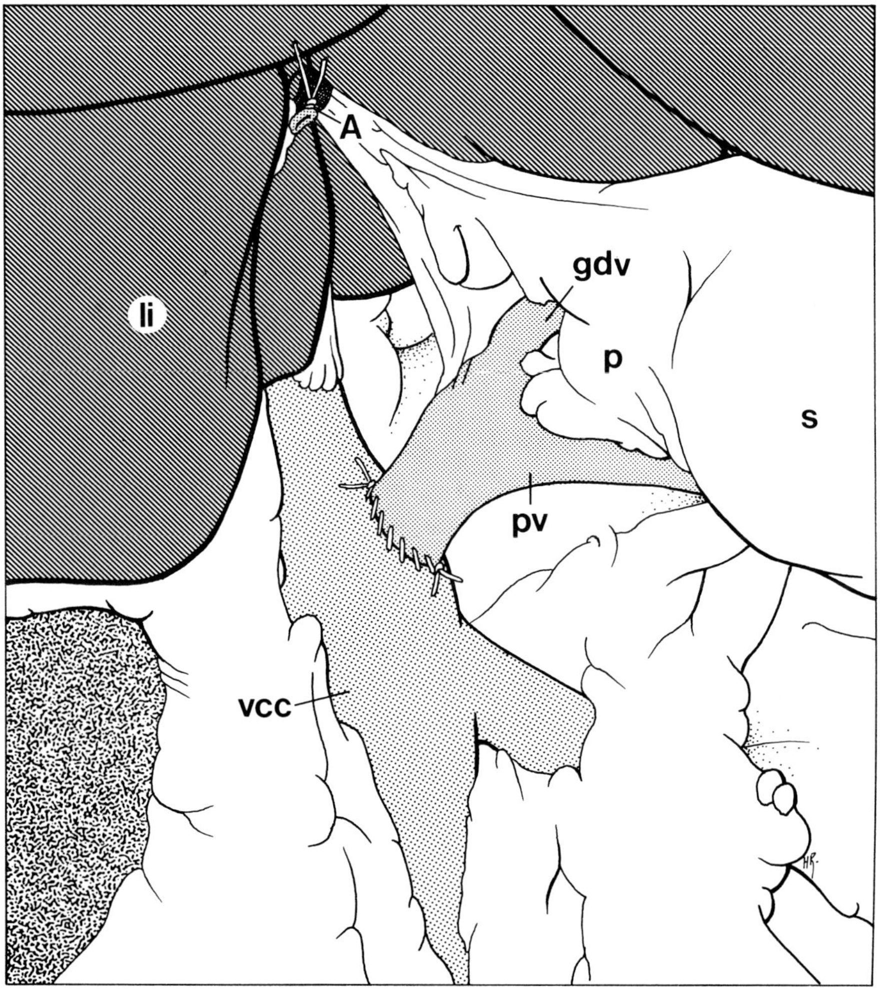

Figure 9.2.31. The final result.
A functioning portacaval shunt by means of an end-to-side anastomosis, according to Sun Lee.
A. Ligature on the portal vein.

vcc	Vena cava caudalis.
s	Stomach.
pv	Portal vein.
p	Pancreas.
li	Liver.
gdv	Gastroduodenal vein.

Manual of Microsurgery on the Laboratory Rat, Part I
Van Dongen, Remie, Rensema and Van Wunnik (eds)
© 1990 Elsevier Science Publishers B.V. (Biomedical Division)

CHAPTER 10

Permanent double bile fistula (with intact enterohepatic circulation)

R. REMIE, J.W. RENSEMA, G.H.J. VAN WUNNIK and J.J. VAN DONGEN

10.1 Introduction

The bile duct is fairly translucent and about 1 mm in diameter. It runs from the hilum of the liver, where the hepatic ducts meet, through the pancreatic tissue, where it collects the excretory ducts of the pancreas, into the lower end of the duodenum (Figure 10.2.1.). At this point the duct is surrounded by a muscular structure, the sphincter of Oddi. The laboratory rat has no gall bladder.

The enterohepatic circulation (EHC) points to the phenomenon that several substances excreted by the liver, are reabsorbed in the gut. They are transported back to the liver via the portal blood, they participate in liver metabolism, and are re-excreted into the bile and so on. In this way an optimal concentration of for example bile acids at the sites of their physiologic action, is guaranteed.

In the last three decades a number of techniques have been developed (Fisher and Vars, 1955; van Zyl, 1959; Light et al. (1959); Duane et al. (1979); Enderlin and Honohan (1977); Vonk et al. (1978); Weis and Barth (1978); Balabaud et al. (1981); Tse et al. (1982); Kuipers et al. (1985a)). Van Zyl (1959) was the first to use a double cannulation of the bile duct to restore the EHC. He used polyethylene catheters which were exteriorized in the middle of the animal's back. Light et al. (1959) used a cannula for restoration of the EHC, which was introduced from an opening in the greater curvature of the stomach and pushed into the duodenum.

Our technique is based upon the one described by Vonk et al. (1978). The method used by Kuipers et al. (1985a), which is an extension of Vonk's technique, compared with our's varies only in the area where the bile is led back into the body (approximately 2 cm distally from the pylorus, directly into the duodenum).

Kuipers et al. (1985b) describe the effects of interruption and restoration of the

EHC on several parameters, such as food intake, body weight, plasma glycocholate and cholesterol concentration, and concluded that their model was an excellent tool for studying the bilary excretion process and the effects of bile on intestinal absorption.

Using the technique described below we are able amongst other things, to study the pharmacokinetic properties of compounds that are cleared or metabolized by the liver and excreted into the bile. The animals can be followed for several weeks or even months. In combination with the permanent jugular vein cannula, the model enables excellent kinetic profiling of drugs and other substances of course, in the absence of anaesthetics, which are known to affect the process of bile formation as well as the bile acid absorption (Kuipers et al. 1985a).

10.2. The operation

Anaesthesia

The animal should preferably be anaesthetized with N_2O/O_2/halothane. If this type of anaesthesia is not available, then FFM (i.p.) should be used (see Chapter 6).

The operation can be divided into six parts:

10.2.1. Preparation of the crown of the head.
10.2.2. Opening of the abdominal wall.
10.2.3. Double cannulation of the bile duct.
10.2.4. Closure of the abdominal wall.
10.2.5. Subcutaneous tunnelling to the head.
10.2.6. Fixation of the cannulae.

Parts 10.2.1., 10.2.2., 10.2.4., 10.2.5. and 10.2.6. are described in Chapter 7 (General techniques).

10.2.3. Double cannulation of the bile duct

After opening the abdominal wall, the intestines should be lifted out and laid next to the animal (on the right side, as viewed by the surgeon) on gauze moistened with warm saline solution. Using jewellers forceps the bile duct should be stripped of its surrounding tissue. The duct should be ligated with a 7–0 silk suture. Subsequently the duct should be placed under tension using artery forceps, enabling easier handling during cannulation.

A second 7–0 silk ligature should be loosely placed around the duct (Figure 10.2.1.). With the aid of greater magnification, a V-shaped hole should be made using jewellers forceps and iridectomy scissors. Figure 10.2.2. shows the position of the hands and instruments during this procedure. A sterile silicon cannula (for its preparation, see General techniques, Chapter 7) should be inserted into the duct. To enable this to happen the duct wall should be lifted using jewellers forceps, thereby facilitating easy cannulation (Figures 10.2.3. and 10.2.4.).

The ligature should be tied and pulled tautly ensuring that the cannula is not obstructed. If this part of the operation has been completed successfully, the bile will be driven into the cannula by the force of the respiratory pulse. Subsequently, the first ligature should be released from the artery forceps, and the threads tied behind the silicon ring, again ensuring the free passage of bile through the cannula (Figure 10.2.5.). The rat should then be turned clockwise through 90°, and the ligature reclamped, thereby putting the distal part of the duct under tension. A third ligature should be loosely introduced around the duct, distal to the first ligature. Following the procedure described earlier another V-shaped opening should be made between the third and the first ligature using jewellers forceps and iridectomy scissors (Figures 10.2.6. and 10.2.7.).

The preparations have now been made for the introduction of the second cannula. As described in Chapter 7 (General techniques) this cannula differs from the previous one with regard to the diameter of the tip. Figures 10.2.8. and 10.2.9. show how the cannula is inserted into the distal part of the bile duct. The cotton wool stick can be very useful in absorbing pancreatic juices, thus allowing an unimpeded view at the place of insertion. The third ligature should be tied and pulled taut, and the first ligature should be re-released from the artery forceps and tied around the second cannula behind the silicon ring. All the loose threads should now be cut close to the knots (Figure 10.2.10.). The animal should be returned to its original position and as shown in Figure 10.2.11. the sections of the cannulae which lie between the silicon rings should be placed "kink-free" in the abdominal cavity. With a 7–0 silk suture the cannulae should be fixed to the abdominal muscle near the xiphoid cartilage as shown in Figure 10.2.11.. Subsequently the abdomen should be closed in two layers (part 10.2.4.), and the cannulae should be tunnelled subcutaneously (part 10.2.5.) as described in Chapter 7 (General techniques).

With a 5 cm piece of polyethylene tubing (0.75 × 1.45 mm), the two long ends of the 20G, L-shaped stainless steel adapters (see Chapter 7) should be connected. Using a piece of adhesive tape, the polyethylene tube should be fixated in the position shown in Chapter 7, Figure 7.9.8.. The short ends of the L-shaped adapters should be connected to the bile cannulae. It is good to form the habit of always having the proximal bile cannula (the one taking the bile from the liver) on the same side of the head. This will prevent you from making mistakes when you connect the animals to the swivelled sampling cannula prior to the experiment.

The cannulae together with the angled tubing should be fixated to the skull as described in Chapter 7. Figure 7.9.8. shows the final result before the acrylic glue has been applied.

10.3. Collection of bile

The animal should be housed in an individual cage (see Chapter 7). When bile has to be collected, the animal is attached to a long swivelled PE-cannula (0.75 × 1.45 mm). The end of the cannula must be just below the bottom of the cage. This will provide enough underpressure to let the bile flow into the cannula.

References

Balabaud, C., Saric, J., Conzalez, P. and Delphy, C. (1981) Bile collection in free moving rats. Lab. Animal Sci. 31: 273–275.

Duane, W.C., Gilberstadt, M.L. and Wiegand, D.M. (1979) Diurnal rhythms of bile acid production in the rat. Am. J. Physiol. 236: 175–179.

Enderlin, F.E. and Honohan, T. (1977) Long term bile collection in the rat. Lab. Animal Sci. 27: 490–493.

Fisher, B. and Vars, H.M. (1955) A method of collecting bile in rats: normal values in rat bile. Amer. J. Med. Sci. 222: 116.

Kuipers, F., Dijkstra, T., Havinga, R., van Asselt, W. and Vonk, R. (1985a) Acute effects of pentobarbital-anaesthesia on bile secretion. Biochem. Pharmacol. 34: 1731–1736.

Kuipers, F., Havinga, R., Bosschieter, H., Toorop, G.P., Hindriks, F.R. and Vonk, R. (1985b) Enterohepatic circulation in the rat. Gastroenterology 88: 403–411.

Light, H.C., Witmer, C. and Vars, H.M. (1959) Interruption of the enterohepatic circulation and its effect on rat bile. Am. J. Physiol. 197: 1330–1332.

Tse, F.L.S., Ballard, F., and Jaffe, J.M. (1982) A practical method for monitoring drug excretion and enterohepatic circulation in the rat. J. Pharmacol. Methods 7: 139–144.

Vonk, R.J., van Doorn, A.B.D. and Strubbe, J.H. (1978) Bile secretion and bile composition in the freely moving, unanaesthetized rat with a permanent biliary drainage: influence of food intake on bile flow. Clin. Sci. Mol. Med. 55: 253–259.

Weis, E.E. and Barth C.A. (1978) The extracorporeal bile duct: a new model for determination of bile flow and bile composition in the intact rat. J. Lipid Res. 19: 856–862.

Zyl, A. van (1959) Thyroid function in relation to bile lipids and bile acids: an experimental approach by cannulation of the bile duct of rats so that the entero-hepatic circulation is maintained. S. Afr. Med. J. 33: 618.

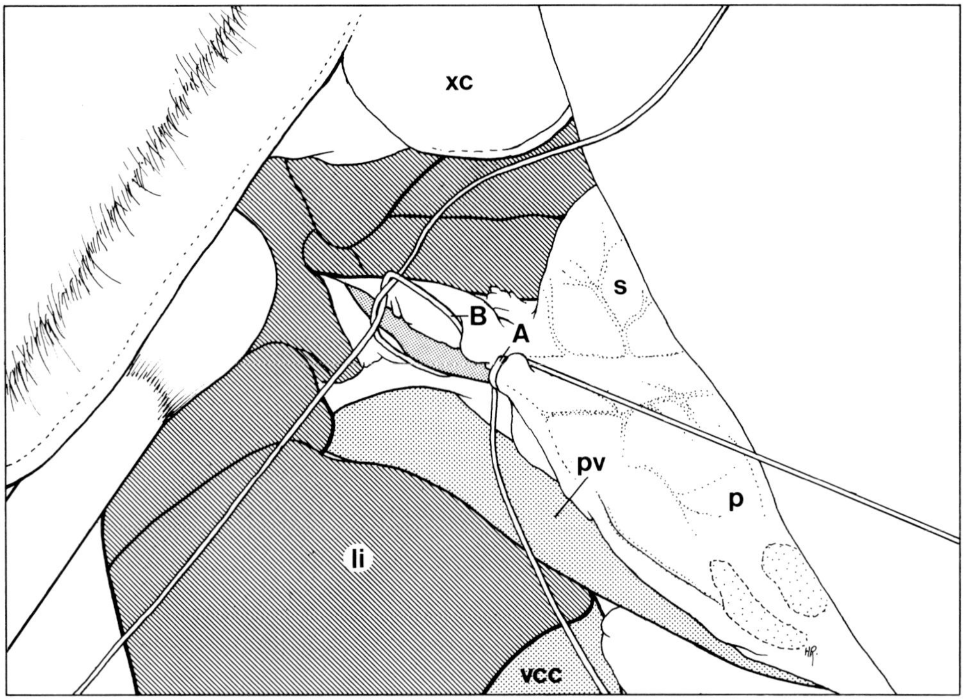

Figure 10.2.1. Ligation of the bile duct.
The common bile duct is made visible, freed of its surrounding tissue by sharp dissection. A distal ligature is placed and tied. The proximal ligature is placed loosely around the duct.

A. Distal ligature.
B. Proximal ligature.

li Liver
pv Portal vein.
p Pancreas.
vcc Vena cava caudalis.
s Stomach.
xc Xiphoid cartilage.

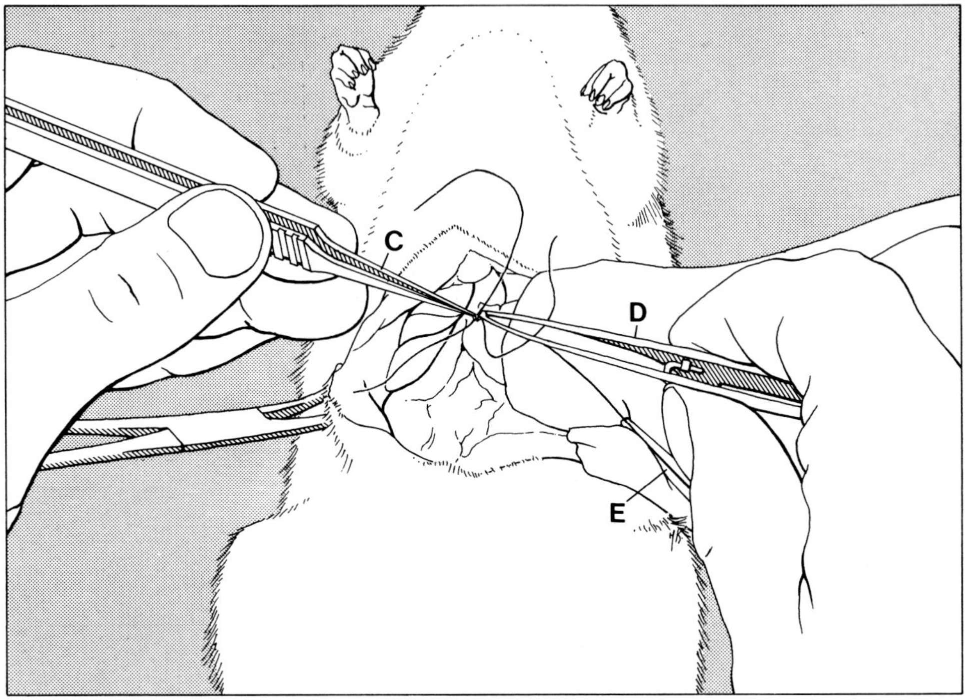

Figure 10.2.2. Cutting a V-shaped hole.
A V-shaped hole is cut in the wall of the common bile duct, using iridectomy scissors, and jewellers forceps. The bile duct is distended by the caudal ligature, which is clamped with artery forceps.
C. Jewellers forceps.
D. Iridectomy scissors.
E. Artery forceps.

→

Figure 10.2.3. Insertion of the proximal cannula (I).
The hole in the bile duct is exposed. The cannula is handled just behind the silicon ring and can be inserted into the duct.
F. Cannula.
F^1. Silicon ring.
G. V-shaped hole.
H. Angled jewellers forceps.
I. Anatomical forceps.

Figure 10.2.4. Insertion of the proximal cannula (II).
The Silastic cannula is inserted into the bile duct.

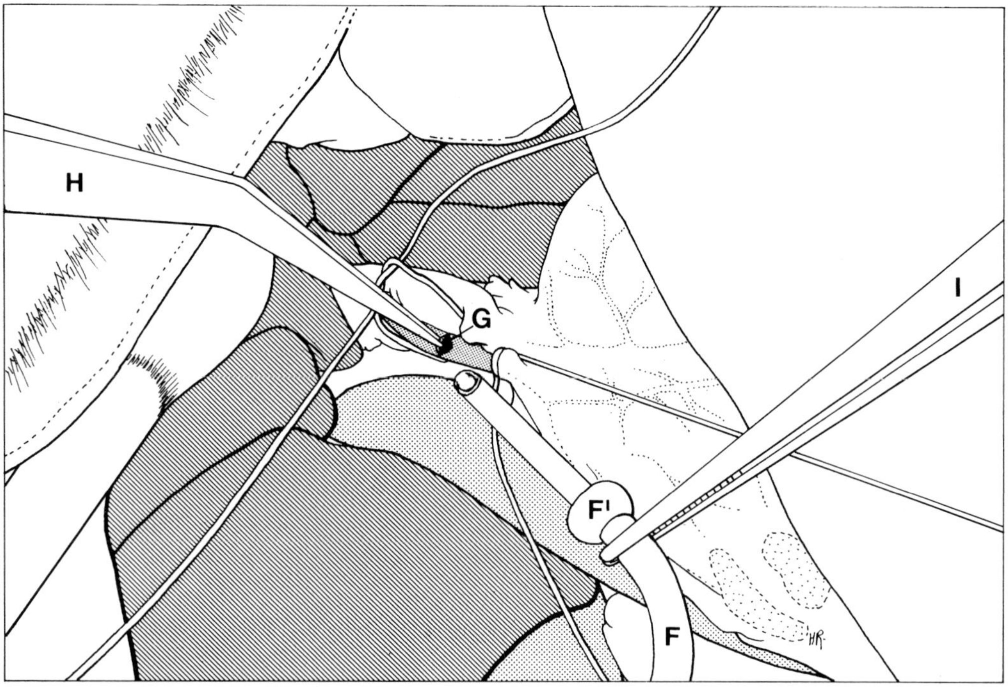

Fig. 10.2.3.

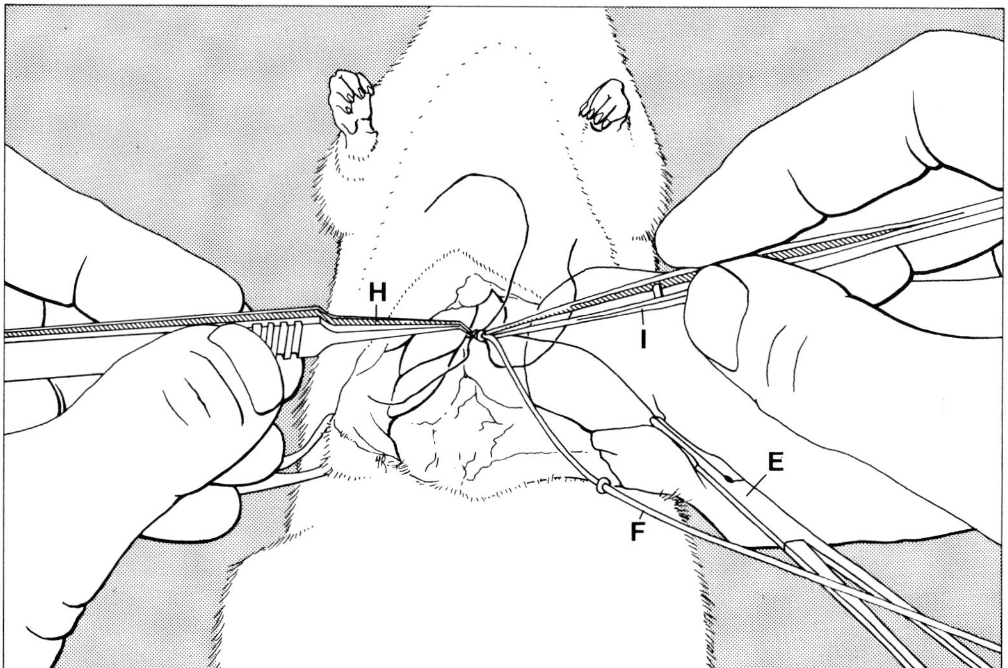

Fig. 10.2.4.

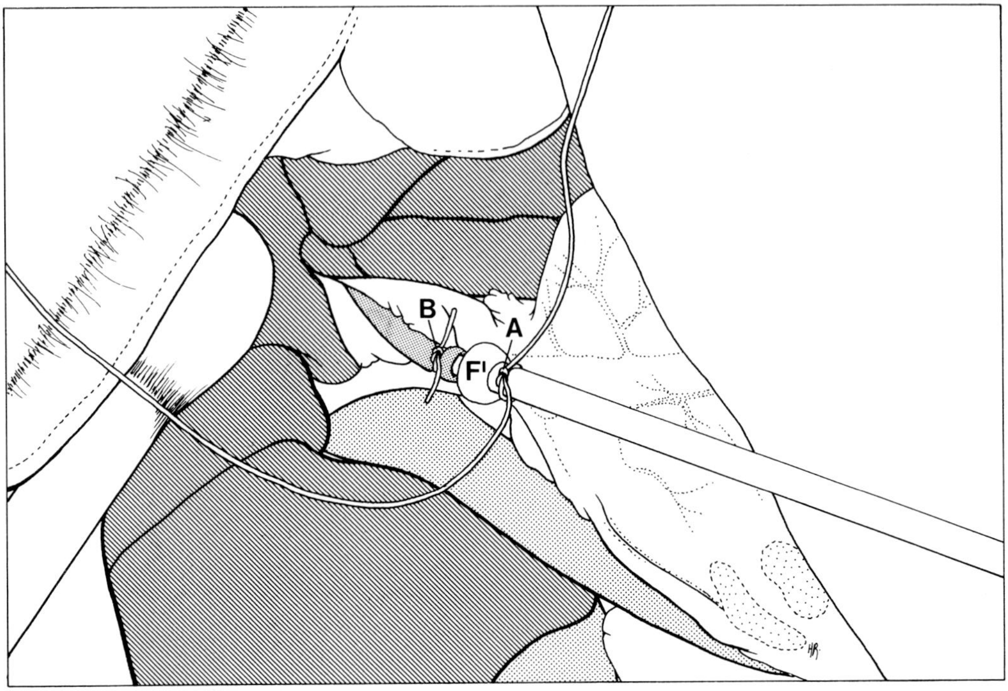

Figure 10.2.5. Fixation of the proximal cannula.
The proximal ligature is pulled taut and tied, thus securing the inserted cannula, and the strings are cut. The distal ligature is tied behind the first silicon ring.

A. Distal ligature.
B. Proximal ligature.
F^1. Silicon ring.

→

Figure 10.2.6. Cutting the second hole.
The animal is turned through a 90° angle. The cannula is bent, thus exposing the distal part of the bile duct. A second aperture is cut after clamping the distal ligature with artery forceps.

D. Iridectomy scissors.
H. Angled jewellers forceps.
F. Cannula.

Figure 10.2.7. Detail of the second hole.
A third ligature is placed loosely around the duct, and V-shaped hole is made.

F. Proximal cannula.
A. Distal ligature.
J. The third ligature.

li	Liver.	vcc	Vena cava caudalis.
pv	Portal vein.	s	Stomach.
p	Pancreas.	xc	Xiphoid cartilage.

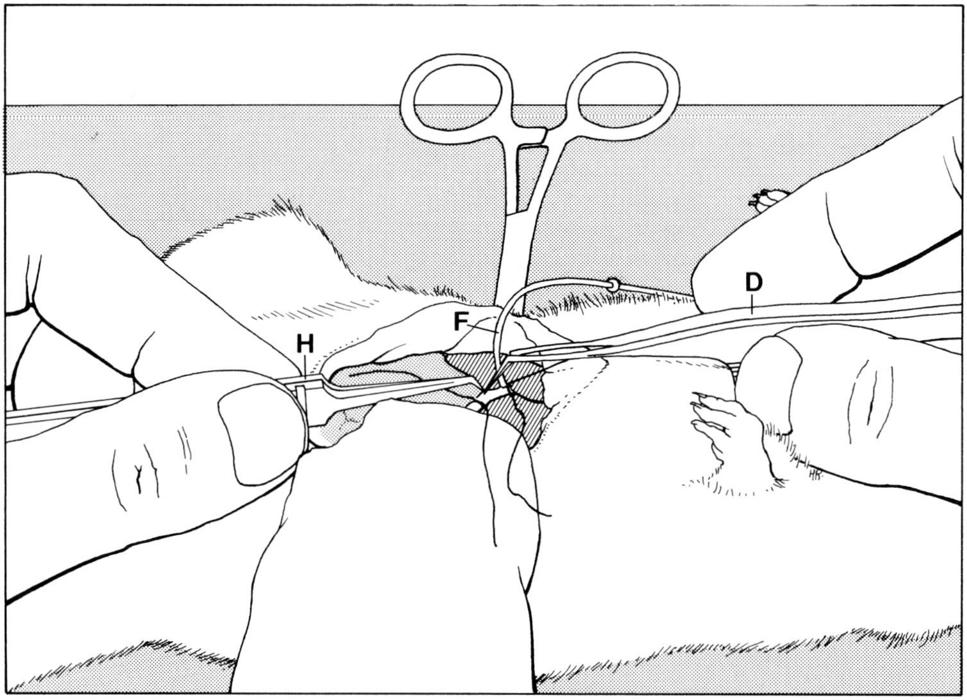

Fig. 10.2.6.

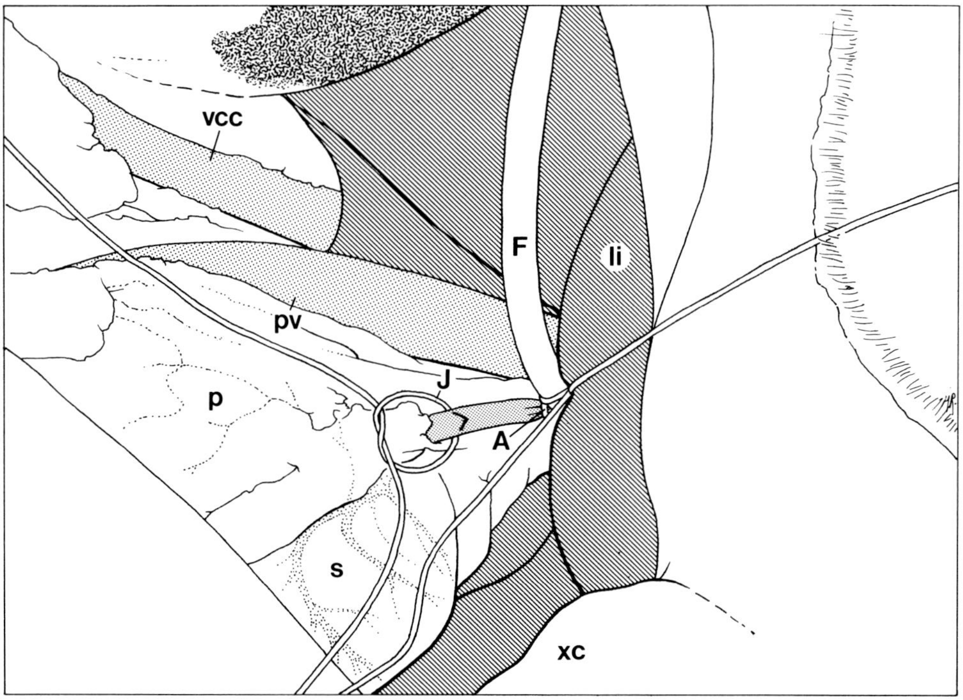

Fig. 10.2.7.

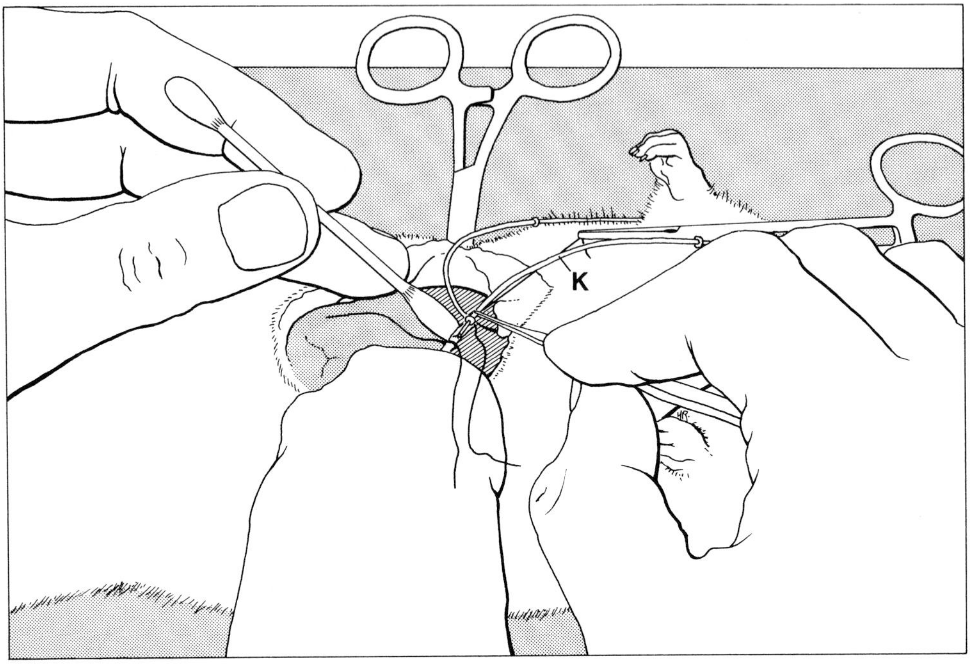

Figure 10.2.8. Insertion of the distal cannula (I).
The distal cannula is inserted towards the duodenum, while the pancreatic juices are absorbed by the cotton wool stick.
K. Distal cannula.

→

Figure 10.2.9. Insertion of the distal cannula (II).
Detail of the insertion of the cannula.
K. Distal cannula.

Figure 10.2.10. Fixation of the cannulae.
The distal cannula is fixed by tightening the third ligature. The distal ligature is tightened just behind the silicon ring, and the threads are cut.
A. The third ligature.

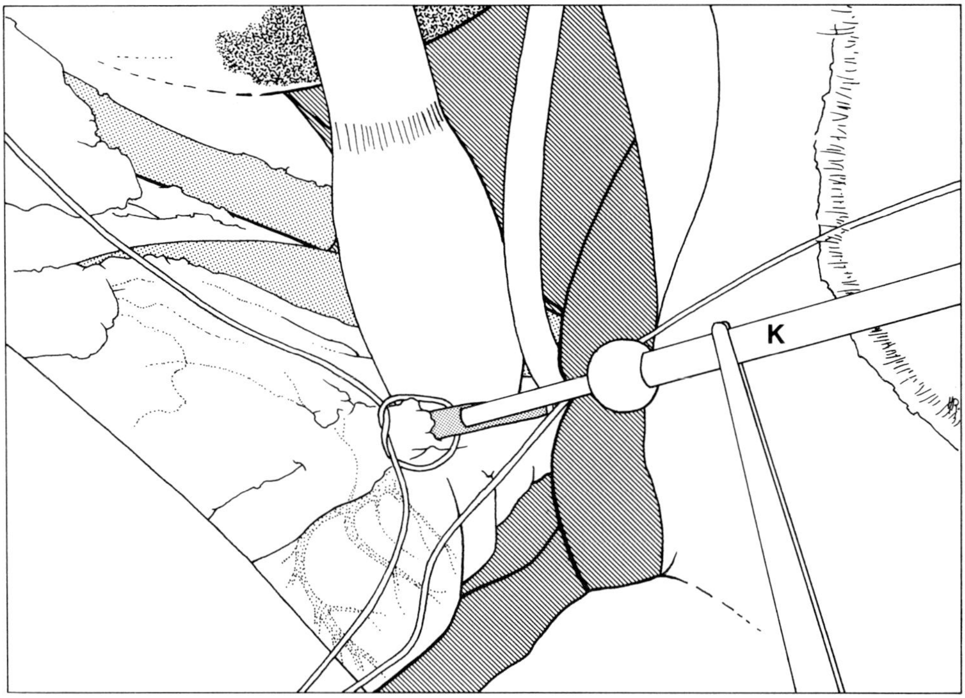

Fig. 10.2.9.

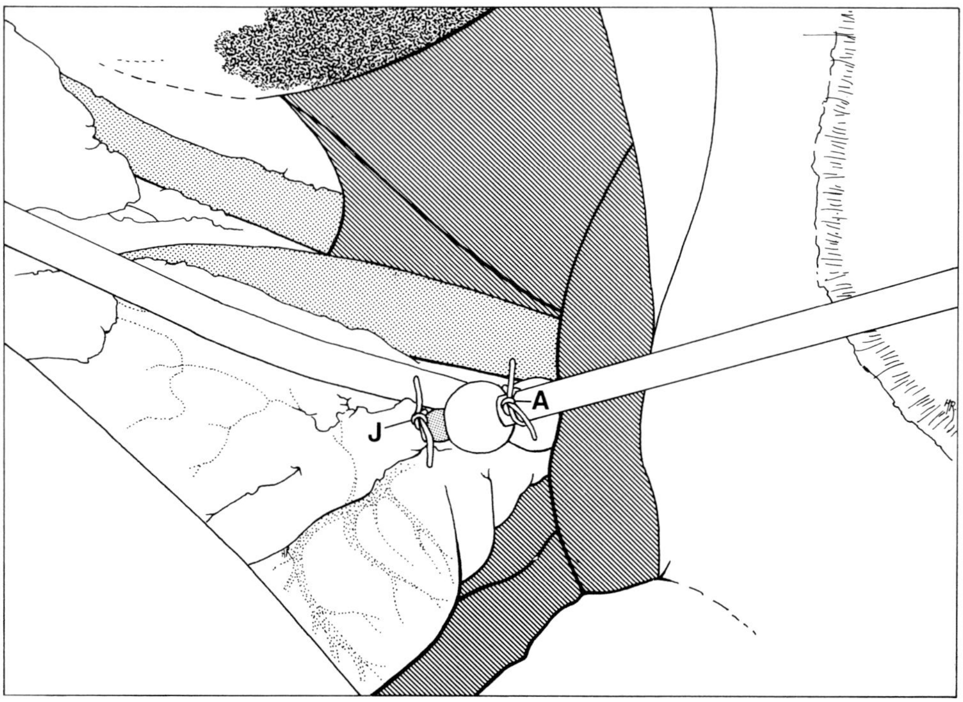

Fig. 10.2.10.

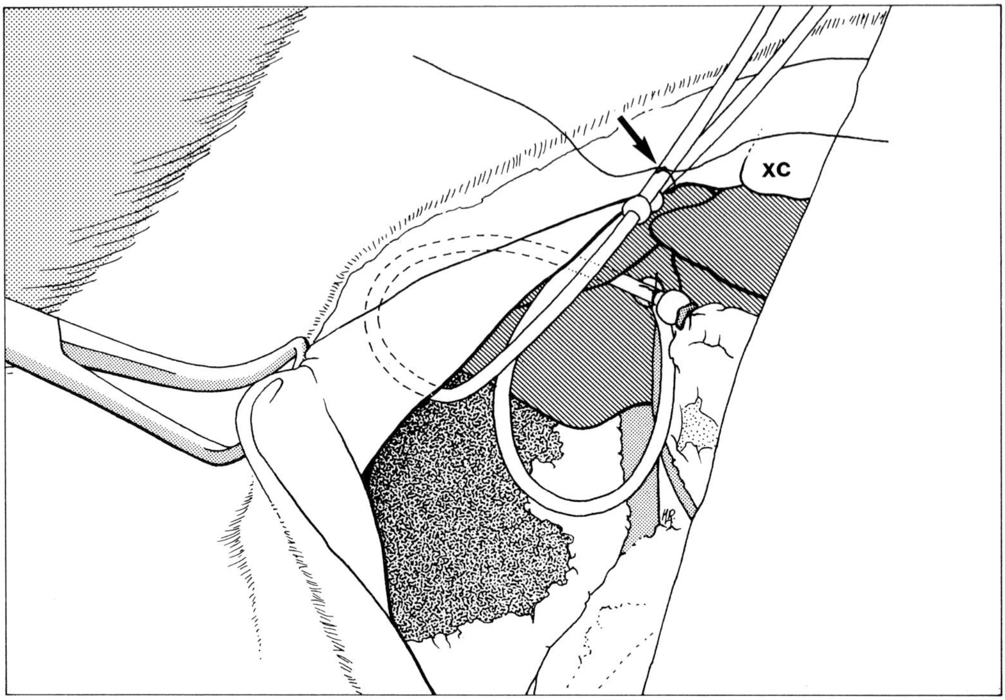

Figure 10.2.11. Fixation of the cannulae to the internal abdominal muscle.
The portal area is repositioned and the two cannulae are placed "kink-free" in the abdominal cavity. Both cannulae are anchored to the internal abdominal muscle near the xiphoid cartilage (arrow).

xc Xiphoid cartilage.

Manual of Microsurgery on the Laboratory Rat, Part I
Van Dongen, Remie, Rensema and Van Wunnik (eds)
© *1990 Elsevier Science Publishers B.V. (Biomedical Division)*

CHAPTER 11

Permanent cannulation of the portal vein

R. REMIE, J.J. VAN DONGEN, J.W. RENSEMA and
G.H.J. VAN WUNNIK

11.1 Introduction

Repeated blood sampling, or infusion in the general circulation and the portal vein in unanaesthetized freely moving rats is of major interest for pharmacological and physiological studies. In the past, several cannulation techniques have been described (Hyun et al., 1967; Pelzmann and Havemeyer, 1971; Suzuki T. et al., 1973; Russell and Mogenson, 1975; Sable-Amplis and Abadie, 1975; Helman et al., 1984). Sable-Amplis and Abadie (1975) described a T-shaped cannula of Clay-Adams polyethylene tubing inserted in the portal vein between the gastroduodenal vein and the splenic vein. Helman et al. (1984) used the left portal branch to enter the vein, due to their lack of success with the T-shaped cannula. Russell and Mogenson (1975) used the rostral mesenteric vein to accomplish cannulation of the portal vein. All the above mentioned methods suffered from a limited long-term patency of the catheter.

In this chapter a technique is described in which the catheter patency was significantly lengthened. Post-operative weight loss was low and amounted to between 3 and 5% on the third day, and pre-operative weight was reached after 5–7 days. After two months, sampling was still feasible in 60% of the rats, and several animals could be used for experiments for over 5 months. An additional application of platinum electrodes around the portal vein in close proximity to the catheter tip in the same freely moving animals, resulted in a model highly suited to the study of presynaptic regulation of neurotransmitter release from noradrenergic nerve terminals (Remie and Zaagsma, 1986; Remie et al., 1988a,b, 1989, 1990).

11.2. The operation

Anaesthesia
The animal should preferably be anaesthetized with N_2O/O_2/halothane. If this type of anaesthesia is not available, then FFM (i.p.) should be used.

Two operations will be described:
11.2.1. Single cannulation of the portal vein.
11.2.2. Portal sample cannula and an infusion cannula combined with stimulation electrodes.

11.2.1. Single cannulation of the portal vein

The first operation can be divided into seven parts:
11.2.1.1. Preparation of the crown of the head.
11.2.1.2. Opening of the abdominal wall.
11.2.1.3. The purse-string suture.
11.2.1.4. Cannulation of the portal vein.
11.2.1.5. Closure of the abdominal wall.
11.2.1.6. Subcutaneous tunnelling to the head.
11.2.1.7. Fixation of the cannula.

Parts 11.2.1.1., 11.2.1.2., 11.2.1.5., 11.2.1.6. and 11.2.1.7. are described in Chapter 7 (General techniques).

11.2.1.3. The purse-string suture
After opening the abdominal wall the intestines should be lifted out and laid next to the animal (on the right side, as viewed by the surgeon) on gauze moistened with warm (30° C) saline solution. This will provide an excellent view of the portal vein area.

Using a micro needle holder and a cotton-wool stick, a four or five, fine-stitch purse-string suture (7–0 silk suture armed with a BV-1 needle) should be placed in the wall of the portal vein at the side opposite the gastroduodenal vein (Figure 11.2.1). The diameter of the purse-string should be approximately 1 mm. The needle and thread should be guided through the vessel paying special attention to the rules given in Chapter 7 about suture techniques (anastomosis). After each stitch, bleeding (if any) should be arrested immediately by applying light pressure on the bleeding spot, using the cotton-wool stick. After the suture has been completed a single knot is made with the drawstrings (Figure 11.2.1.).

11.2.1.4. Cannulation of the portal vein
The portal vein should be clamped with a small curved haemostatic bulldog clamp,

modified to resemble a Satinsky vascular clamp (Figure 11.2.2.). Using iridectomy scissors and a pair of jewellers forceps the centre of the purse-string should be cut (Figure 11.2.3.). Subsequently, the cannula which is filled with heparinized saline (50 IU/ml) should be inserted into the vessel and pushed in until the silicon ring reaches the vein (Figure 11.2.4.). Next the purse-string should be gently tightened, taking care not to obstruct the cannula, which can be controlled by slight aspiration of blood into the syringe followed by an injection of some heparinized saline solution. The drawstrings of the suture are used to anchor the cannula behind the first silicon ring. This is shown in Figure 11.2.5.

In experienced hands the total clamping time is less than 1 min (when the surgeon has assistance, the clamping time can be reduced to 20–30 sec). The second silicon ring is used to anchor the cannula to the internal abdominal muscle, near the xiphoid cartilage (see Figure 10.2.11 in Chapter 10). To complete the operation, steps 11.2.5., 11.2.6. and 11.2.7. must be followed. These steps are described in Chapter 7.

11.2.2. Portal sample cannula and an infusion cannula combined with stimulation electrodes

The model described above can be extended to do research on the presynaptic modulation of the noradrenergic neurotransmission (Remie et al. 1988a,b, 1989, 1990).

A second cannula, used for the infusion of drugs, should be placed into the portal vein 10 mm distally from the first, in the same manner as the first one (see Chapter 7.4. for a complete description of the cannula). Using 8–0 Ethilon a three to four fine-stitch purse-string suture is made in the wall of the portal vein. The vessel should be clamped with the same clamp as used for the first cannula. The portal wall in the purse-string suture should then be punctured with a 23G needle, to make the hole as small as possible, and the cannula is pushed into the lumen of the portal vein, followed by closure of the purse-string suture. The cannula is anchored in the same way as described above.

After completion of both cannulations the stimulation electrodes should be placed around the portal vein. To facilitate this the portal vein is mobilized (blunt dissection) between the gastroduodenal vein and the rostral pancreaticoduodenal vein. This segment should be lifted with straight forceps, and the electrodes put in place. The circles should then be closed to give an optimal vessel fit (Figure 11.2.6). The electrodes may be anchored to the portal vein with two 9–0 Ethilon sutures (not shown).

Before the second layer of the abdominal wall is closed, the free end of the cannulae and the insulated wire should be driven subcutaneously to emerge at the crown of the head. Each cannula should be slid over the short end of a 20G stainless steel L-shaped adapter. The heparinized saline should now be replaced by the viscous PVP-solution. The L-shaped adapters should be anchored to the skull with three small stainless steel screws and dental acrylic glue. These procedures are described in Chapter 7.

References

Helman A., Castaing D., Morin J., Pfister-Lemaire N. and Assan R. (1984) A new technique for hepatic portal vein catheterization in freely moving rats. Am. J. Physiol. 246 (Endocrinol. Metab. 9): E544–E547.

Hyun S.A., Vanhouny G.V. and Treadwell C.R. (1967) Portal absorption of fatty acids in lymph and portal vein cannulated rats. Biochim. Biophys. Acta 137: 296–305.

Pelzmann K.S. and Havemeyer R.N. (1971) Portal vein blood sampling in intestinal drug absorption studies. J. Pharm. Sci. 60: 331–332.

Remie R. and Zaagsma J. (1986) A new technique for the study of vascular presynaptic receptors in freely moving rats. Am. J. Physiol. 251: H463–H467.

Remie R., Knot H.J., Kolker H.J. and Zaagsma J. (1988a) Pronounced facilitation of endogenous noradrenaline release by presynaptic β_2-adrenoceptors in the vasculature of freely moving rats. Naunyn-Schmiedeberg's Arch. Pharmacol. 338: 215–220.

Remie R., Knot H.J., Bos E.A. and Zaagsma J. (1988b) Characterization of presynaptic β-adrenoceptors facilitating endogenous noradrenaline release in the portal vein of permanently cannulated, freely moving rats. Eur. J. Pharmacol. 157: 37–43.

Remie R., Coppes R.P. and Zaagsma J. (1989) Presynaptic muscarinic receptors inhibiting endogenous noradrenaline release in the portal vein of the freely moving rat. Br. J. Pharmacol. 97: 586–590.

Remie R., Coppes R.P., Meurs H., Roffel A.F. and Zaagsma J. (1990) Characterization of vascular muscarinic receptors inhibiting endogenous noradrenaline release in the portal vein of the freely moving rat. Br. J. Pharmacol. 99: 223–226.

Russell P.J.D. and Mogenson G.J. (1975) Drinking and feeding induced by jugular and portal infusions of 2-deoxy-D-glucose. Am. J. Physiol. 229: 1014–1018.

Sable-Amplis R. and Abadie D. (1975) Permanent cannulation of the hepatic portal vein in rats. J. Appl. Physiol. 38: 358–359.

Suzuki T., Sattoh Y., Isozaki S. and Ishida R. (1973) Simple method for portal vein infusion in the rat. J. Pharm. Sci. 62: 345–347.

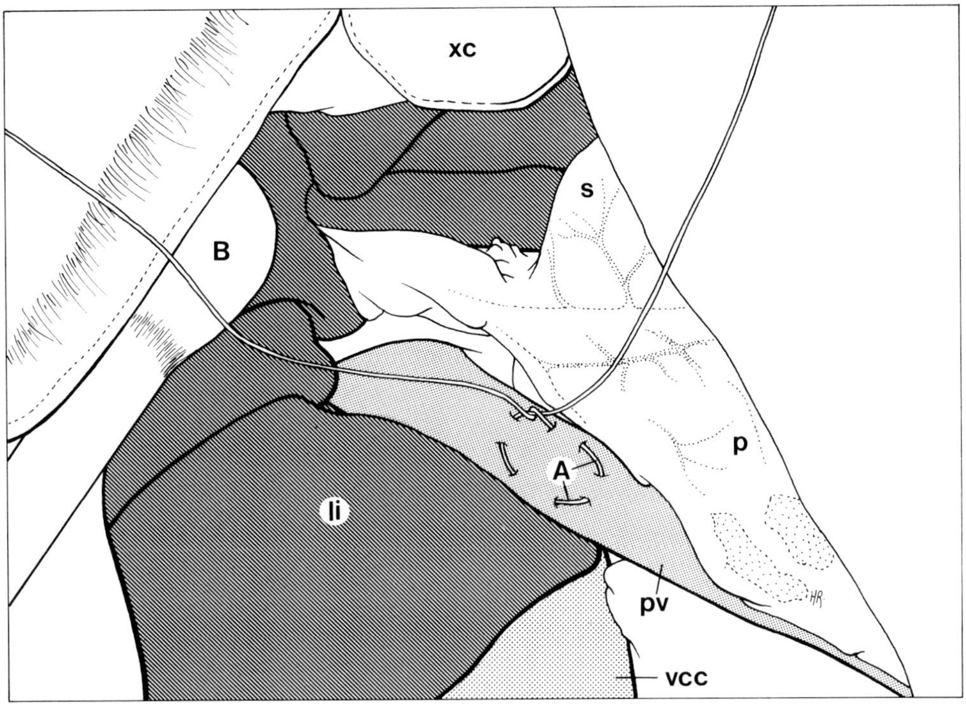

Figure 11.2.1. The purse-string suture.

The purse-string suture placed in the wall of the portal vein is finished.

A. The purse-string suture.

B. Cotton-wool stick.

li Liver.

p Pancreas.

vcc Vena cava caudalis.

pv Portal vein.

s Stomach.

xc Xiphoid cartilage.

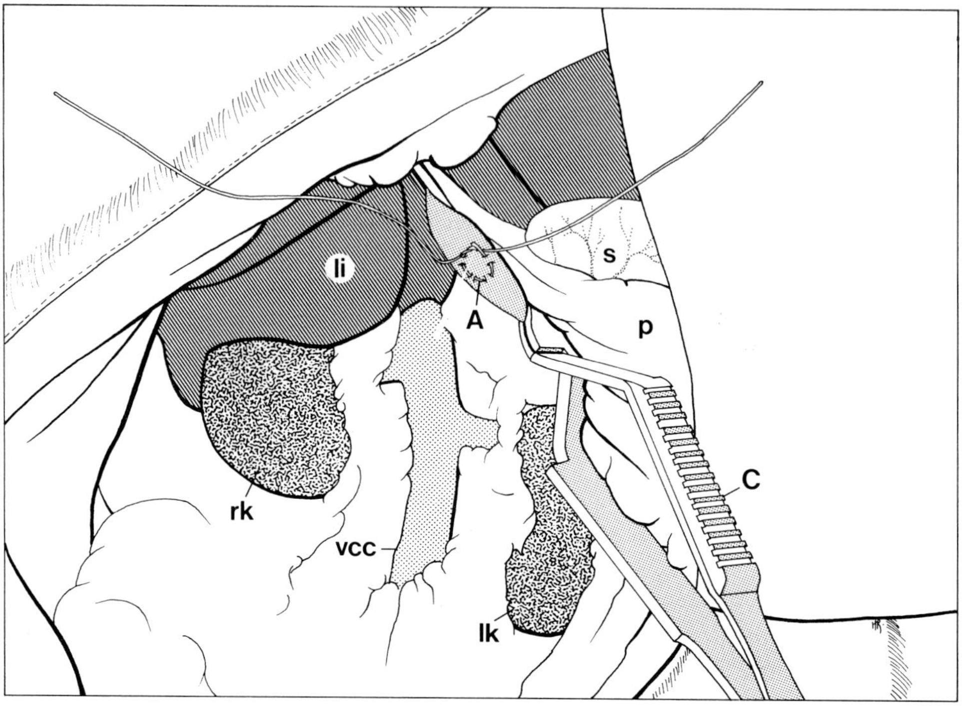

Figure 11.2.2. Clamping the vessel.
A modified bulldog clamp is placed on the portal vein, while the purse-string is lifted, making the vessel bulge out after clamping.
A. The purse-string suture.
C. Bulldog clamp.
li Liver.
p Pancreas.
rk Right kidney.
lk Left kidney.
vcc Vena cava caudalis.
s Stomach.

Figure 11.2.3. Cutting the aperture. →
An aperture is cut in the purse-string suture using iridectomy scissors and jewellers forceps.
D. Iridectomy scissors.
E. Jewellers forceps.
F. Towel clip.

Figure 11.2.4. Insertion of the cannula.
The cannula is inserted into the portal vein towards the liver.
G. Anatomical forceps.
H. Cannula.

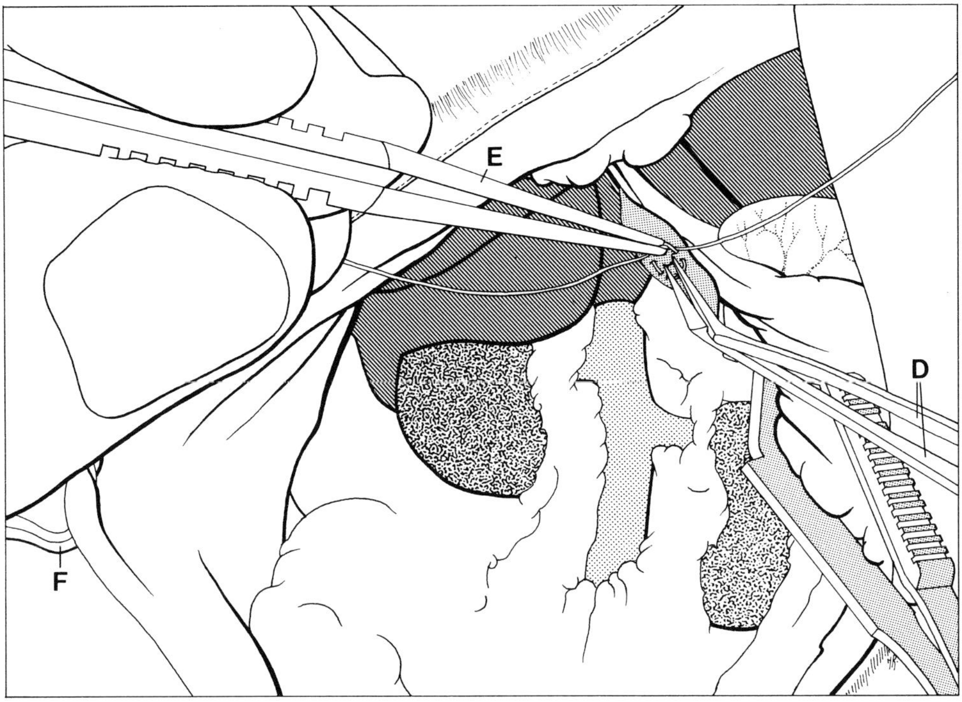

Fig. 11.2.3.

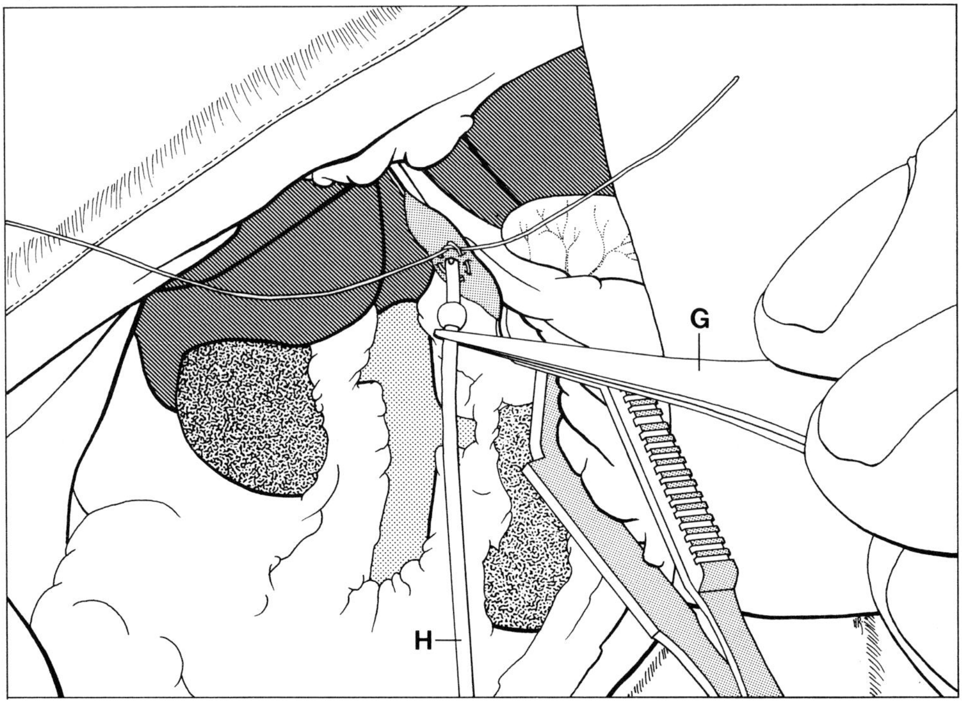

Fig. 11.2.4.

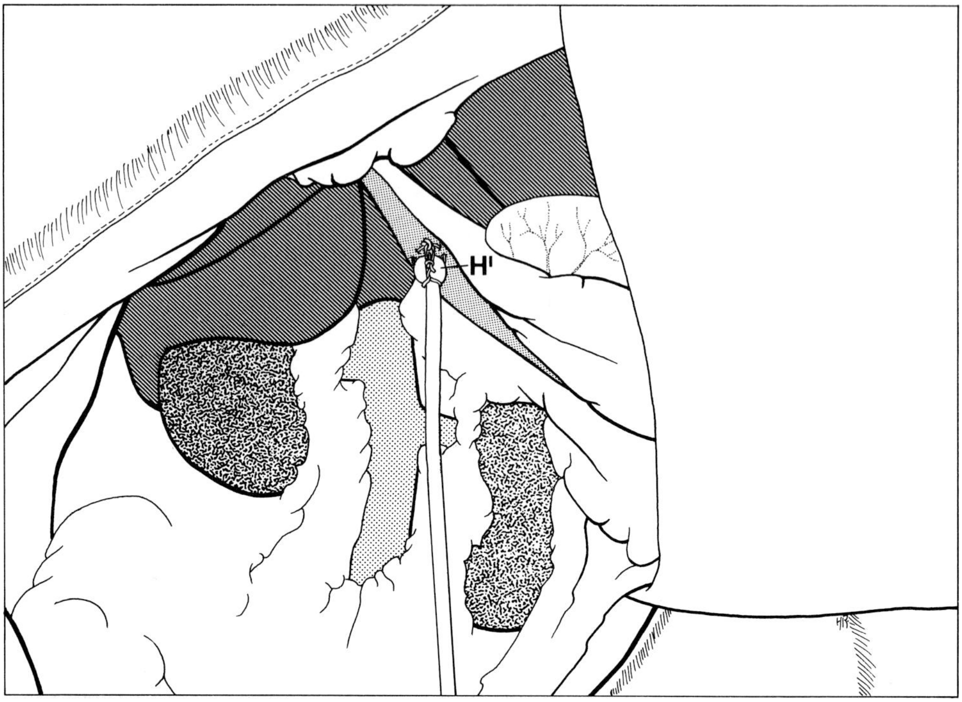

Figure 11.2.5. Tying the purse-string suture.
After removing the clamp, the purse-string suture is tied, the cannula is fixed behind the silicon ring, and the strings are cut.
H[1]. Silicon ring.

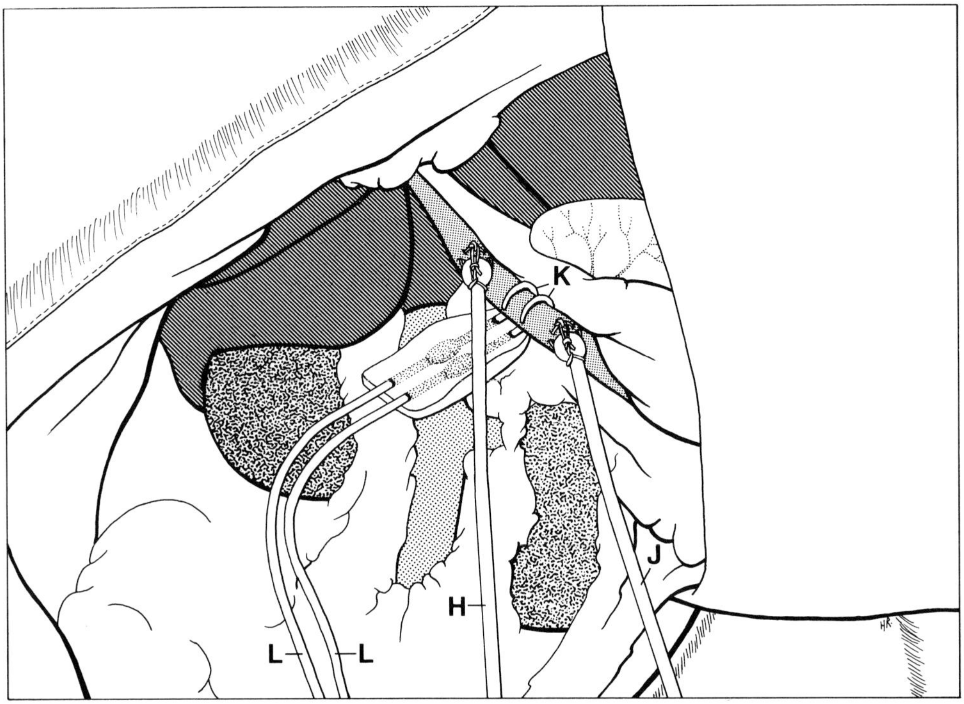

Figure 11.2.6. Portal vein with sample cannula, infusion cannula and stimulation electrodes. After placement of the sample cannula (H) a second cannula (J) is inserted in the same way. Finally the stimulation electrodes, which are held together with acrylic glue, are placed around the vessel.

H. Sample cannula.
J. Infusion cannula.
K. Stimulation electrodes.
L. Insulated wires.

Manual of Microsurgery on the Laboratory Rat, Part I
Van Dongen, Remie, Rensema and Van Wunnik (eds)
© 1990 Elsevier Science Publishers B.V. (Biomedical Division)

CHAPTER 12

Permanent cannulation of the renal vein

R. REMIE, J.W. RENSEMA and J.J. VAN DONGEN

12.1 Introduction

To the best of our knowledge no permanent catheterization techniques have been described on the renal vein.

Samples from the general circulation are usually taken from thoracic vena cava at the level of the right atrium by means of a permanent jugular vein catheter. When kinetic studies for example are performed on drugs which are mainly cleared from the body by the kidneys, or when renal transport mechanisms are to be studied, it may be necessary to cannulate the renal vein. Samples taken from the renal vein will contain a higher amount of the drug to be studied or of its metabolites, compared with blood samples taken from the caudal vena cava.

The technique described below was devised to study renal transport mechanisms, and has been used successfully for several years. Catheters remained patent for relatively long periods of up to a maximum of six weeks. The main cause of the obstruction was the formation of fibrogenous tissue around the catheter tip.

12.2 The operation

Anaesthesia

The animal should preferably be anaesthetized with N_2O/O_2/halothane. If this type of anaesthesia is not available, then FFM (i.p.) should be used (see Chapter 6).

The operation can be divided into eight parts:

12.2.1. Preparation of the crown of the head.
12.2.2. Opening of the abdominal wall.
12.2.3. Exposure of the caudal vena cava and the renal vein.
12.2.4. The purse-string suture.
12.2.5. Cannulation of the renal vein.
12.2.6. Closure of the abdominal wall.
12.2.7. Subcutaneous tunnelling to the crown of the head.
12.2.8. Fixation of the cannula.

Parts 12.2.1., 12.2.2., 12.2.5., 12.2.6, 12.2.7. and 12.2.8. are described in detail in Chapter 7 (General techniques).

12.2.3. Exposure of the caudal vena cava and the renal vein

After opening the abdominal wall, the intestines should be lifted out and laid next to the animal (on the right side, as viewed by the surgeon) on gauze moistened with warm (30° C) saline solution.

This will provide an excellent view of the caudal vena cava (Figure 12.2.1.). At its confluence with the vena cava, the right renal vein should be stripped of its adipose tissue and the peritoneum should be opened. Using small anatomical forceps (one straight and one curved) the peritoneum should be detached from the vena cava by making small spreading movements with the forceps just beneath the peritoneum. Subsequently, the vena cava and the renal vein should be mobilized for approximately 1.5 cm, to allow for the clamping of the vessel. Small pieces of adipose tissue and peritoneum can easily be removed by rubbing gently with a cotton-wool stick. It is important that the area shown in Figure 12.2.1. is clean.

12.2.4. The purse-string suture

Without clamping, a four or five fine-stitch purse-string suture should be placed in the vessel wall at the confluence of the vena cava and the right renal vein (the left kidney as viewed by the surgeon). Using a Barraquer needle holder and a cotton-wool stick, the 7–0 silk suture, armed with a BV-1 needle, should be guided through the vessel, paying special attention to the rules set out in Chapter 7.5 regarding suture techniques (anastomosis). After each stitch, any bleeding should be immediately arrested by applying light pressure on the area in question, using a cotton-wool stick. Having completed the suture a single knot should be made with the drawstrings (Figure 12.2.2.). As depicted, the drawstrings should be joined at the lateral part of the purse-string suture. Three microvascular clips should then be placed on the vena cava and the renal vein, as shown in Figure 12.2.3. The proximal clip on the vena cava should be placed first, followed by the clip on the renal vein and finally the distal vena cava clip.

12.2.5. Cannulation of the renal vein

A small aperture should be cut immediately inside the purse-string suture (Figure 12.2.3.) using iridectomy scissors and jewellers forceps. Blood clots, if present, have to be removed by directing a fine jet of saline solution from a 2 ml syringe with a cut 23G needle at the opening in the purse-string suture. The cannula, which is filled with a heparinized saline solution (50 IU/ml) should be pushed into the opening as far as possible. Subsequently, the purse-string suture should be pulled taut and the clip on the renal vein removed, while pushing the cannula further until the first silicon ring reaches the vessel wall. The proximal clip on the vena cava should now be removed as quickly as possible, to avoid congestion and bleeding from the purse-string suture. The cross-clamping time should be kept as short as possible. The patency of the cannula should be checked and the drawstrings of the purse-string suture used to anchor the cannula behind the first silicon ring (Figures 12.2.4. and 12.2.5.).

The cannula should be laid "kink-free" in the abdominal cavity (Figure 12.2.6.) and should be sutured to the internal abdominal muscle near the xiphoid cartilage. Subsequently, the abdomen should be closed in two layers (part 12.2.6.), and the cannula should be tunnelled subcutaneously (part 12.2.7.). The cannula together with the L-shaped adapter should be fixed to the skull (part 12.2.8.) as described in Chapter 7.

Blood samples can be taken from the animal using the procedure described in Chapter 7 (blood sampling). Sampling speed, however, should be reduced, because rapid aspiration would lead to a reflux of blood from the vena cava into the renal vein, thereby diluting the sample.

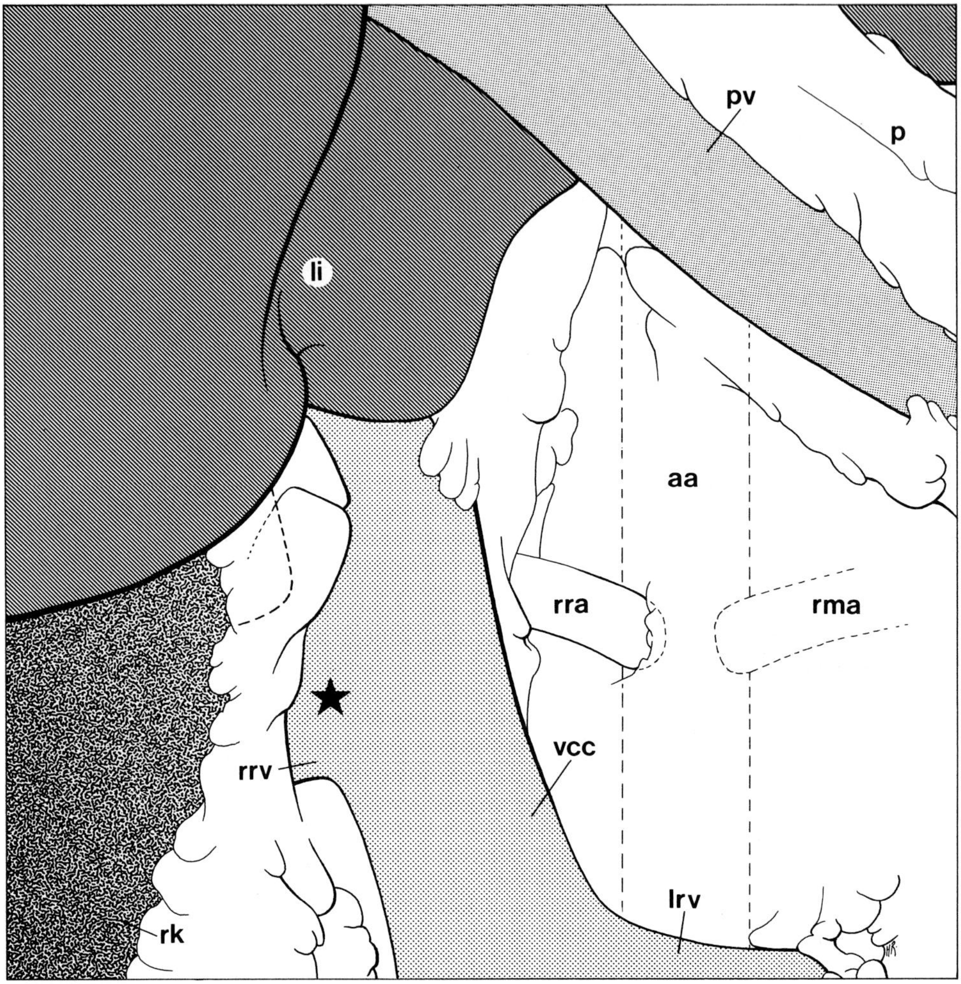

Figure 12.2.1. Anatomy of the portal-renal area.
The spot marked with an asterisk indicates the place of the purse-string suture at the entrance of the right renal vein.

rra	Right renal artery.
rma	Rostral mesenteric artery.
rrv	Right renal vein.
vcc	Vena cava caudalis.
lrv	Left renal vein.
aa	Abdominal aorta.
li	Liver.
p	Pancreas.
pv	Portal vein.
rk	Right kidney.

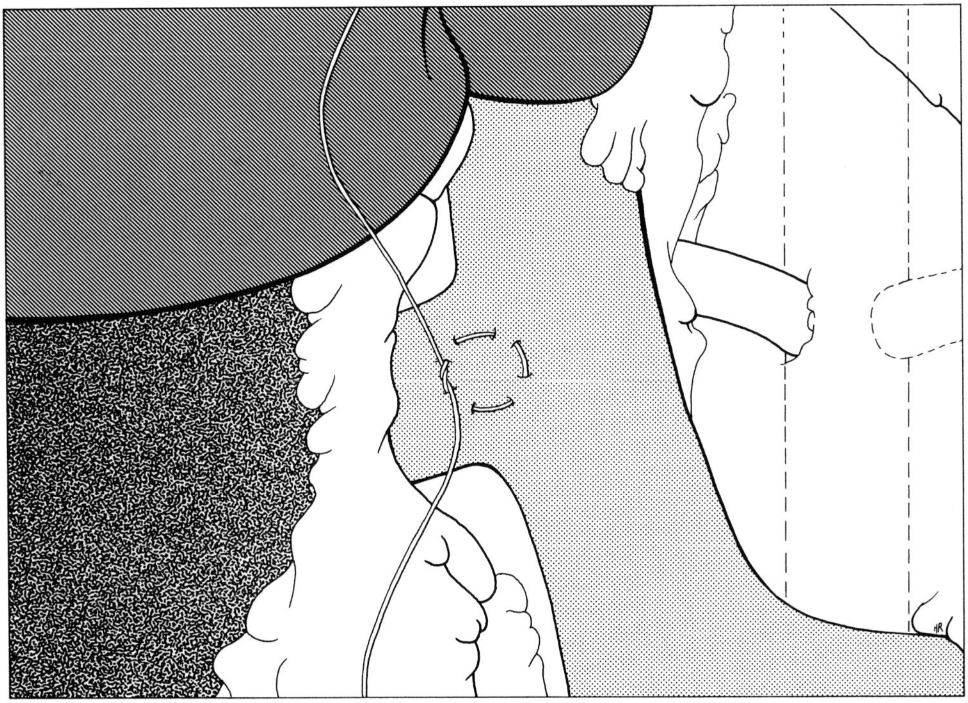

Figure 12.2.2. The purse-string suture.
The purse-string suture in the wall of the vena cava/renal vein is finished.

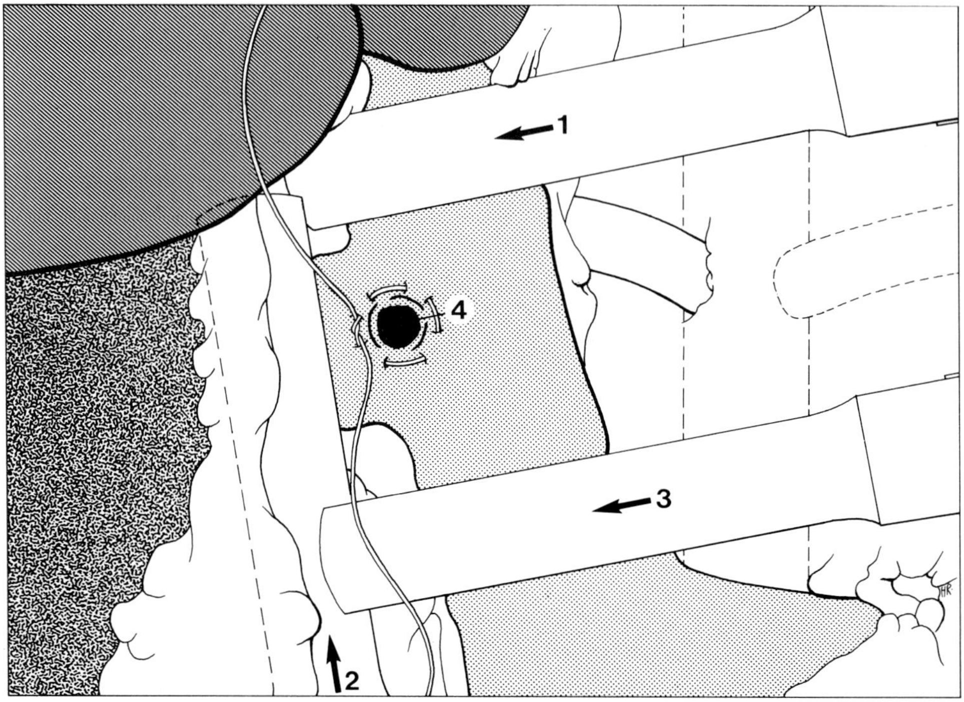

Figure 12.2.3. Clamping of the vessels.
Three Heifetz clips are placed. The first on the proximal part of the vena cava (1), the second on the right renal vein (2), and the third on the vena cava just distally from the right renal vein (3).
After the clamps have been placed, an aperture is cut in the purse-string suture.

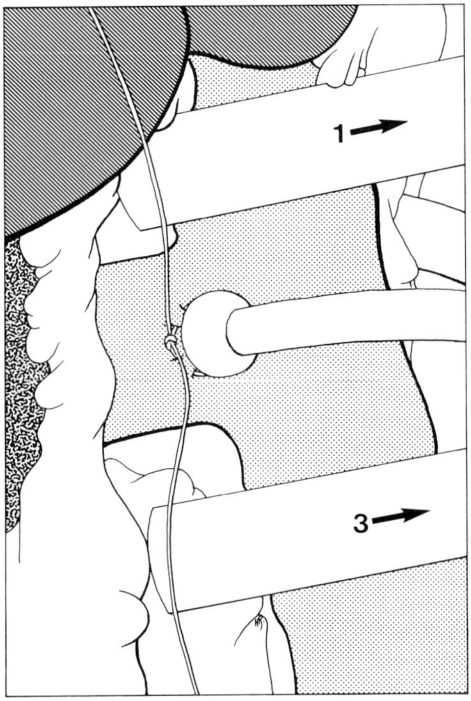

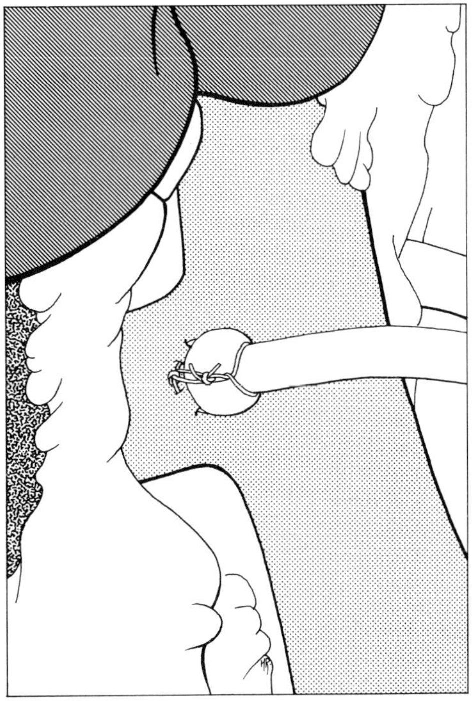

Figure 12.2.4. Insertion of the cannula.
Immediately after cutting the hole, the cannula is inserted into the vein in the direction of the kidney, after which the clamp on the renal vein is removed allowing the cannula to be pushed in further till the silicon ring reaches the vessel and the purse-string suture is pulled taut. Next the proximal clamp (1) is removed followed by the distal clamp (3).

Figure 12.2.5. Fixation of the cannula.
The cannula is fixed by tightening the purse-string suture, and the strings are used to anchor the cannula behind the silicon ring.

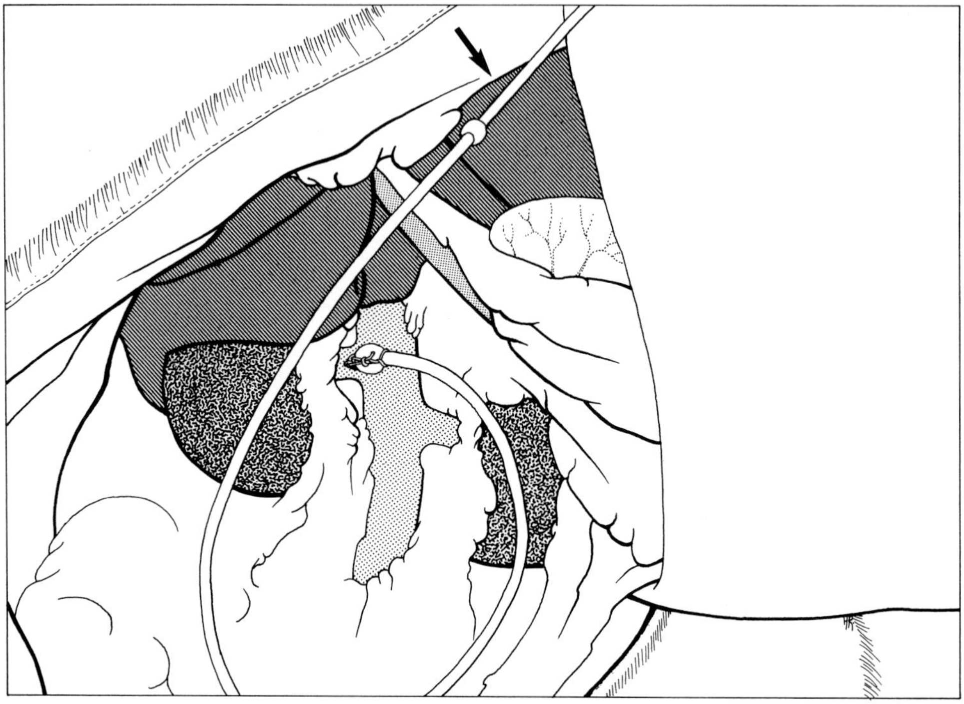

Figure 12.2.6. Placing the cannula in the abdomen.
The cannula is placed "kink-free" in the abdominal cavity and is anchored to the internal abdominal muscle near the xiphoid cartilage (arrow).

Manual of Microsurgery on the Laboratory Rat, Part I
Van Dongen, Remie, Rensema and Van Wunnik (eds)
© 1990 Elsevier Science Publishers B.V. (Biomedical Division)

CHAPTER 13

Permanent cannulation of the iliolumbar artery

R. REMIE, J.J. VAN DONGEN and J.W. RENSEMA

13.1. Introduction

The majority of physiological and pharmacological knowledge about blood pressure, its regulation and the influence of drugs on the cardiovascular system, has been derived from experiments with acutely prepared, anaesthetized or immobilized rats. This information, although valuable, is obscured by the direct effects of anaesthesia and surgical intervention. General anaesthesia for example, has a considerable impact on base-line blood flow and myocardial function. Surgery can amongst other things, introduce local vasomotion, thus disturbing the normal haemodynamic parameters. In several areas, for example the study of the relationship between social behaviour and blood pressure, it is simply impossible to use either restrained or anaesthetized rats. Restraining the animal, or restricting its freedom of movement by technical means will strongly influence the parameters which are to be measured. Commonly employed techniques such as plethysmographic, or cuff methods have several limitations. The animals have to be handled, restrained and trained before experiments can be performed. Moreover, the method itself introduces variations in blood pressure, and there seems to be an inconsistency between the direct blood pressure value and the one measured by the cuff method (Bunag, 1971; Bunag et al. 1971).

Apart from measuring blood pressure, sampling of arterial blood or infusion into the arterial system may also be of interest.

Direct measurement of blood pressure is usually done by cannulation of one of the carotid arteries. This, however, can interfere with the proper functioning of the pressure receptors in the carotid sinus. Several techniques have been described (Weeks and Jones, 1960; Buckingham, 1976; Sloop and Krause, 1981); most of them, however, are unclear about the percentage of success, and/or the long-term patency of the cannula. We have been using the technique we devised for several years now, and in its final form it has proved to have a low (less than 5%) mortality rate during surgery, a high patency rate of more than 85% after two weeks, and more than 65% after four weeks. Some animals could be used for up to three months.

13.2. The operation

Anaesthesia

The animal should preferably be anaesthetized with N_2O/O_2/halothane. If this type of anaesthesia is not available, then FFM (i.p.) should be used (see Chapter 6).

The operation can be divided into six parts:

13.2.1. Preparation of the crown of the head.
13.2.2. Opening of the abdominal wall.
13.2.3. Cannulation of the iliolumbar artery.
13.2.4. Closure of the abdominal wall.
13.2.5. Subcutaneous tunnelling to the head.
13.2.6. Fixation of the cannula.

Parts 13.2.1., 13.2.2., 13.2.4., 13.2.5. and 13.2.6. are described in detail in Chapter 7 (General techniques).

13.2.3. Cannulation of the iliolumbar artery

To enable easy cannulation, the aorta and the iliolumbar artery should be dissected free from the iliolumbar vein and vena cava, to a distance of 1 and 2 cm respectively. This is achieved with a standard preparation technique as described in Chapter 3. Figure 13.2.1. shows the ligatures that are placed around the iliolumbar artery. The first ligature (7–0 silk) is placed approximately 6 mm from the bifurcation. A second ligature (7–0 silk) is then placed about 2 mm proximal to the first. Both ligatures should be drawn tight. Subsequently, two clamps are placed on the abdominal aorta. When you first position the distal clamp, the segment will be filled with blood under pressure, making it easier to place the third ligature. This ligature is a monofilament suture (8–0, Ethilon) which should be applied in the muscular layer of the iliolumbar artery at the place shown in Figure 13.2.2. Using angled jewellers forceps and iridectomy scissors, a V-shaped hole should be made in the wall. Figure 13.2.3. shows clearly the position of the hands and instruments, and the place of the incision is shown in Figure 13.2.4. The sterile cannula which is filled with heparinized saline solution (50 IU/ml) should be inserted into the aorta as shown in Figures 13.2.5. and 13.2.6. Next the 8–0 Ethilon suture should be pulled taut, but not tight, in order to avoid obstruction of the cannula. The second ligature should be tightened just behind the silicon ring, making it impossible for the cannula to be pushed out of the vessel. After the iliolumbar artery has been cut, between the first and the second ligature (Figure 13.2.7.), allowing for the cannula to be placed in line with the aorta, the clamps should be released. The distal clamp should be released first (lower pressure), followed by the proximal clamp.

The cannula should be laid "kink-free" in the abdominal cavity and then sutured to the internal abdominal muscle, near the xiphoid cartilage. Subsequently, the abdomen should be closed in two layers (part 13.2.4.), and the cannula tunnelled subcutaneously (part 13.2.5.). The cannula, together with the L-shaped adapter, should be fixed to the skull (part 13.2.6.), as described in Chapter 7.

References

Buckingham, R.E. (1976) Indwelling catheters for direct recording of arterial blood pressure and intravenous injection of drugs in the conscious rat. J. Pharm. Pharmac. 28: 459–461.

Bunag, R.D. (1971) Pressor effects of the tail-cuff method in awake normotensive and hypertensive rats. J. Lab. Clin. Med. 78: 675–682.

Bunag, R.D., McCubbin, J.W. and Page, I.H. (1971) Lack of correlation between direct and indirect measurement of arterial pressure in unanaesthetized rats. Cardiovasc. Res. 5: 24–31.

Sloop, C.H. and Krause, B.R. (1981) Portal and aortic blood sampling technique in unrestrained rats. Physiol. Behav. 26(3): 529–533.

Weeks, J.R. and Jones, J.A. (1960) Routine direct measurement of arterial pressure in unanesthetized rats. Proc. Soc. Exp. Biol. Med. 104 (1): 646–648.

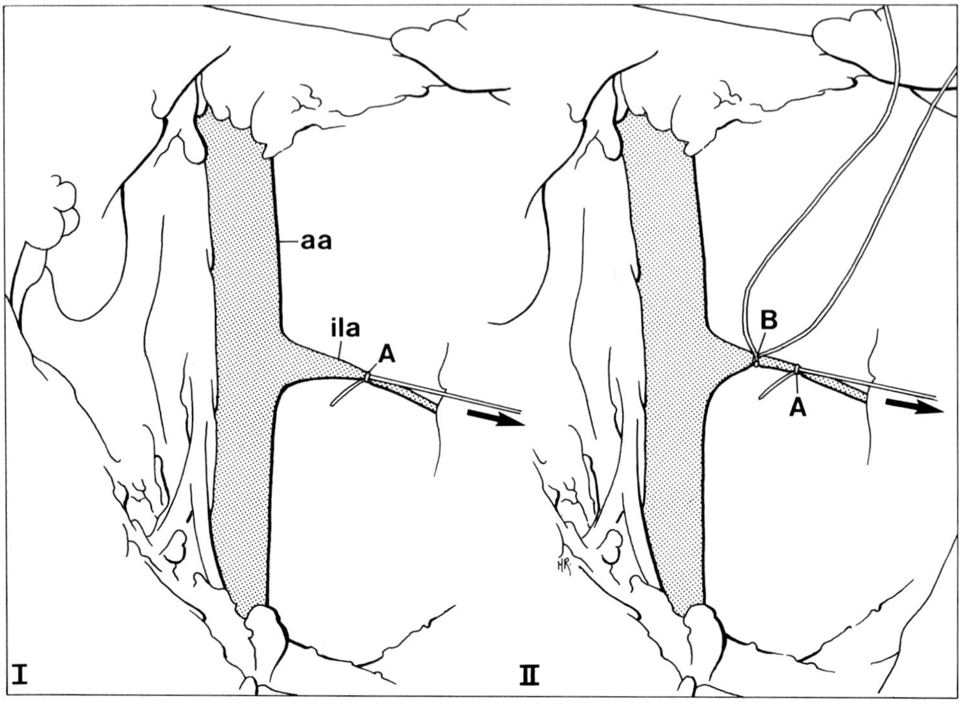

Figure 13.2.1. Ligation of the iliolumbar artery.

I. The abdominal aorta and the iliolumbar artery are stripped of their surrounding tissue. The iliolumbar artery is mobilized over a distance of 5 mm from the aorta, and a ligature (A) is placed and tied. One string of the ligature is placed under tension (arrow) using a bulldog clamp.

II. A second ligature (B) is placed.

A. First ligature.

B. Second ligature.

aa Abdominal aorta.

ila Iliolumbar artery.

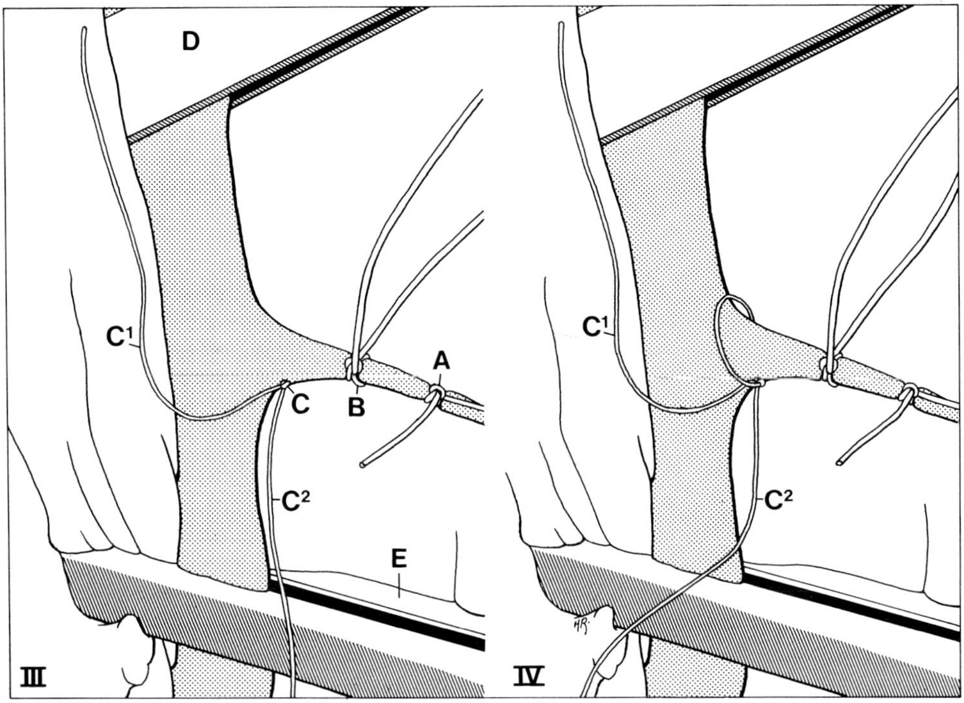

Figure 13.2.2. Clamping the aorta.

III. Two clamps are placed on the infra-renal abdominal aorta (D and E). A third ligature (8-0, Ethilon suture) is placed in the muscular layer of the iliolumbar artery (C).

IV. The drawstring C^2 is turned around the vessel and a single knot is placed (not tied).

C. Third ligature (8-0, Ethilon).

D. Heifetz clip.

E. Small atraumatic bulldog clamp.

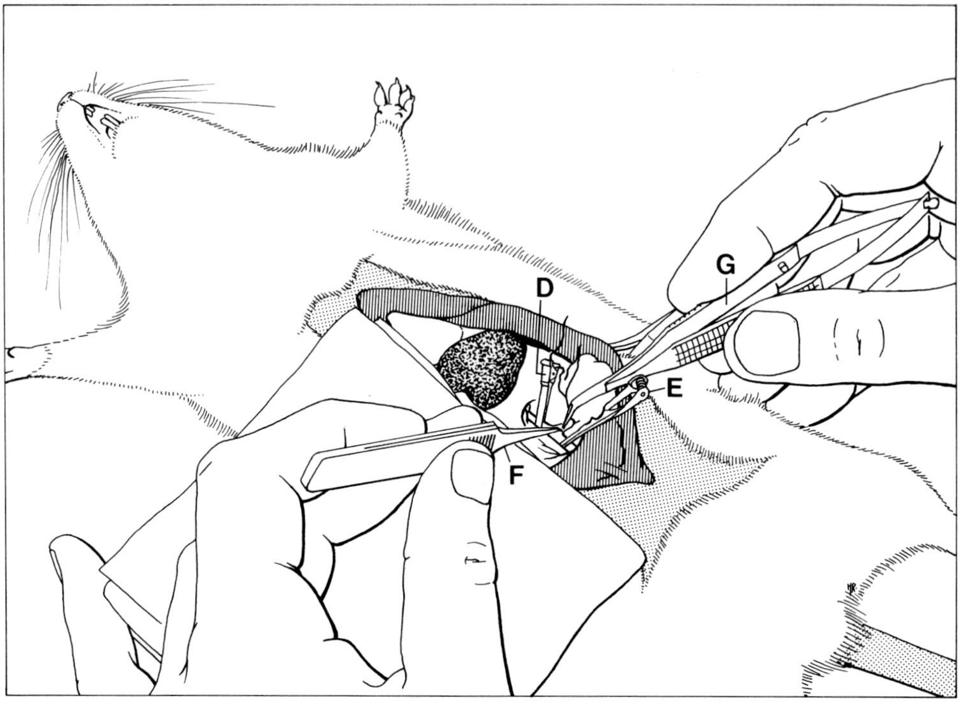

Figure 13.2.3. Making a hole.

Using angled jewellers forceps and iridectomy scissors a V-shaped hole is cut in the wall of the iliolumbar artery.

D. Heifetz clip.

E. Small atraumatic bulldog clamp.

F. Angled jewellers forceps.

G. Iridectomy scissors.

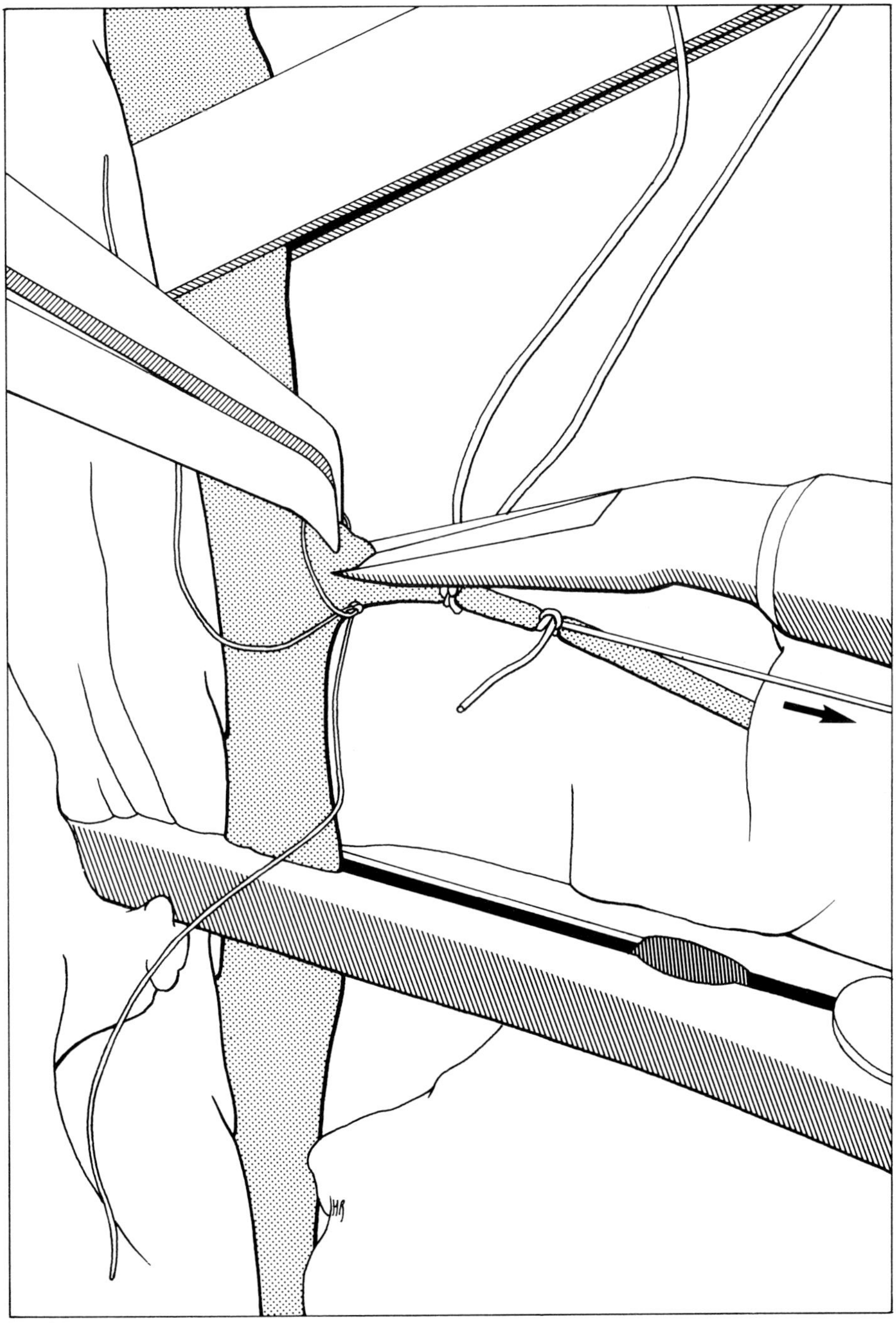

Figure 13.2.4. Detail of the cutting of the V-shaped hole.

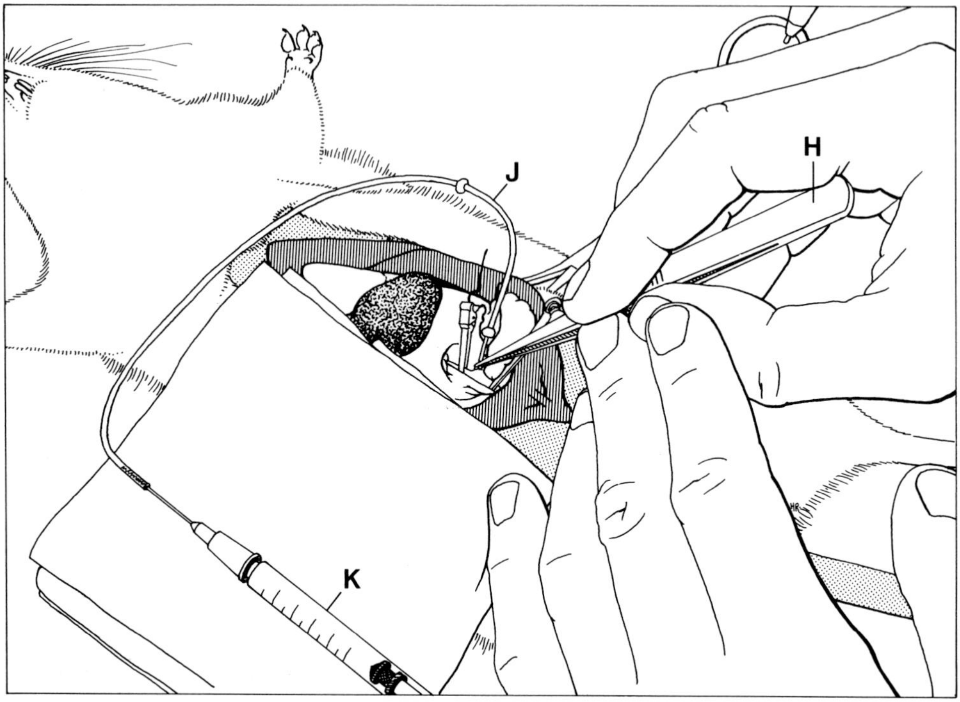

Figure 13.2.5. Insertion of the cannula (I).
Using jewellers forceps the cannula is held near the tip, while the left hand serves as a support to simplify insertion.
H. Jewellers forceps.
J. Cannula.
K. Syringe filled with heparinized saline.

→

Figure 13.2.6. Insertion of the cannula (II).
After the tip of the cannula has been inserted it is held near the silicon ring for further insertion.
H. Jewellers forceps.
J. Cannula.
J^1. Silicon ring.

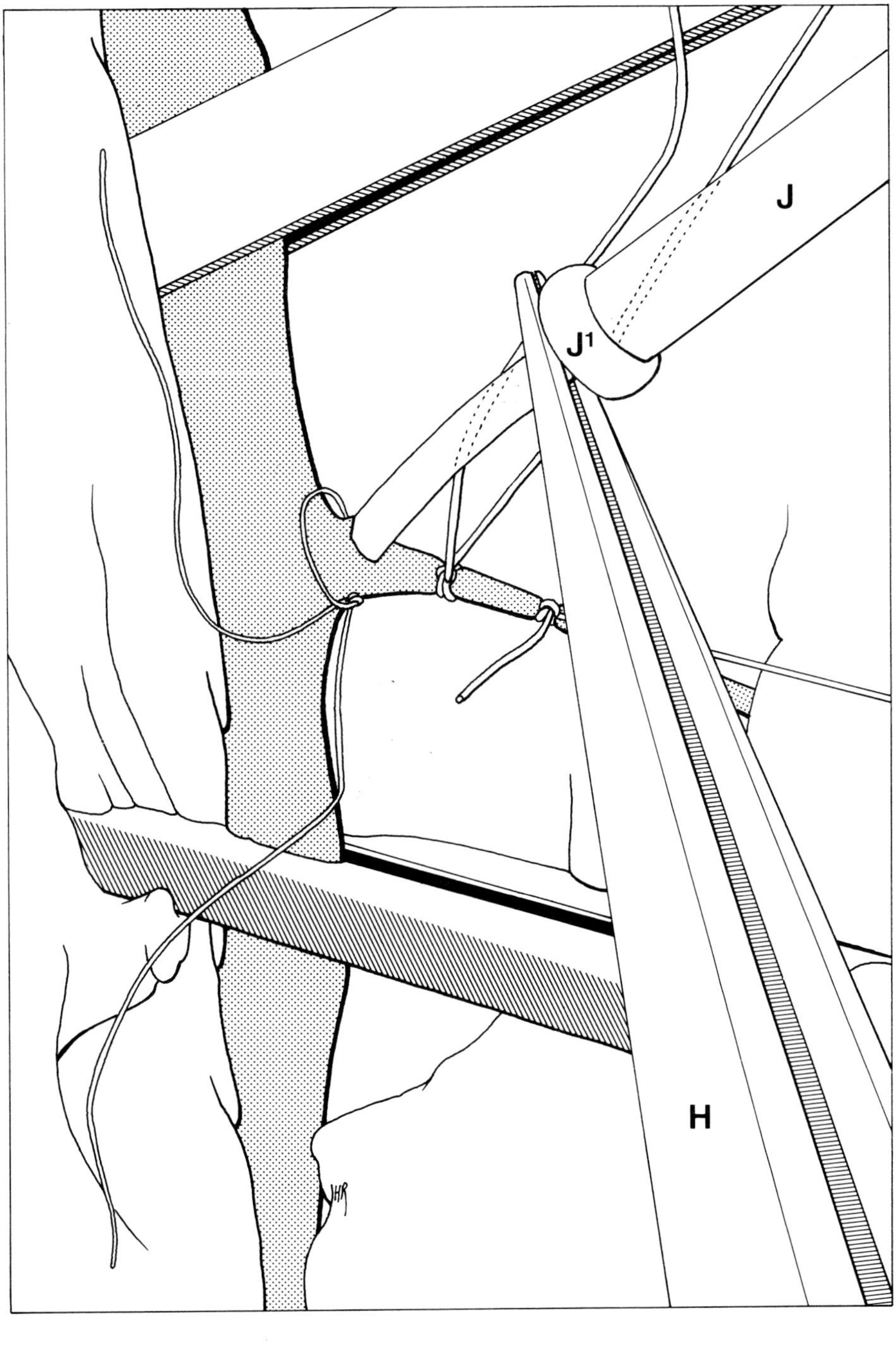
J
J1
H
HR

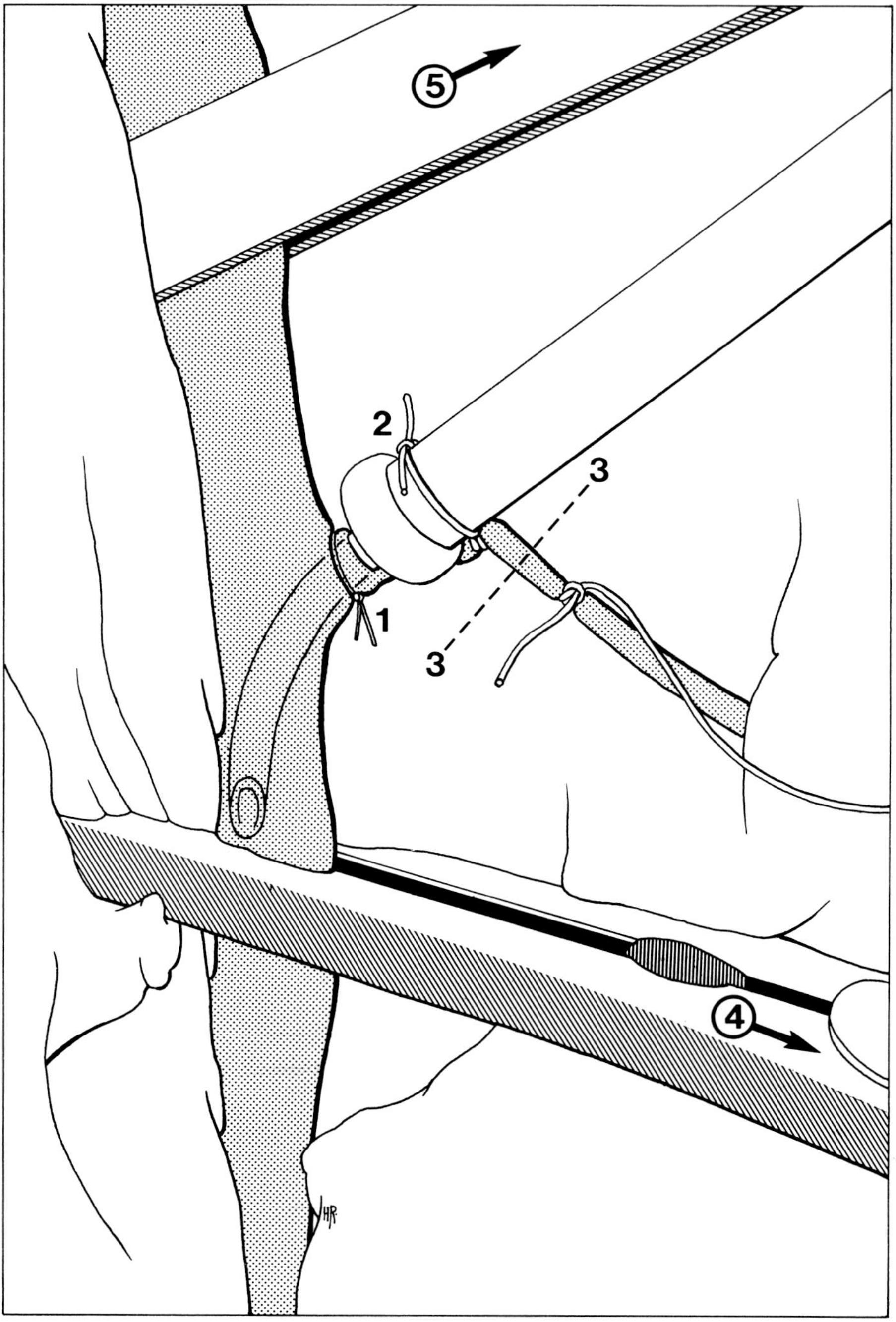
5
2
3
1
3
4
HR

←

Figure 13.2.7. Finishing the cannulation.

1. Tension on the artery is discontinued, and the third ligature is tightened.
2. The second ligature is tied to anchor the cannula behind the silicon ring.
3. The iliolumbar artery is cut between the first and the second ligature.
4. The distal clamp is removed.
5. The proximal clamp is removed.

Manual of Microsurgery on the Laboratory Rat, Part I
Van Dongen, Remie, Rensema and Van Wunnik (eds)
© *1990 Elsevier Science Publishers B.V. (Biomedical Division)*

CHAPTER 14

Permanent cannulation of the thoracic duct

R. REMIE, J.J. VAN DONGEN and J.W. RENSEMA

14.1. Introduction

Cannulation of a lymphatic vessel is used for example in studies on lymphocytes in immunology, in pharmacokinetic studies, and in nutrition research.

Collection of lymph is rather difficult, due to the delicate nature of the lymphatic vessels. In addition, the lymphatic flow rate is low (0.3–0.7 ml/h), and the formation of lymph clots can present serious problems. The most suitable place for the collection of lymph is the thoracic duct.

The thoracic duct rises from the cisterna chyli, which is a thin-walled ampullar sack attached to the lumbar muscles and the abdominal aorta, running rostrally just left of the aorta towards the diaphragm. It enters the thorax through the aortic hiatus. The thoracic duct is very delicate and often virtually transparent, which makes it hard to distinguish it from the surrounding tissues. A fatty meal, for example condensed or creamy milk, given 2 hours prior to the operation will result in white-coloured lymph, which makes the ductus easily identifiable.

In the past, several techniques have been described (Bollman et al., 1948: Girardet, 1975). We have chosen not to totally obstruct the duct by placing a purse-string suture in the wall of the duct, by which the cannula is secured. By so doing, the animal's lymph can be collected during the experiment, and after refilling the cannula with a PVP-solution (see Chapter 8) the lymph flow remains undisturbed.

14.2. The operation

Anaesthesia

The animal should preferably be anaesthetized with N_2O/O_2/halothane. If this type of anaesthesia is not available, then FFM (i.p.) should be used (see Chapter 6).

The operation can be divided into six parts:

14.2.1. Preparation of the crown of the head.
14.2.2. Opening of the abdominal wall.
14.2.3. Cannulation of the thoracic duct.
14.2.4. Closure of the abdominal wall.
14.2.5. Subcutaneous tunnelling of the cannula.
14.2.6. Fixation of the cannula to the crown of the head.

Parts 14.2.1., 14.2.2., 14.2.4., 14.2.5. and 14.2.6. are described in Chapter 7 (General techniques).

14.2.3. Cannulation of the thoracic duct

After opening the abdominal cavity, the intestines should be packed in gauze moistened with warm saline (30° C), and laid to the left of the animal (as viewed by the surgeon). The suprarenal abdominal aorta should be located and mobilized by gently tearing the connective tissue. Using blunt dissection technique, the thoracic duct is mobilized along the dorsolateral surface of the aorta as shown in Figure 14.2.1. A small three to four fine-stitch purse-string suture should be placed in the wall of the duct, using a 9–0 Ethilon suture (Figure 14.2.2.). As shown in Figures 14.2.3. and 14.2.4., a hole should be cut inside the purse-string with a very fine pair of scissors, while holding the wall with angled jewellers forceps. The cannula which is filled with a heparinized saline solution (25 IU/ml), should then be inserted into the duct as shown in Figures 14.2.5. and 14.2.6., using anatomical forceps. After the tip of the cannula has been inserted into the thoracic duct, the curved forceps are removed (Figure 14.2.7.) and the total tip is pushed into the duct. The ligature should then be closed and some lymph will flow into the cannula (Figure 14.2.8.). The cannula should be secured within the abdominal cavity by attaching it to the abdominal muscle near the xiphoid cartilage with a 7–0 silk suture (see Chapter 10). Following the closure of the abdominal wall and the tunnelling of the cannula to the crown of the head, the L-shaped adapter is placed on the cannula. It is filled with a PVP-solution and closed with a heat sealed polyethylene-cap (PE).

As already mentioned, one of the major threats to the patency of the catheter is clot formation. To minimize this risk an additional jugular vein cannula should be positioned (see Chapter 8), to be used for the infusion of heparinized saline (50 IU/ml) at a rate of 0.1 ml/h. Alternatively a Model 2ML2 or 2ML4 osmotic mini-pump

(Alzet) filled with heparin can be used to prevent clotting during approximately 14 and 28 days respectively.

Collection of lymph
The animal should be housed in an individual cage (see Chapter 7). When lymph has to be collected, the animal is attached to a long swivelled PE-cannula (0.75 × 1.45 mm). The end of the cannula must be between 5–10 cm below the bottom of the cage, in order to provide sufficient underpressure to let the lymph flow into the cannula, without additional aspiration.

References

Bollman, J.L., Cain, J.C. and Grindlay, J.H. (1948) Techniques for the collection of lymph from the liver, small intestine, or thoracic duct of the rat. J. Lab. Clin. Med. 33: 1349–1352.
Girardet, R.E. (1975) Surgical technique for long-term studies of thoracic duct circulation in the rat. J. Appl. Physiol. 39: 682–688.

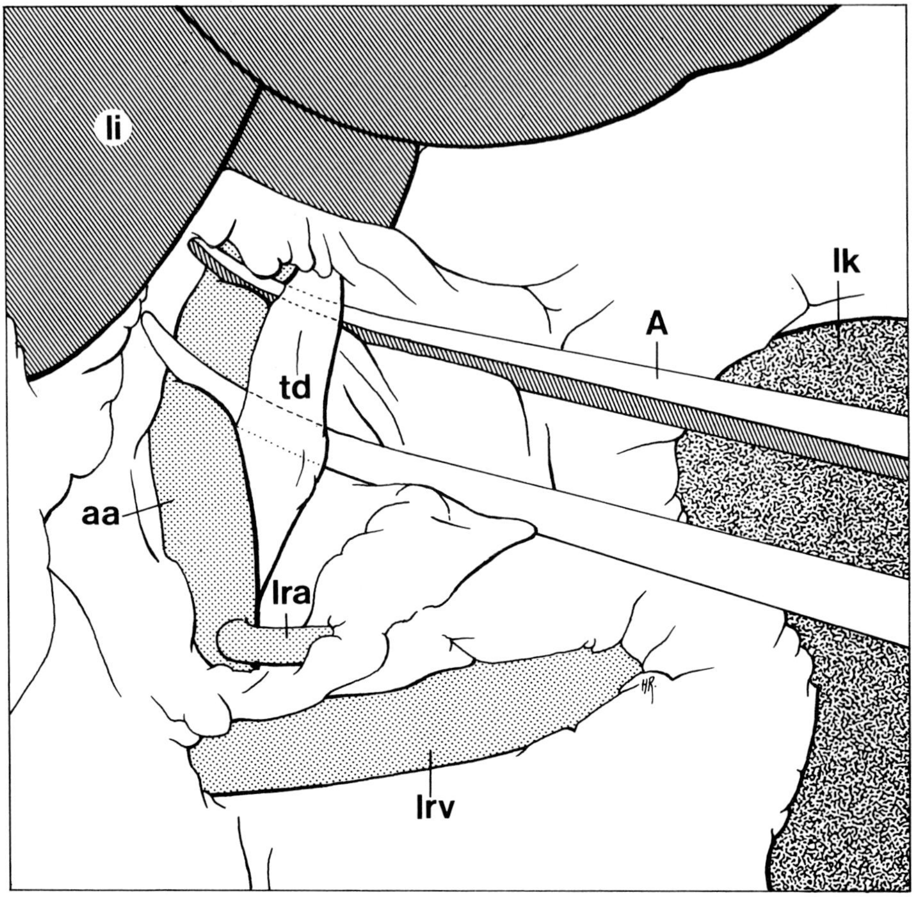

Figure 14.2.1. Mobilization of the thoracic duct.
The thoracic duct is carefully mobilized and curved anatomical forceps are used to keep the lymphatic duct in position lateral of the abdominal aorta.

A. Curved anatomical forceps.
aa Abdominal aorta.
td Thoracic duct.
lra Left renal artery.
lrv Left renal vein.
lk Left kidney.
li Liver.

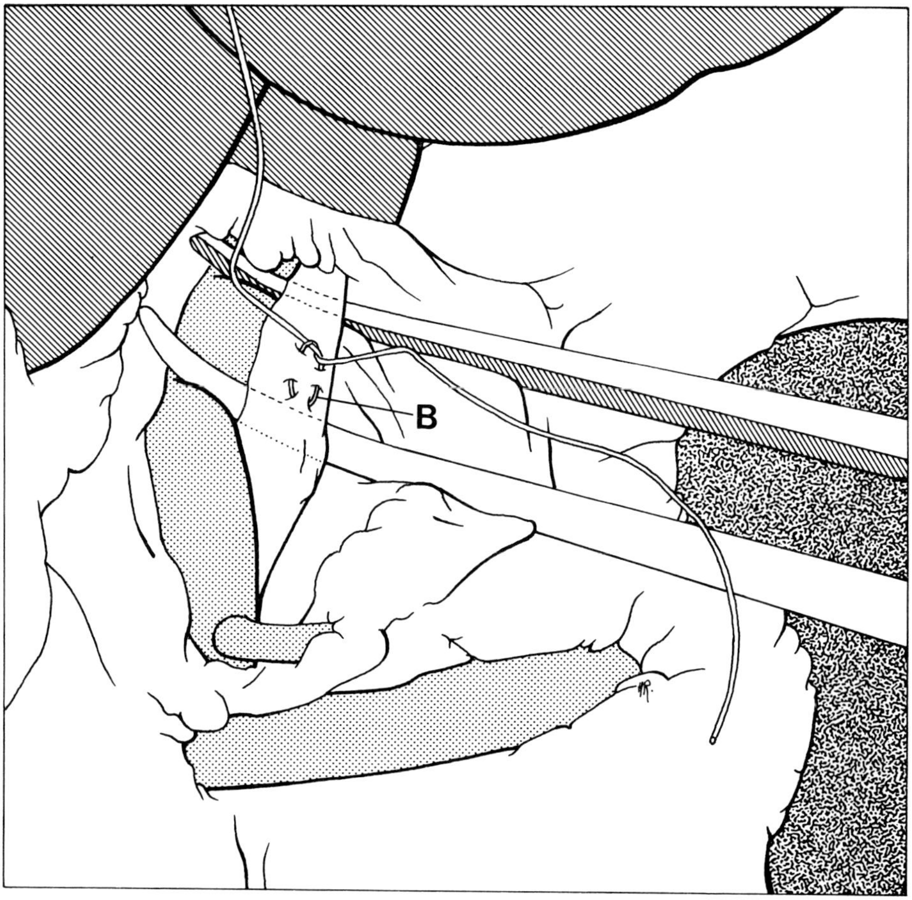

Figure 14.2.2. The purse-string suture.
A purse-string suture (B) is placed in the wall of the thoracic duct.

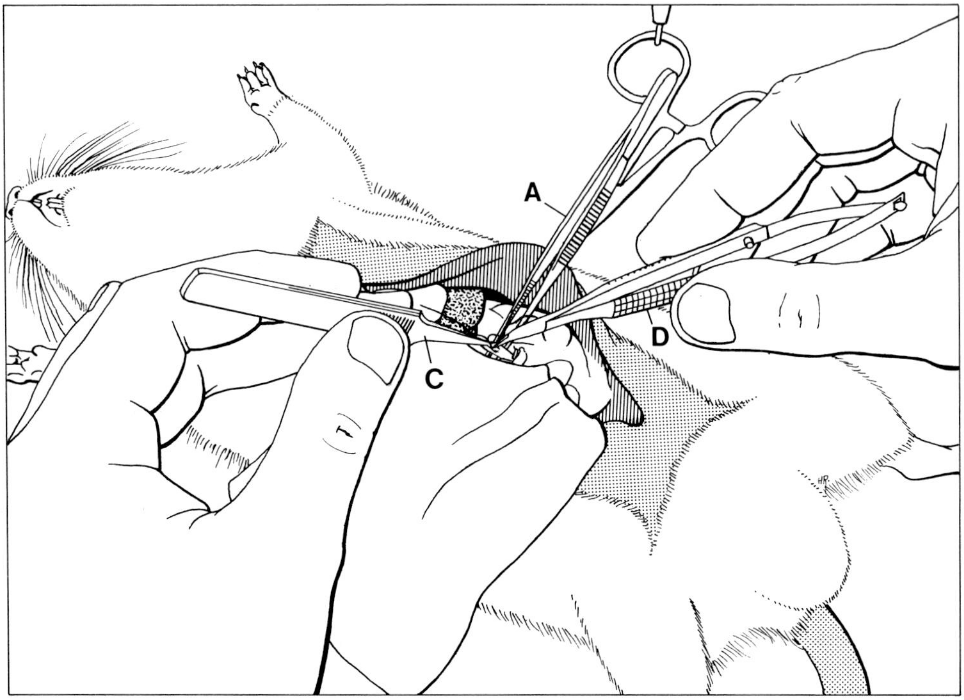

Figure 14.2.3. Cutting the hole (I).
Using iridectomy scissors an aperture is cut inside the purse-string suture.
A. Curved anatomical forceps.
C. Angled jewellers forceps.
D. Iridectomy scissors.

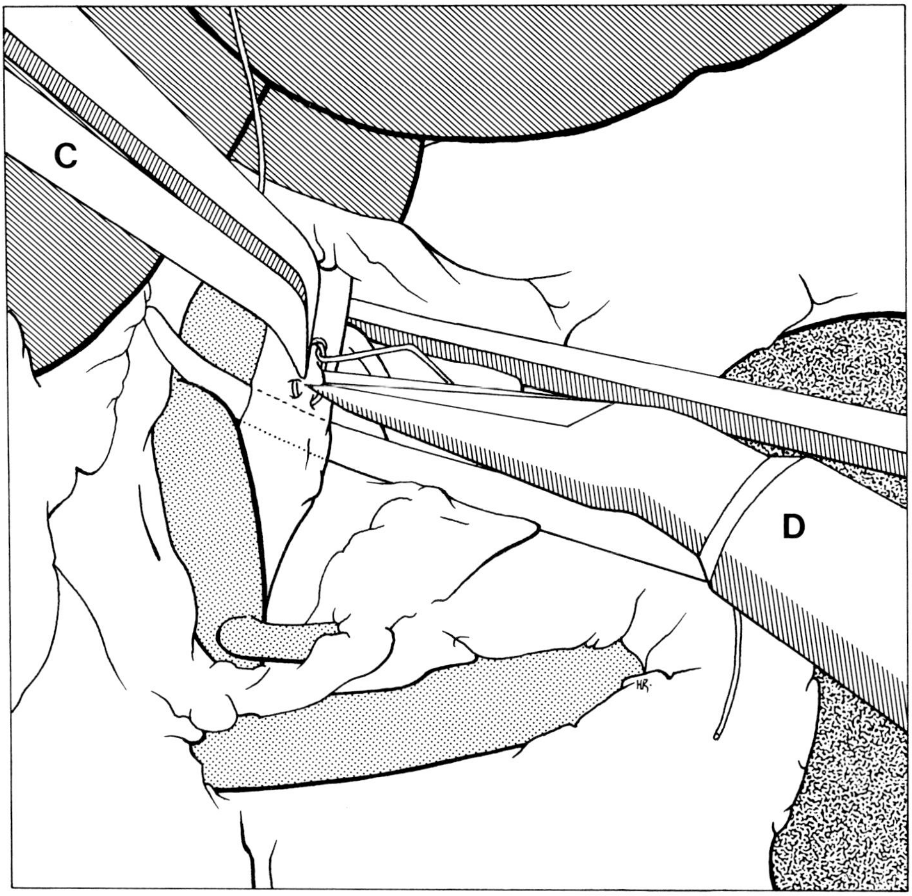

Figure 14.2.4. Cutting the hole (II).
Detail of the cutting of the aperture in the purse-string suture.
C. Angled jewellers forceps.
D. Iridectomy scissors.

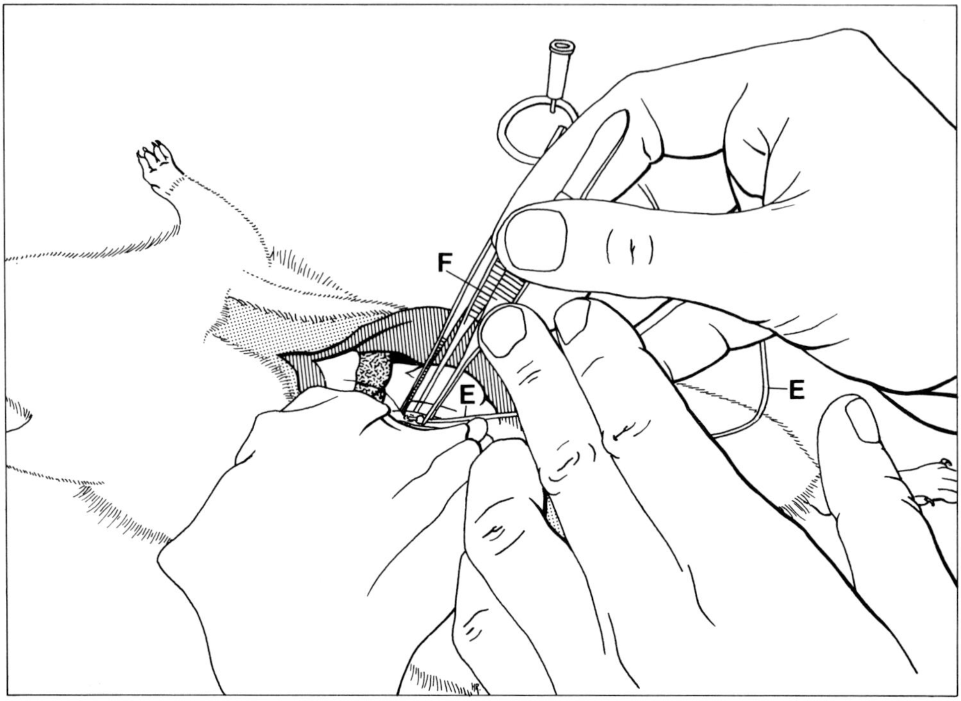

Figure 14.2.5. Insertion of the cannula (I).
Position of the hands during insertion of the cannula using straight anatomical forceps.
E. Cannula.
F. Straight anatomical forceps.

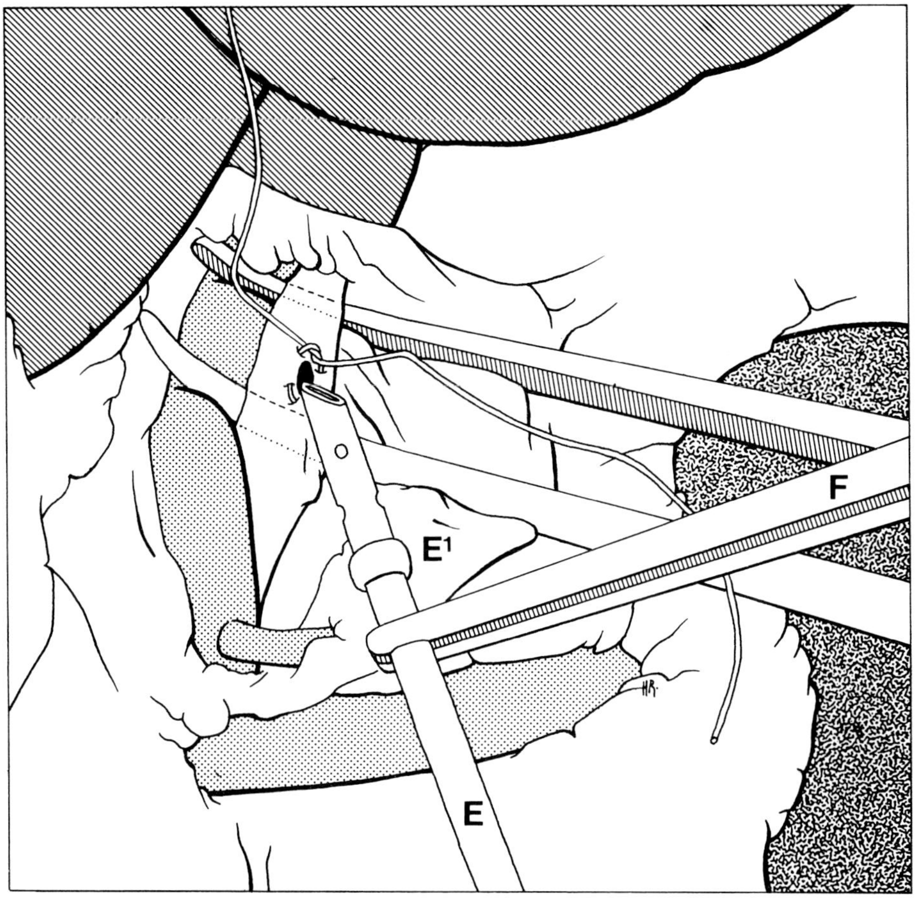

Figure 14.2.6. Insertion of the cannula (II).
Detail of the insertion of the tip of the cannula.
E[1]. Silicon ring.
F. Straight anatomical forceps.

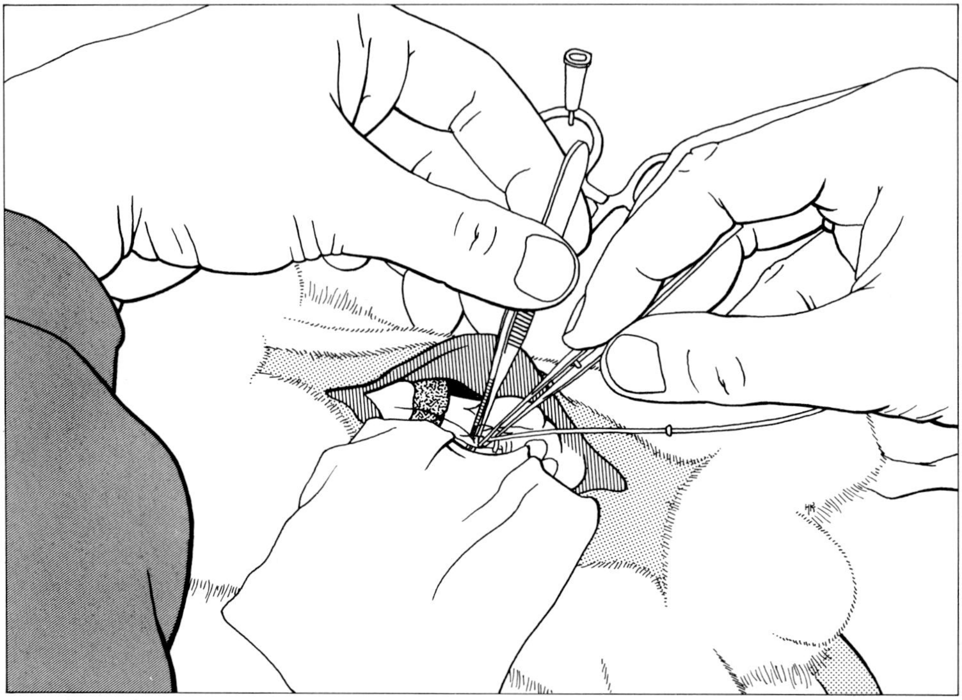

Figure 14.2.7. Insertion of the cannula (III).
The cannula is pushed in further with the straight anatomical forceps, while the left hand is used to lift the curved anatomical forceps. The latter is removed when the silicon ring has reached the wall of the thoracic duct.

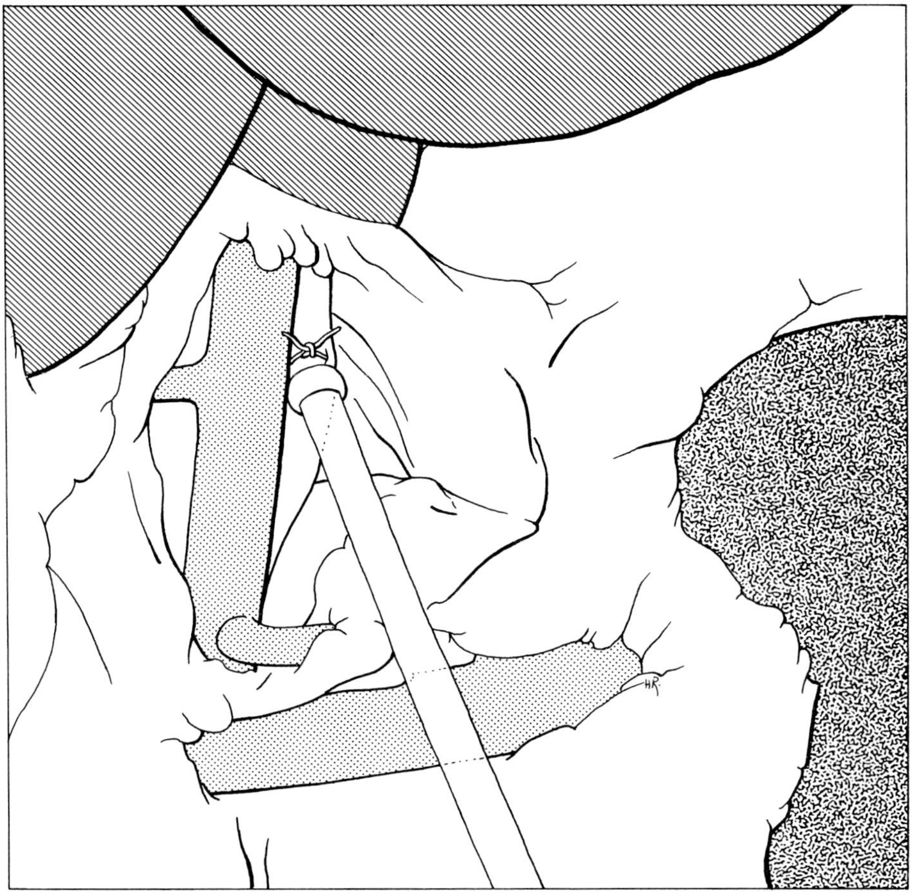

Figure 14.2.8. Fixation of the cannula.
The purse-string suture is tied and the draw strings are cut.

Manual of Microsurgery on the Laboratory Rat, Part I
Van Dongen, Remie, Rensema and Van Wunnik (eds)
© *1990 Elsevier Science Publishers B.V. (Biomedical Division)*

CHAPTER 15

Perfusion of the isolated gut in vivo

R. REMIE, J.W. RENSEMA and J.J. VAN DONGEN

15.1. Introduction

The intestinal tract is a very important route for drug administration. Intestinal preparations are needed not only in order to study intestinal secretion, absorption and motility, but also to study intestinal control of the liver, the pancreas and the stomach. It is also a well known fact that the transport rate varies in different sections of the gastrointestinal tract.

One of the major difficulties one encounters, when working with isolated segments of the intestinal tract, is their tendency to deteriorate both functionally and morphologically, which can only be partially remedied by instilling liquid nutrients into the lumen of the relevant segment.

In the 19th century Thiry, and later Vella were the first to describe the isolation of an intestinal segment. In this chapter we will describe two modifications of the so-called "Thiry-Vella loop". Before commencing the operation we must pay attention to some surgical approaches required at the end-to-end anastomosis of the gut. Basically two types of stitches can be used:
- The transfixing stitch.
- The invaginating or Lembert stitch.

The former passes through all layers from the serous to the mucosa (Figure 15.1.1.). The latter enters and leaves the gut wall on either side of the anastomosis, without passing through the mucosal layer (Lembert, 1826) (Figure 15.1.1.). Both stitches can be used as continuous or interrupted sutures. The continuous suture with invaginating stitches is somewhat difficult to carry out, and rather time consuming. Lambert

(1965) prefers interrupted invaginating stitches for standard end-to-end anastomosis. Our preference, however, is for the continuous transfixing suture as it takes less time to perform and produces excellent results.

15.2. The operation

Anaesthesia
The animal should preferably be anaesthetized with N_2O/O_2/halothane. If this type of anaesthesia is not available, then FFM (i.p.) should be used (see Chapter 6).

Two techniques will be described:
15.2.1. Isolation and cannulation of a gut loop
15.2.2. The modified Thiry-Vella loop

15.2.1. The isolation and cannulation of a gut loop

This can be divided into eight parts:
15.2.1.1. Preparation of the crown of the head.
15.2.1.2. Opening of the abdominal wall.
15.2.1.3. Isolation of a gut segment.
15.2.1.4. End-to-end anastomosis of the gut.
15.2.1.5. Cannulation of the gut segment.
15.2.1.6. Closure of the abdominal wall.
15.2.1.7. Subcutaneous tunnelling of the cannulae to the head.
15.2.1.8. Fixation of the cannulae to the crown of the head.

Parts 15.2.1.1., 15.2.1.2., 15.2.1.6., 15.2.1.7. and 15.2.1.8. are described in Chapter 7 (General techniques).

15.2.1.3. Isolation of a gut segment
As mentioned above the transport rate varies in the different sections of the gastrointestinal tract. Therefore the part of the gastrointestinal tract to be cannulated must be located accurately. Figure 15.2.1. shows how to manipulate the gut, using cotton-wool sticks, so as not to damage the tissue. The segment to be isolated should be kept moist with warm saline solution (30° C), and the remaining part of the tract should also be covered with moistened gauze.

Figure 15.2.2. shows the segment to be isolated including the sides where the gut has to be divided. To begin with, the blood vessels (the arcade) have to be ligated. Figure 15.2.3. shows how a 7–0 silk suture is placed around both the artery and the vein (only the vein is depicted in the drawings) using angled jewellers forceps. The distance between the ligatures should be at least 2 mm, to allow for both easy and safe cutting of both the gut wall and the blood vessels (Figure 15.2.4.). Prior to cutting the gut wall, iodine solution must be put on that area. Figures 15.2.5. and 15.2.6. depict the situation after ligation and cutting. After cutting the wall you will see that it curls, exposing the mucosa. Again iodine solution must be applied to both ends.

Parts A and C must then be approximated, and part B must be swung over. Figures 15.2.7. and 15.2.8. show how segment B is carefully moved using cotton wool sticks. Subsequently, segment B is covered with saline moistened gauze.

15.2.1.4. End-to-end anastomosis of the gut

The end-to-end anastomosis of the intestine resembles the one used for blood vessels. However, no triangulation is required as two stay sutures will do the job sufficiently. There are four distinguishable stages:

a. The stay sutures

The first stay suture (7–0 silk armed with a BV-1 needle) is placed as a transfixing stitch opposite the mesentery as shown in Figure 15.2.9. Again no forceps are used, merely a cotton-wool stick. The second stay suture is placed in the same way, but is inserted 180° away from the first one, close to the mesentery (Figure 15.2.10.). This will result in an anterior and a posterior suture line of equal length. The ends of the sutures with the numbers 1 and 3 are armed, and will be used to complete the anastomosis. The ends with the numbers 2 and 4 are left about 6 cm long, and will be used to put some tension on the anastomosis using small bulldog type haemostatic clamps.

b. The anterior suture line

The armed part of the first stay suture (thread number 1) is used for the anterior suture. Our preference is for a continuous suture technique with transfixing stitches. However, care must be taken not to put too much tension on the suture as this will result in a rigid anastomosis. When the anterior wall has been finished the suture is tied to the loose end of the second stay suture (thread number 3) and the result is shown in Figure 15.2.11.

c. Reversal of the anastomosis

In order to get the posterior suture line into view, the small bulldog clamps must be released and the anastomosis has to be reversed. Using anatomical forceps which are slid behind the anastomosis from the mesenteric side towards the opposite side, thread number 2 is picked up and brought through to the other side. Subsequently both the stay suture (number 4) and the armed suture (number 3) are swung over to the other side, the anterior wall will now become posterior. Both bulldog clamps are replaced and the stay sutures are put under tension, resulting in a clear view of the posterior suture line. At this point one can ideally inspect the posterior suture from the inside (Figure 15.2.12.). If necessary, corrections must be performed.

d. The final suture line

This suture is carried out in exactly the same way as the previous one. Again, do not pull the sutures too tight, just sufficiently to approximate the mucosae without leakage. Figure 15.2.13. shows the completed anastomosis with both stay sutures still in place.

15.2.1.5. Cannulation of the gut segment

Two cannulae are inserted into gut segment B and are secured with 6–0 silk sutures as shown in Figure 15.2.14. The preparation of these cannulae is described in Chapter 7. The cannulae and the gut segment should be flushed with warm saline solution, and placed "kink-free" in the abdominal cavity. With a 7–0 silk suture the cannulae should be fixed to the abdominal muscle near the xiphoid cartilage as shown in Figure 15.2.15. Subsequently the abdomen should be closed in two layers (part 15.2.6.), and the cannulae should be tunnelled subcutaneously (part 15.2.7.) to the crown of the head and glued to the skull with acrylic glue (part 15.2.8.) as described in Chapter 7 (General techniques).

15.2.2. The modified Thiry-Vella loop

This can be divided into five parts:

15.2.2.1. Opening of the abdominal wall.
15.2.2.2. Isolation of a gut segment.
15.2.2.3. End-to-end anastomosis of the gut.
15.2.2.4. The fistulae.
15.2.2.5. Closure of the abdominal wall.

Parts 15.2.2.1. and 15.2.2.5. are described in detail in Chapter 7 (General techniques). Parts 15.2.2.2. and 15.2.2.3. are described above.

15.2.2.4. The fistulae

Using a pair of sharp-sharp scissors a hole is made in both the abdominal muscle layer and the skin, as shown in Figure 15.2.16. Subsequently, standard end-to-side anastomosis technique is used to sew the gut to the internal abdominal muscle, using 7–0 silk sutures. As shown in Figure 15.2.17. the two stay sutures are at 180° (biangulation) and the posterior wall is sutured first. Figure 15.2.18. shows the result of both anastomoses. Following this the skin is sutured to the abdominal muscle, using a running suture (7–0, monofilament suture) (Figure 15.2.19.).

Alternatively one may pull the gut through the hole in the abdominal muscle, and suture the gut directly to the skin and the abdominal muscle, again using a continuous suture (7–0 silk). The latter technique is much quicker, whereas the former is more accurate.

References

Lambert, R. (1965) Surgery of the digestive system in the rat. Charles C. Thomas, Springfield Illinois, USA.

Lembert, A. (1826) Memoire sur l'enterorrhaphie avec description d'un procede nouveau pour practiquer cette operation chirurgicale. Repertoire general d'anatomie et de physiologie pathologique et de clinique chirurchicale. 2: 104.

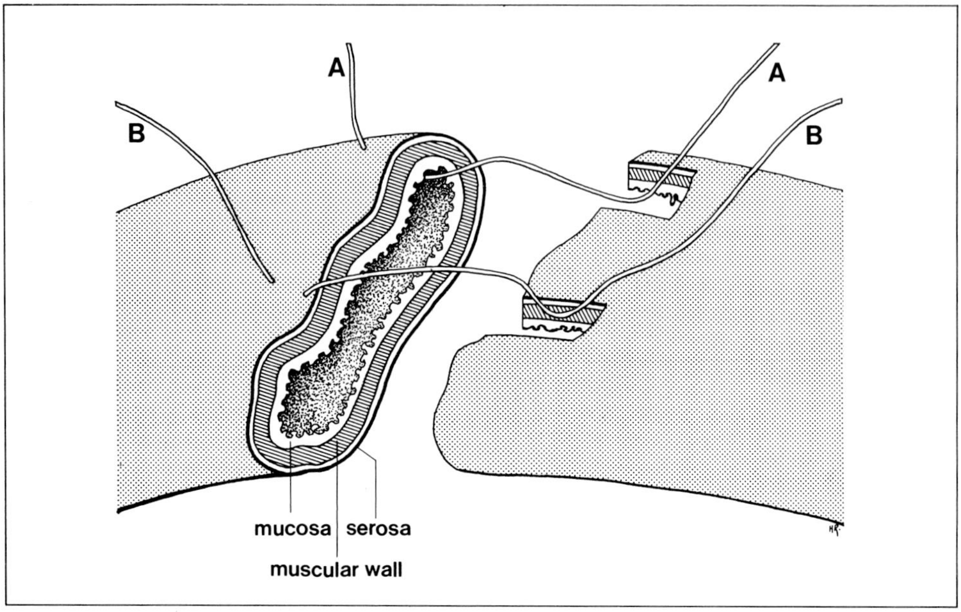

Figure 15.1.1. Stitches used in bowel surgery.
Two types of stitches that can be used in the end-to-end anastomosis of the gut.
A. Transfixing stitch.
B. Invaginating, or Lembert stitch.

→

Figure 15.2.1. Handling the intestine.
An intestinal loop is exposed carefully, using a cotton-wool stick for manipulation.
D. Cotton wool stick.
si Small intestine.

Figure 15.2.2. Location of the segment.
A segment of the small intestinal loop to be cannulated (B) is located; The segment should be vascularized by two or more tributary arteries. For reasons of clarity only the venous arcades are drawn.
B. Segment to be isolated.
1 and 2. Sides where the gut will be divided.
var Venous arcade.

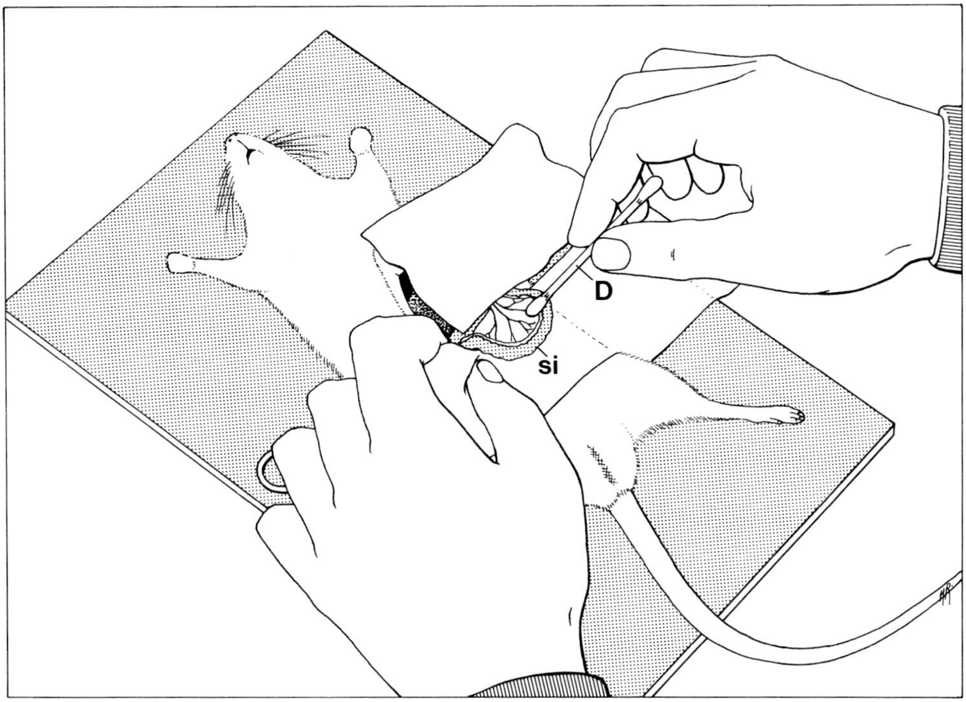

Fig. 15.2.1.

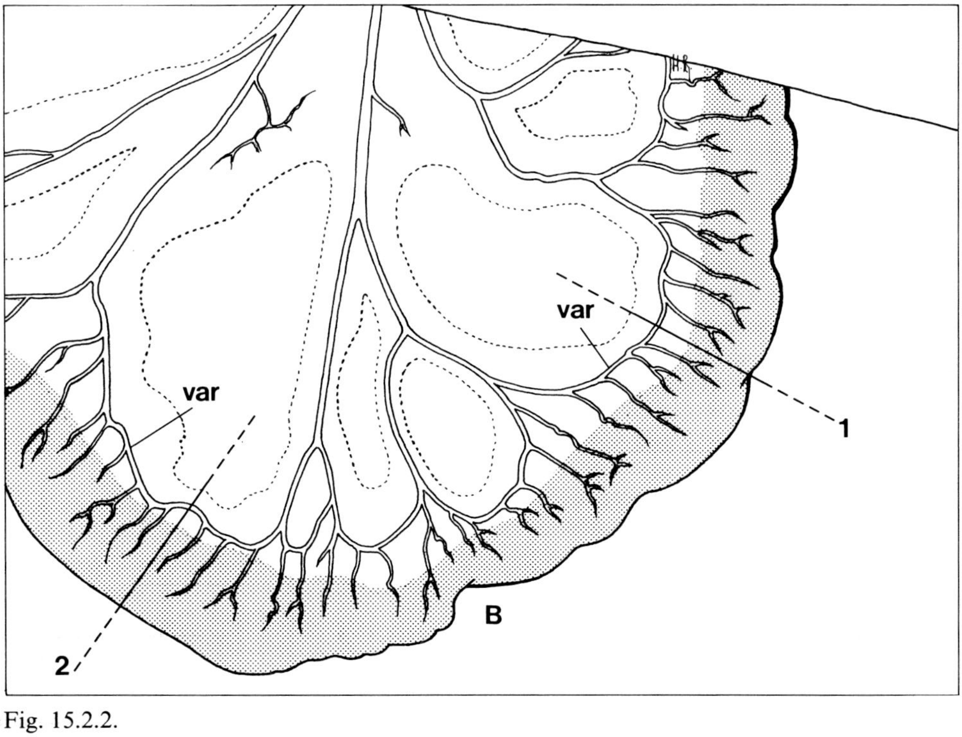

Fig. 15.2.2.

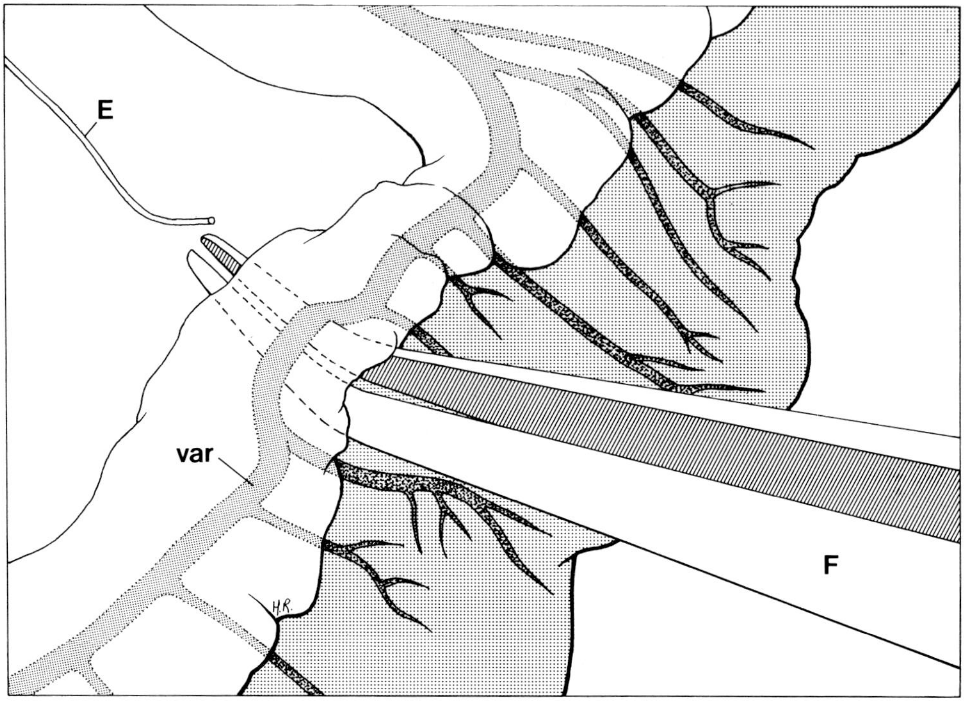

Figure 15.2.3. Ligation of the arcade (I).
A 7-0 silk suture is collected from under the artery (not shown) and the vein of the arcade, using angled jewellers forceps.
E. 7-0 silk suture.
F. Angled jewellers forceps.
var Venous arcade.

→

Figure 15.2.4. Ligation of the arcade (II).
Two ligatures are placed around the blood vessels at 2-3 mm from each other.
E. 7-0 silk sutures.

Figure 15.2.5. Ligation of the arcade (III).
The two ligatures are tightened, the gut wall is disinfected with iodine solution, and both the vessels of the arcade and the gut wall are cut.

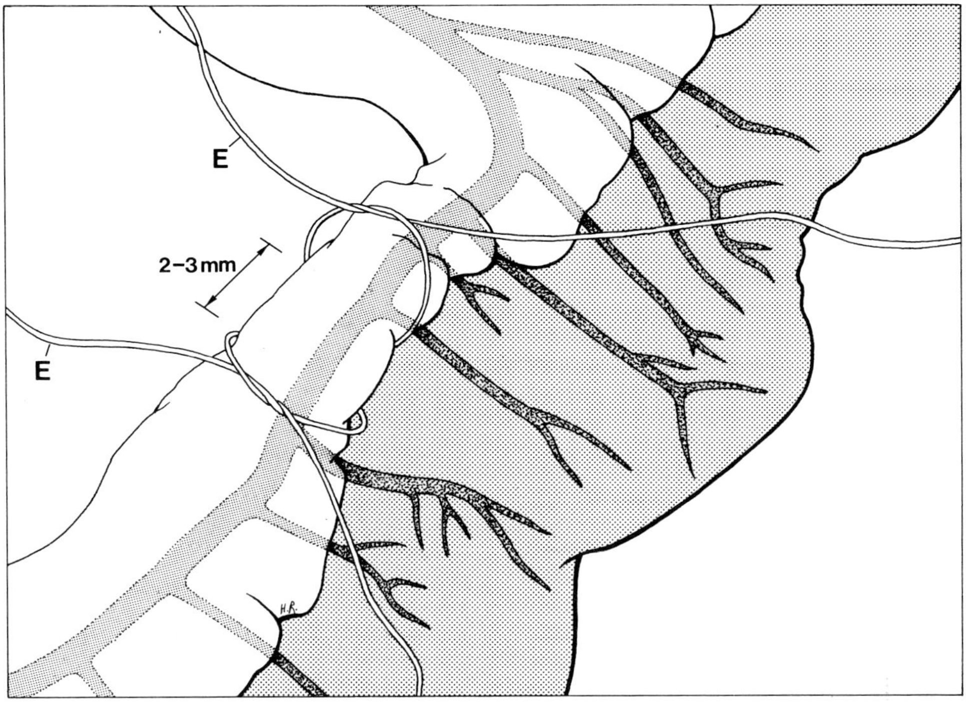

Fig. 15.2.4.

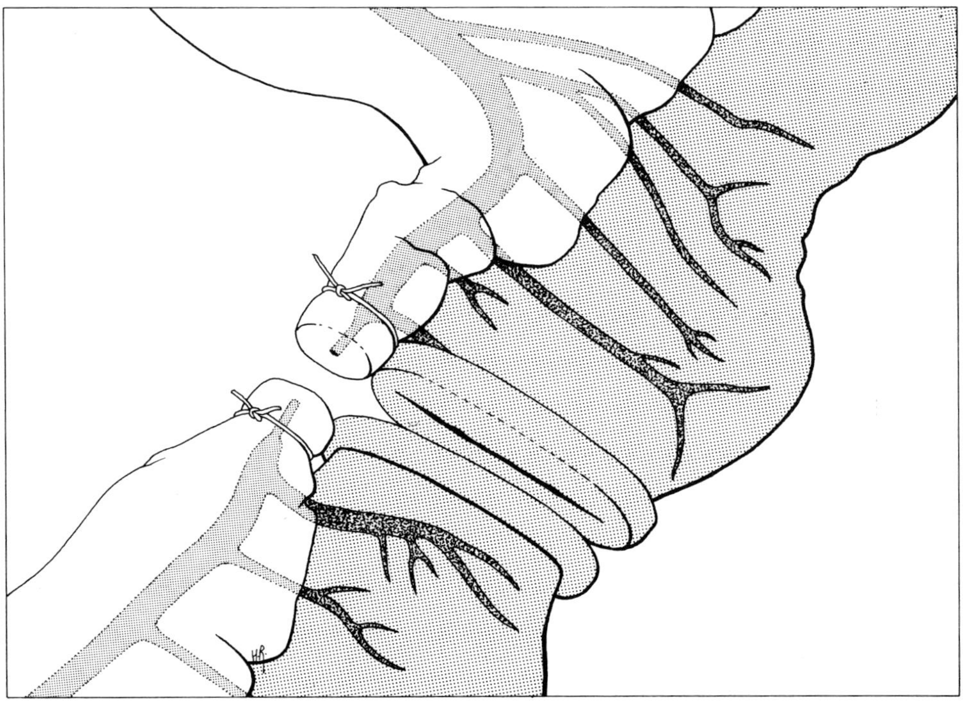

Fig. 15.2.5.

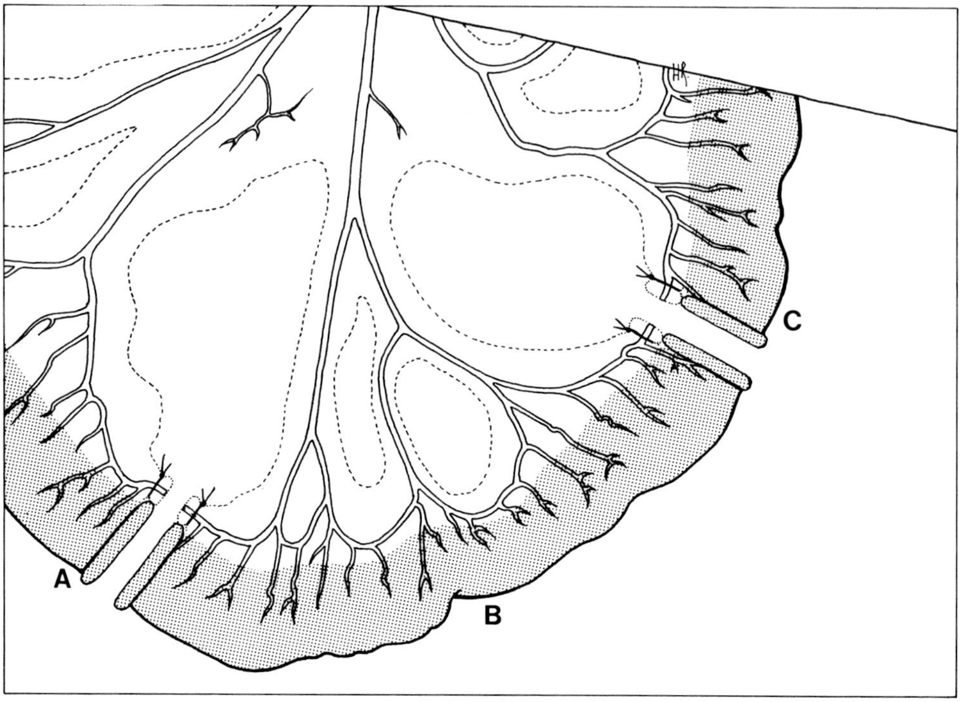

Figure 15.2.6. Ligation of the arcade (IV).
Situation after ligation and cutting.

→

Figure 15.2.7. Preparing the gut for the end-to-end anastomosis (I).
The isolated segment is turned over in a rostral direction, using cotton wool sticks.

Figure 15.2.8. Preparing the gut for the end-to-end anastomosis (II).
Segment B is laid on gauze moistened with warm saline avoiding torsion of the vessels, and the segments A and C can be approximated.

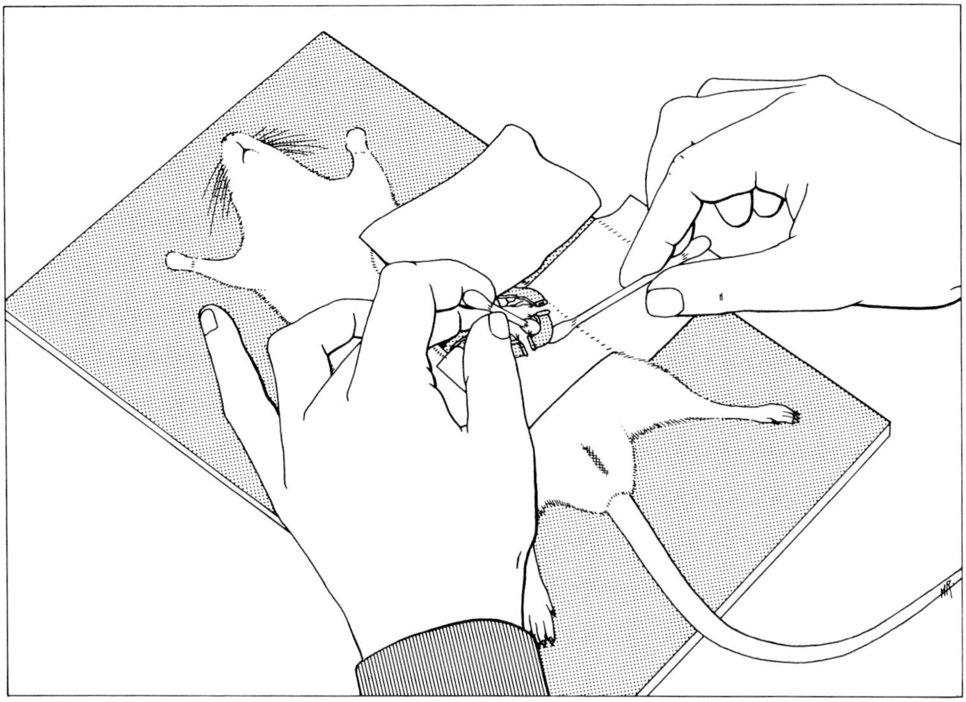

Fig. 15.2.7.

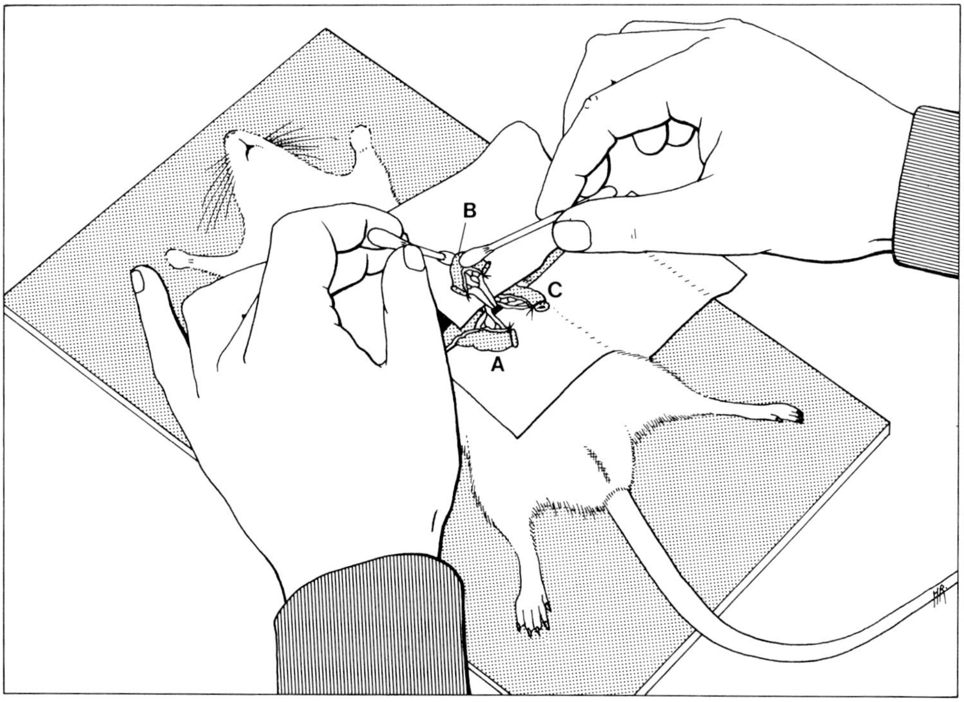

Fig. 15.2.8.

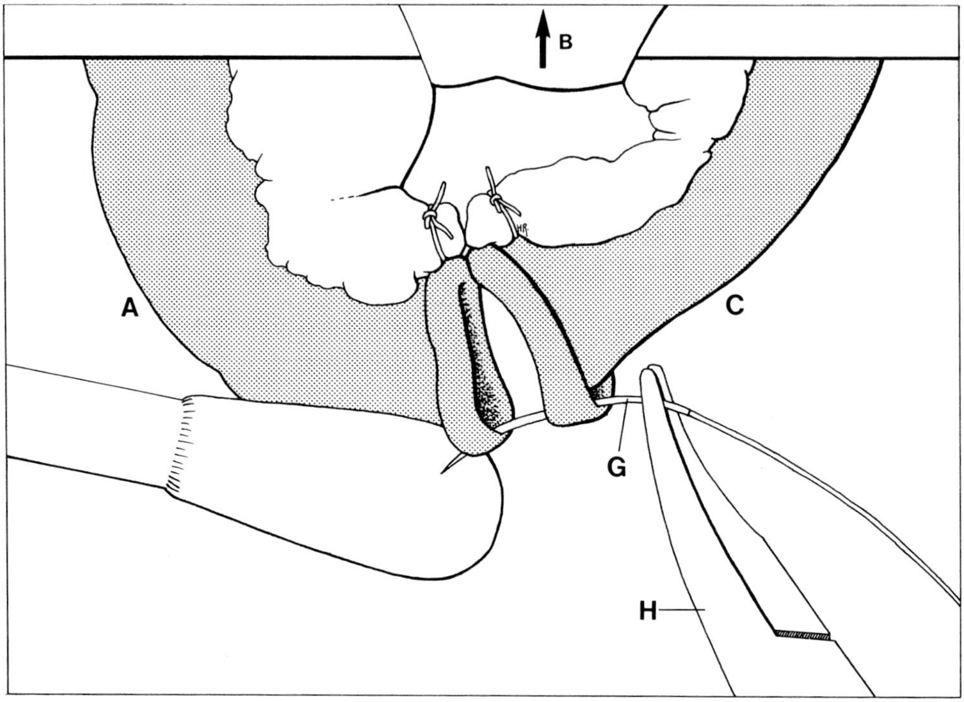

Figure 15.2.9. End-to-end anastomosis of the gut (I).
After approximation of the remaining parts A and C, the first stay suture is placed.
G. Needle of a 7-0 silk suture.
H. Needle holder.

→

Figure 15.2.10. End-to-end anastomosis of the gut (II).
The two corner sutures are placed. The ends of the sutures 1 and 3 are armed with the BV-1 needle. Threads 2 and 4 will be put under some tension in order to expose the anastomosis.
J. Knot in the first corner suture.
K. Knot in the second corner suture.

Figure 15.2.11. End-to-end anastomosis of the gut (III).
Using the armed thread number 1, a continuous suture with transfixing stitches is placed in the anterior wall. After completion of the anterior wall suture thread number 1 is tied to the loose end of the second corner suture (thread number 3).

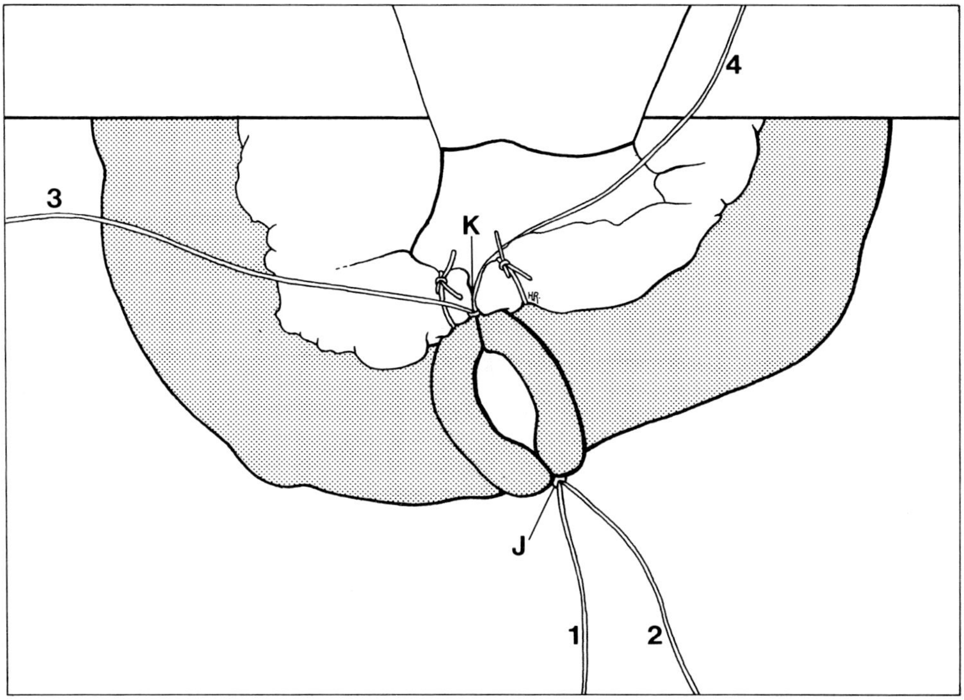

Fig. 15.2.10.

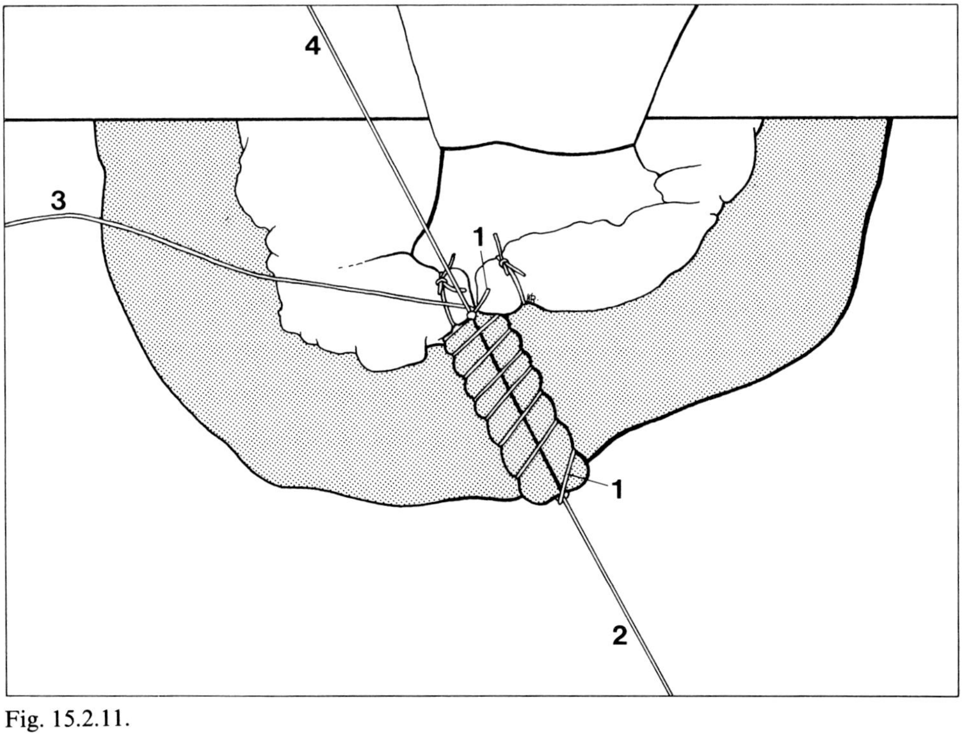

Fig. 15.2.11.

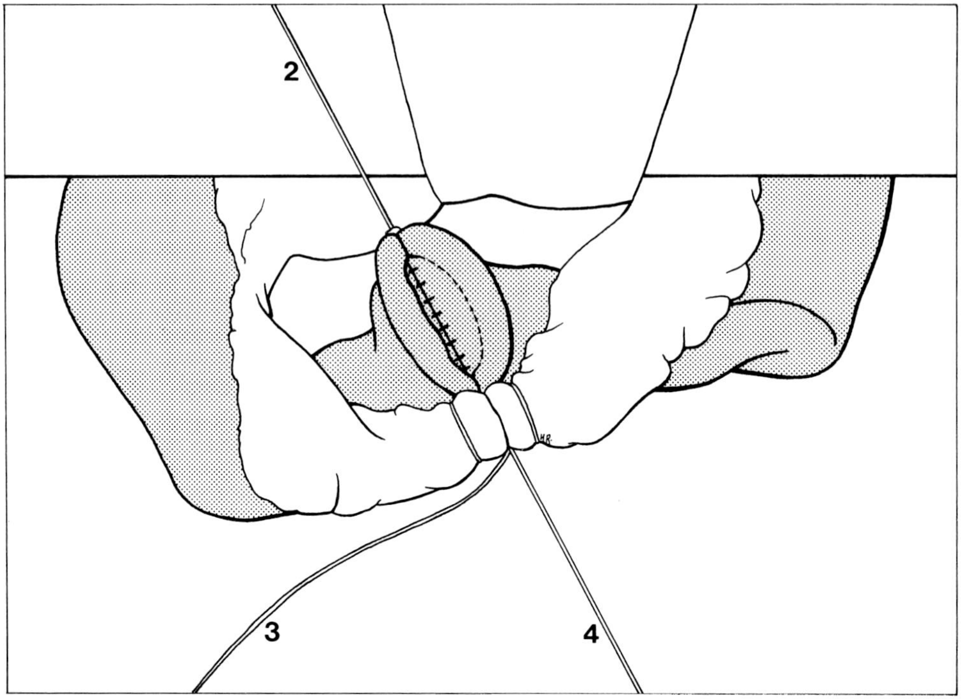

Figure 15.2.12. End-to-end anastomosis of the gut (IV).
Reversal of the anastomosis. The stitches of the former anterior side can be inspected.

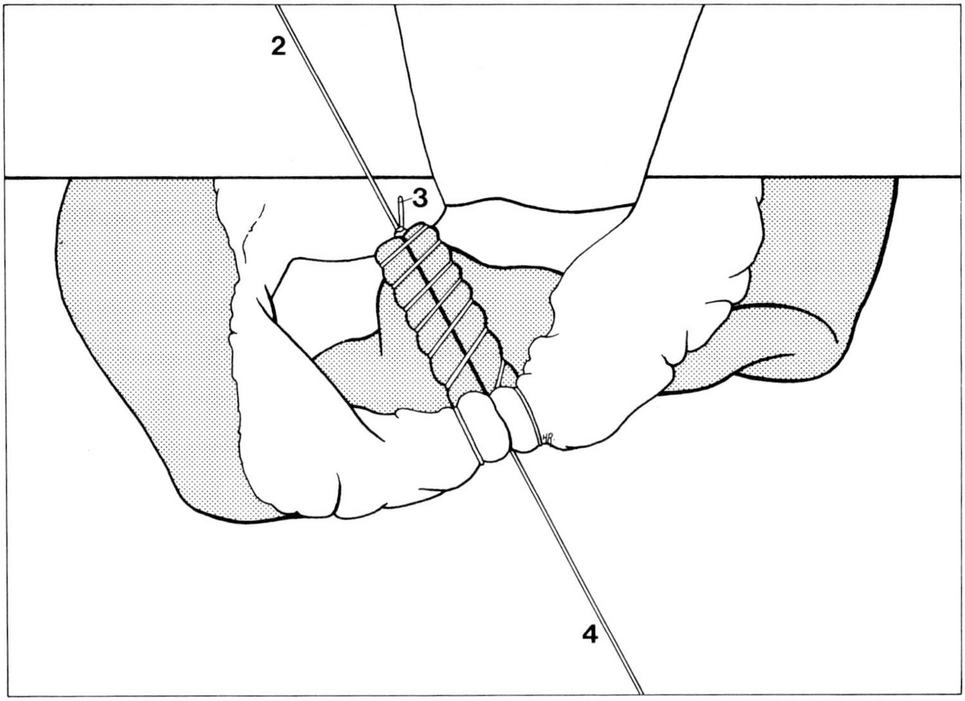

Figure 15.2.13. End-to-end anastomosis of the gut (V).
The armed thread number 3 is used for the posterior wall (now anterior) using the same technique. Finally threads number 2 and 3 are tied together.

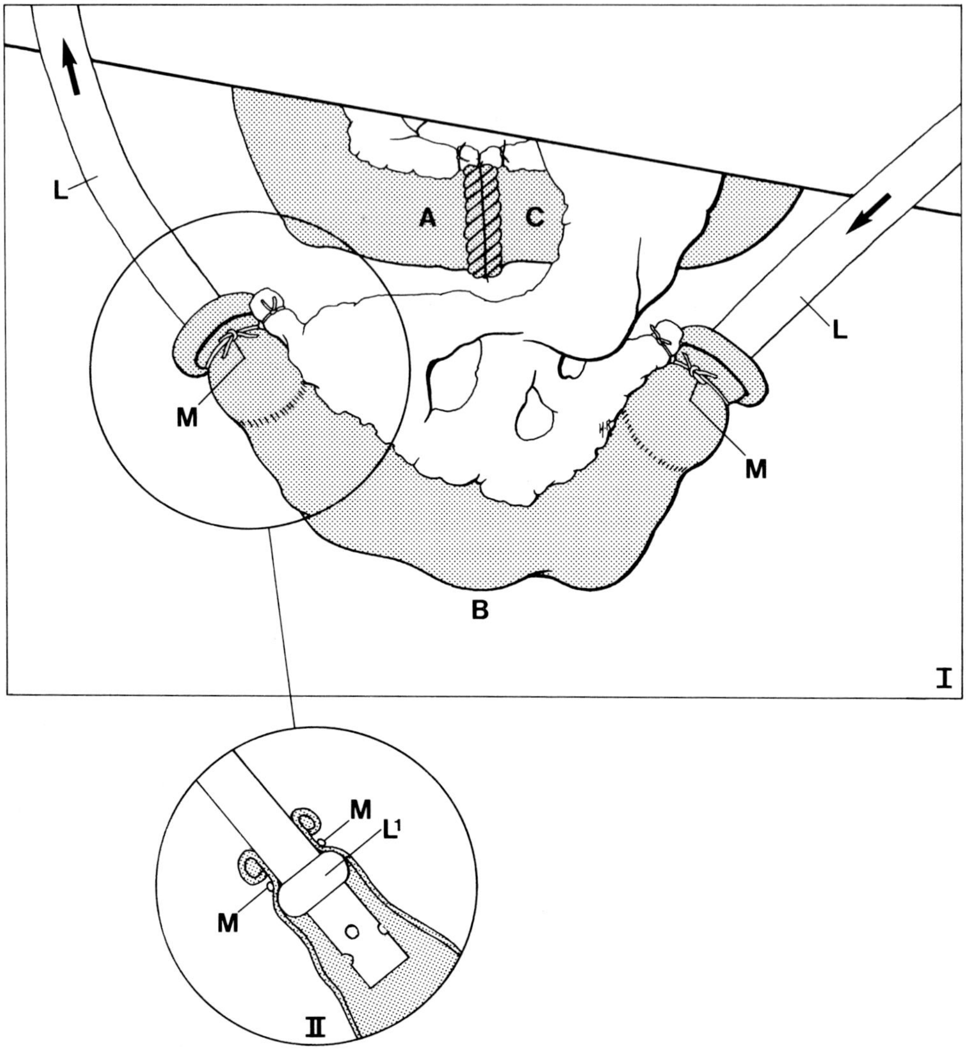

Figure 15.2.14. Cannulation of the gut segment (I).

I. Two cannulae are inserted into the gut segment B, secured behind the silicon ring, and flushed with warm saline solution (arrows).

II. Detail of the tip of the cannula insertion into the gut lumen.

L. Cannula.

L^1. Silicon ring.

M. Ligatures to secure the cannula.

→

Figure 15.2.15. Cannulation of the gut segment (II).

Both cannulae are placed "kink-free" in the abdominal cavity and are secured to the internal abdominal muscle near the xiphoid cartilage (arrow).

B. Gut segment.

L. Cannulae.

xc Xiphoid cartilage.

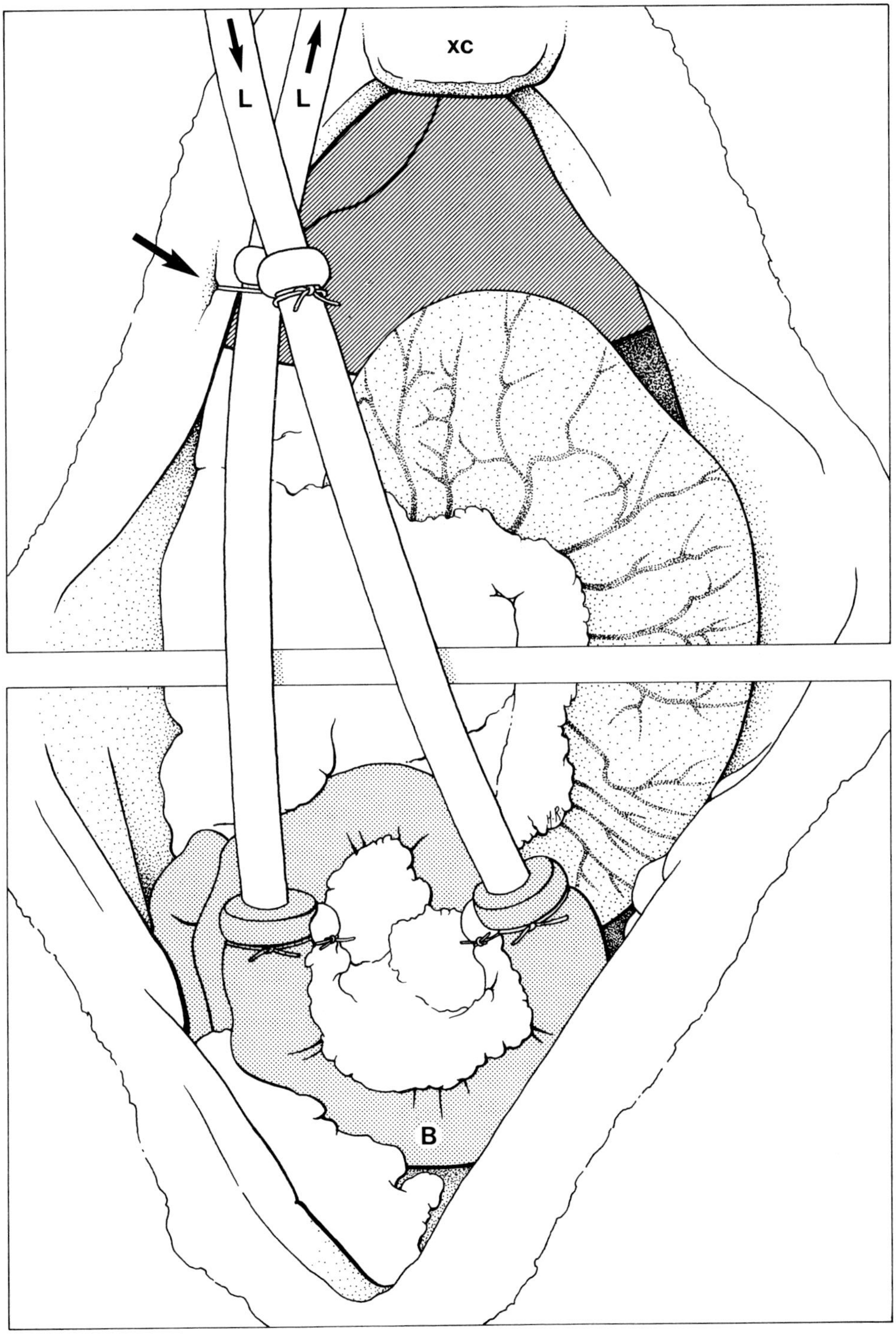
xc
L
L
B

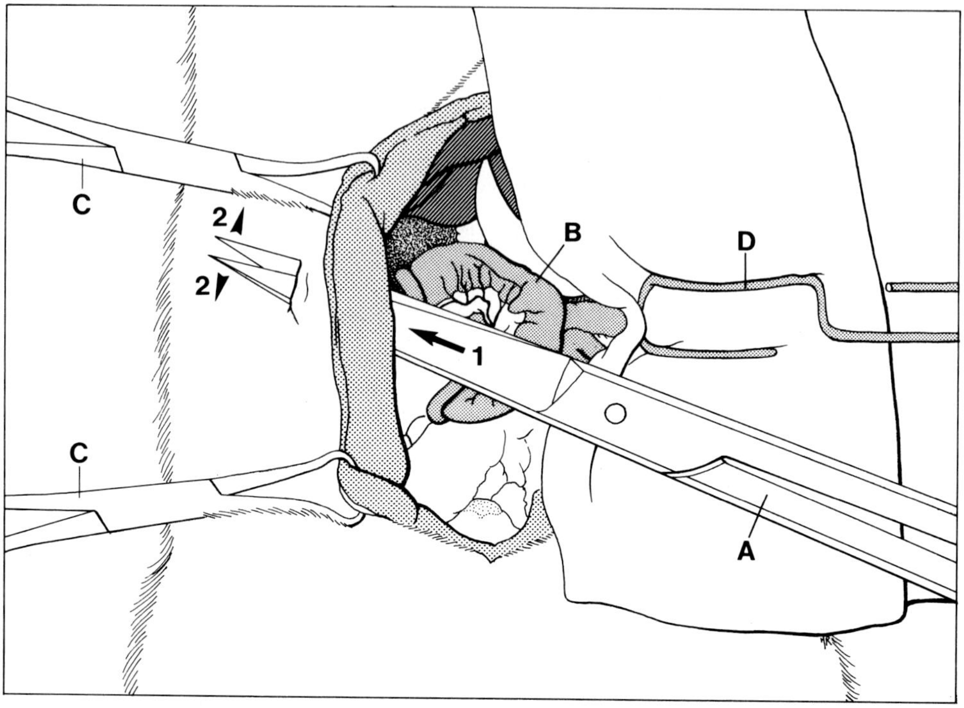

Figure 15.2.16. The fistula (I).
Using a pair of sharp-sharp scissors, a hole is made in the abdominal wall and the skin. After passage through the wall (1) the scissors are spread slightly)2).
A. Pair of scissors.
B. Isolated gut segment.
C. Towel clamps used as retractors.
D. A large paper clip modified to serve as a retractor.

→

Figure 15.2.17. The fistula (II).
The end-to-side anastomosis between the gut and the abdominal wall is started with two corner sutures placed at 180° from each other. Using small bulldog clamps the anastomosis is put under slight tension.
E. Corner suture.
ub Urinary bladder.
li Liver.
rk Right kidney.
s Stomach.

Figure 15.2.18. The fistula (III).
Both anastomoses are completed.
F. End-to-end anastomoses.

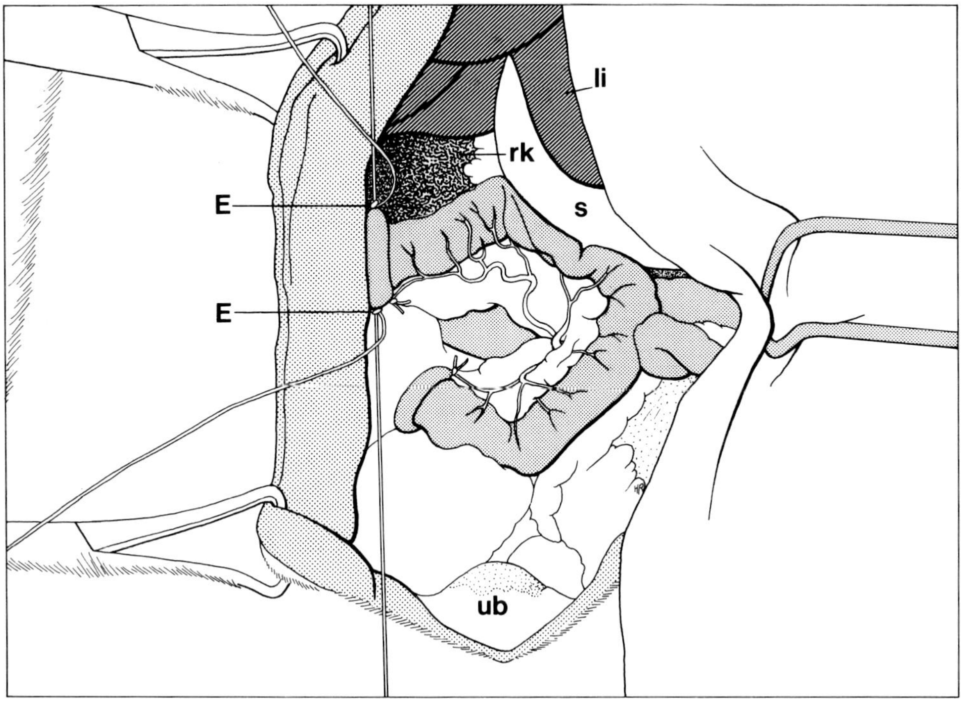

Fig. 15.2.17.

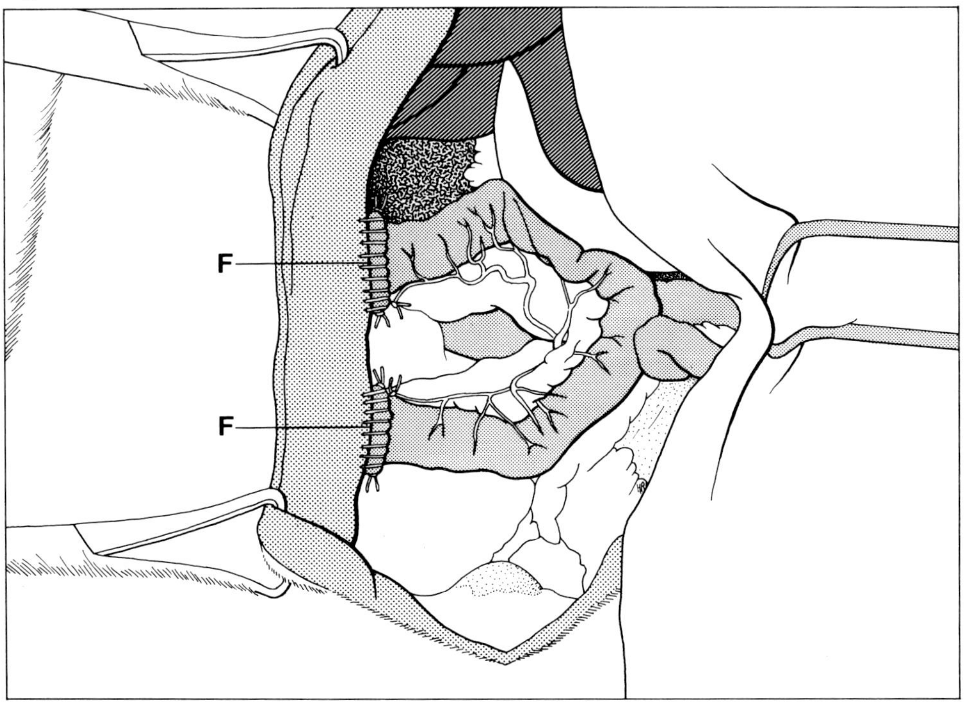

Fig. 15.2.18.

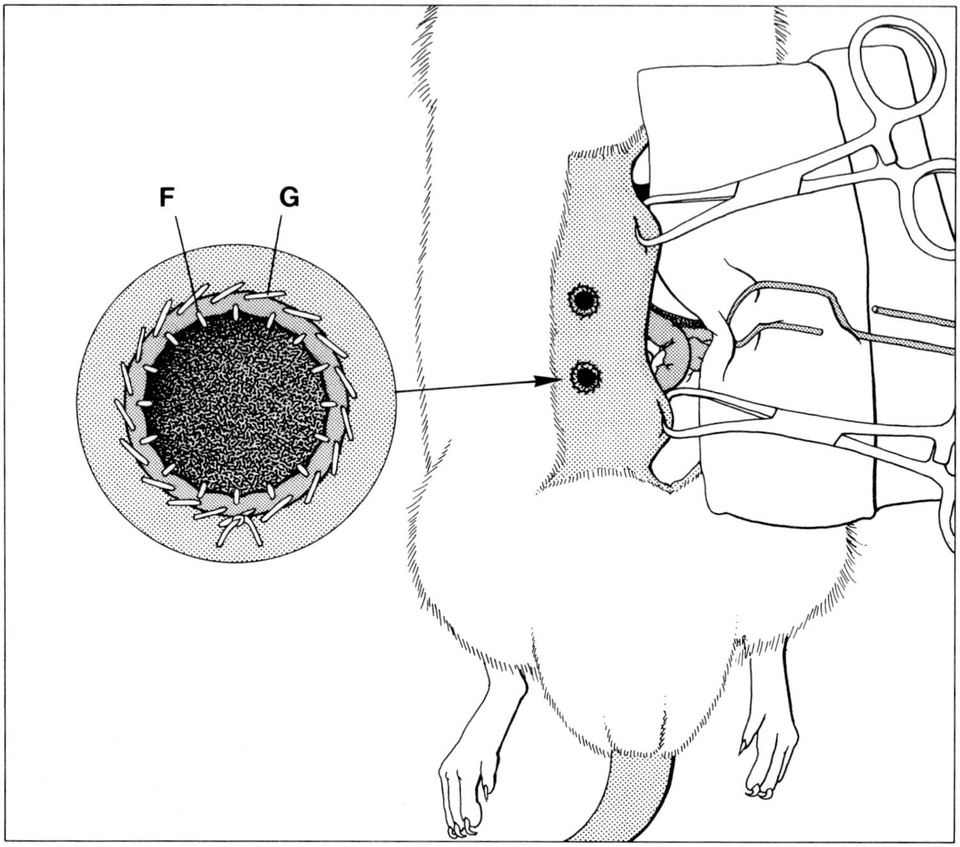

Figure 15.2.19. The fistula (IV).
After turning over the abdominal wall together with the towel clips, the skin is sutured to the external abdominal muscle using a running suture technique.
F. End-to-side anastomosis (the gut against the internal abdominal wall).
G. Running suture (external abdominal wall against the skin).

Manual of Microsurgery on the Laboratory Rat, Part I
Van Dongen, Remie, Rensema and Van Wunnik (eds)
© 1990 Elsevier Science Publishers B.V. (Biomedical Division)

CHAPTER 16

Intra-uterine operations

J.C. VAN DER WAL, J.J. VAN DONGEN, J.W. RENSEMA,
M. EVERSDEN and R. REMIE

16.1. Introduction

Intra-uterine operations are performed on the rat in order to manipulate embryonic or fetal tissues which are useful or sometimes vital for experimental investigations. It may be necessary to collect materials for microscopical study, such as exposing the fetus or embryo to particular experimental circumstances, for example the administration of certain drugs. In such an instance the mother animal will be sacrificed after the removal of the uterus contents or total hysterectomy. Other experiments requiring intra-uterine operations are those where influence of manipulation on the fetus or embryo is to be studied during the prenatal stage of growth. Subsequently, the effects of for example surgery on normal physical development can be studied.

Surgery can vary from resection, for example of an extremity without the necessity of opening the uterus, to an extensive intra-uterine operation like neurotomy. In the former the operation can be adequately performed by carefully squeezing a leg through the wall of the uterus using anatomical forceps.

Another application for an intra-uterine operation is the obtaining of a specific pathogen-free (SPF) colony (see Chapter 2). These SPF animals are obtained by either performing a hysterectomy (total uterus extirpation) or a Caesarian section, both of which are carried out under sterile conditions in pregnant rats at parturition. A hysterectomy should be carried out, and the gravid uterus immersed into an antiseptic fluid (chlorhexidine/cetrimide) kept at body temperature. The uterus passes through a sterile lock into a sterile isolator, after which the fetuses are removed from the uterus and dried with cotton-wool plugs. When spontaneous breathing is initiated, the umbilical cord is rubbed through, as opposed to being cut, so as to avoid bleeding, and the young are placed in an isolator.

In this chapter as an example of an intra-uterine operation a tenotomy operation of extensor tendons of the foreleg will be described (van der Wal and van Dongen, 1986; Zelena, 1963). The aim of this technique is to bring about change in the architecture of the muscle and connective tissue of the extensor tendons by cutting the tendons at the level of the wrist. The underlying hypothesis is that the arrangement of muscle and connective tissue influences the development and spatial arrangement of the mechanoreceptors (van der Wal, 1988; Zelena, 1963 and 1982). This technique allows for the growth of the tenotomized animal to maturity, after which the presence of and the spatial arrangements of the mechanoreceptors will be evaluated in direct comparison with a non-operated animal of the same age.

The surgery is planned for the 18th or 19th day of the pregnancy. It is apparent that the induction of the afferent nerves of these receptors takes place around this time, whilst all distinguishing adult marks of muscle spindles and of Golgi tendon organs are present around the 21st day of pregnancy (Soukop and Zelena, 1977a,b, 1985; van der Wal, 1988; Zelena, 1963, 1982).

The following procedure serves as an example for similar operations which aim to influence experimentally the development of mechanoreceptors. A technique which also could be employed here is an intra-uterine arthrodesis, which is an artificial stiffening of a joint, for example the stiffening of the elbow or the joint between two vertebrae. Another technique is neurotomy, which is the piercing of a nerve, such as the ischiadic nerve of the hindleg (Zelena, 1982). In the case of the described experiment it was apparent that tenotomized tendons of rats which were not fused, affixed again, but this time to the proximal part of the wrist joint. Through this, changes in the muscle and connective tissue architecture of the lateral elbow region of young adult rats will be induced. In other experiments it is sufficient to study the changes postnatally for several days (Soukop and Zelena, 1977a).

16.2. Practical aspects of intra-uterine operations

16.2.1. Breeding and management.
16.2.2. Housing conditions.
16.2.3. Anatomy.
16.2.4. The operation.

16.2.1. Breeding and management

Rats are viviparous and have a very rapid multiplication. Their gestation period lasts for approximately 21 days, and between 6 and 12 young are produced. Depending on the number of test animals required, either a polygamous or monogamous breeding system can be used.

Prior to mating a vaginal swab should be taken in order to determine the stage of the oestrous cycle. In this way the best time can be found for fecundation. Alternatively, a less labour intensive procedure for mating can be followed by placing a male into a cage of females for a period of 24 hours before removing it. The females can then be checked on vaginal plugs for the presence of ejaculated semen. This method has its restrictions because after 24 hours the plug is no longer present and the inspection of vaginal plugs causes stress for the animals. One can assume that every pregnant female is fecundated during the 24 hours of the gathering of the male and females. Therefore every pregnant female can undergo an intra-uterine operation on the 19th day of pregnancy.

16.2.2. Housing conditions

Once the mothers have been operated upon, they must be kept in optimal housing conditions. Experience shows that rats, especially when highly pregnant must not be housed amongst other species. Rats, especially when pregnant, undergo stress when mice are in the vicinity. There are several conditions which are prerequisites in affording the mother animal the opportunity to create its own microclimate. It is vital to maintain the body temperature level, to keep the particular smell of the nest amongst other things, and to avoid dehydration of the young. Unexpected changing of light in the day and night increases aggressiveness. This can be overcome by employing a dimmer switch during the twilight periods. One must also make sure that the light intensity does not rise above 50 lux (F. Schlingmann, personal communication).

Different apparatus and light sources as well as bedding material, heating and ventilation systems which produce ultrasonic sounds, can all have a detrimental effect on the welfare of the mother animal. So as not to alarm the pregnant animal, bedding material should not be cleaned during the 2 days prior to, or the 4 days after the operation. When the cage is cleaned, a part of the old bedding material should be mixed in with the new.

After parturition there is a particular risk of cannibalism towards the young operated animals. This can be reduced by paying proper attention to the afore mentioned detrimental effects of housing circumstances and striving to achieve an optimal climate.

From research with regard to the above mentioned experiment, there appears to be a correlation between the percentage of young tenotomized rats who reach young adulthood and the size of the litter (van der Wal and van Dongen, 1986; van der Wal, 1988). The surviving percentage among operated animals appears to be greater in nests of more than ten animals, than in smaller nests. A possible explanation could be the fact that the young with abnormalities such as scar tissues, deformity of the operated leg, variation of fragrancy or behaviour, escape the mother's attention easier in a large nest. For this reason it is preferable to carry out a maximum of 3 or 4 intra-uterine operations out of ten or more available fetuses.

16.2.3. Anatomy

The placenta of the rat is of an allanto-chorial type, and is not fully established before the end of the second week of pregnancy. Instead a pseudoplacenta is functional some time prior to the completion of the placenta. This implies that transition from the embryonic stage to the fetal stage is marked by the completion of the placental establishment. The form of the placenta is discoidal. The placenta itself is restricted to a particular region of the uterus and consists of both maternal and fetal tissue. In the initial period the vascular system of the mother is completely separate from that of the fetus by a wall of maternal blood vessels, mucosa of the uterus (which consists of epithelial and connective tissues), trophoblast (consisting of ectoderm of the chorionic vesicle), extra-embryonic connective tissue and the wall of the fetal blood vessels (Rowett, 1965). Later on a more specific form will develop along with a substantial degeneration of the above mentioned tissues, but still there will be no integration or direct connection of the bloodstream of the mother animal to the blood of the fetus. There will always be at least one single layer of endothelium of the fetal blood vessels separating the blood circulations. The placenta does ultimately take care of the excretion, nutrition and fetal oxygenation during the prenatal stage.

During the 17th and 21st day of pregnancy the development of the fetus consists mainly of body growth. The formation, development and functional working of the organs is completed after approximately (only) 14 days as is the formation of skin in its primitive stage. An intra-uterine operation to the foreleg of the fetus should only be carried out after the skin is fully grown in order that the fetal skin can be closed. An inadequately closed fetal skin will immediately be recognized by the mother animal which may then lead to cannibalism.

16.2.4. The operation

This operation requires the presence of two microsurgeons sitting opposite each other, preferably using a double binoculair operation microscope. The rat should be placed on a heating mat and its abdomen opened by a midline incision from the pubic bone to the xiphoid cartilage. The gestated uterus should be carefully inspected and exposed (Figure 16.2.1.). Throughout the entire operation the uterus should be covered as far as possible with gauze and regularly moistened with warm saline (35° C). Prior to the incision into the uterus wall, the fetuses, which are recognizable through the wall of the uterus, should be examined in order to select the best placed foreleg with regard to the blood supply of the uterus and the position of the fetus concerned. After defining the operation area the uterus should be covered with gauze and moistened.

Before opening the uterus a purse-string suture should be made involving 6–7 stitches using 7–0 resorbable suture material, in this instance made at the level of the shoulder of the foreleg (Figures 16.2.1. and 16.2.2.). Special care must be paid to the fetus beneath. Subsequently, with the aid of iridectomy scissors an incision should be made within the purse-string suture (Figure 16.2.3.). The incision should be modest yet large enough to permit the foreleg to pass through. Having made the incision in the uterus wall, fetal membranes will bulge through the aperture. Generally, after having divided the amnion membrane (paying special attention to the chorial blood vessels), some amniotic fluid will exude.

Light pressure should be brought upon the elbow of the fetus and to the distal part of the foreleg using two cotton-wool sticks. In this way the leg can be manipulated towards the aperture, through the uterus wall. Subsequently, the cotton-wool stick should be moved to the uterus wall beneath the sole of the foot of the fetus, thereby giving some counter pressure behind the elbow of the fetus (Figure 16.2.4.). Avoid excerting too much pressure especially in the trunk region of the fetus, otherwise you run the risk of the fetus moving. This could result in the foreleg lying in an unfavourable position relative to the aperture in the uterus. Should the foreleg not spontaneously protrude out of the uterus, then, using the least traction possible, squeeze the foreleg out using two cotton-wool sticks until the elbow is exposed outside the uterus cavity. It is sometimes necessary to prevent retraction of the foreleg by pulling on the purse string suture, which is as yet not tied. Having exposed the leg to its shoulder, the foreleg should remain spontaneously outside the incision opening because of the flexion position of the elbow. Therefore traction or fixation of the leg can generally be avoided.

The assistant surgeon should put the wrist of the fetus in flexion with the aid of a cotton-wool stick, whilst supporting the elbow joint with another. In this way the leg is virtually fixated for the incision which is carried out proximal to the wrist at the side of the extensor tendons (Figures 16.2.5. and 16.2.6.). Using appropriate magnification, small subcutaneous blood vessels can be observed, so as to avoid any damage to them. Sometimes haemostasis is however necessary, and is best carried out using a cotton-wool stick.

Using jewellers forceps, the extensor tendons can be held and lifted outside the incised skin one at the time (Figures 16.2.7. and 16.2.8.). The proximal part of the tendon is cut (Figure 16.2.7.), using small iridectomy scissors, causing this tendon to retract in a proximal direction. The remaining part of the tendon should be firmly held between the tips of the forceps, and cut as far as possible distally to the forceps (Figure 16.2.8.). Hereby excision of a certain length of the tendon can be achieved, preventing the reunion of both tendon stumps. Using this method other tendons can then be excised.

Closure of the fetal skin should be made by using histoacrylate glue. Experience has shown that for skin closure there are definite benefits to be reaped from the use of histoacrylate compared with fine suture material, not only during, but also after the operation. In the first place the removal of sutures should be carried out under anaesthesia, and secondly rejection by the mother diminishes when histoacrylate is applied. To apply the histoacrylate, the leg should be dried and the wound edges lined up. Only one drop of histoacrylate is required. During the drying period, repeated checks must be made to ensure that the leg does not get attached to the uterus wall. The leg can then be pushed back into the uterus, using two moistened cotton-wool sticks, and the fetus is then repositioned. The uterus should then be closed by tightening the purse string suture. The area which was operated upon should be covered with gauze and moistened with warm saline as mentioned before to avoid dehydration.

This procedure can be repeated three or four times depending on the number of fetuses present. Subsequently, the uterus should be carefully repositioned within the abdominal cavity and the abdomen closed.

References

Rowett, H.G.Q. (1965) The rat as a small mammal. John Murray, Fifty Albemarle street, London.

Soukop, T. and Zelena, J. (1977a) The number and size of Golgi tendon organs in rats during postnatal development. Pholia Morphol. 25: 79–82.

Soukop, T. and Zelena, J. (1977b) The development of Golgi tendon organs. J. Neurocyt. 6: 171–194.

Soukop, T. and Zelena, J. (1985) Structure of tendon organs of the rat after neonatal de-efferentation. Cell Tissue Res. 241: 229–236.

Wal, J.C. van der and Dongen J.J. van (1986) Intrauterine tenotomy in the rat. A model for studying spatial organization of the morphological substrate of propriocepcis. Proc. 27th Dutch Federation Meeting, April: 342(W12).

Wal, J.C. van der (1988) The organization of the substrate of proprioception in the elbow region of the rat. Thesis, University of Limburg, Maastricht, The Netherlands.

Zelena, J. (1963) Development of muscle receptors after tenotomy. Physiol. Bohemoslov. 12: 30–36.

Zelena, J. (1982) Survival of Pacinian corpuscles after denervation in adult rats. Cell Tissue Res. 224: 673–683.

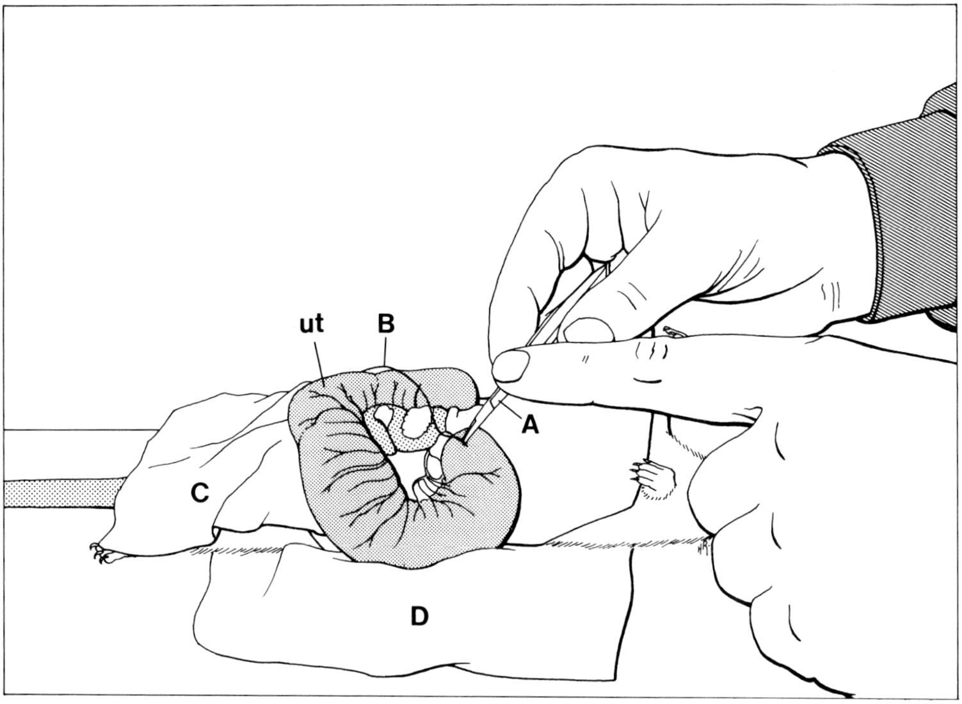

Figure 16.2.1. Placing the purse-string suture (I).
Both uterus horns are exposed, laid on moistened gauzes and a purse-string suture is placed in the wall using a micro needle holder. The index finger of the left hand serves as a support during suturing. For reasons of clarity the uterus is not covered with the moistened gauzes.

A. Needle holder.

B. A 7-0 resorbable suture.

C and D. Moistened gauzes.

ut Uterus.

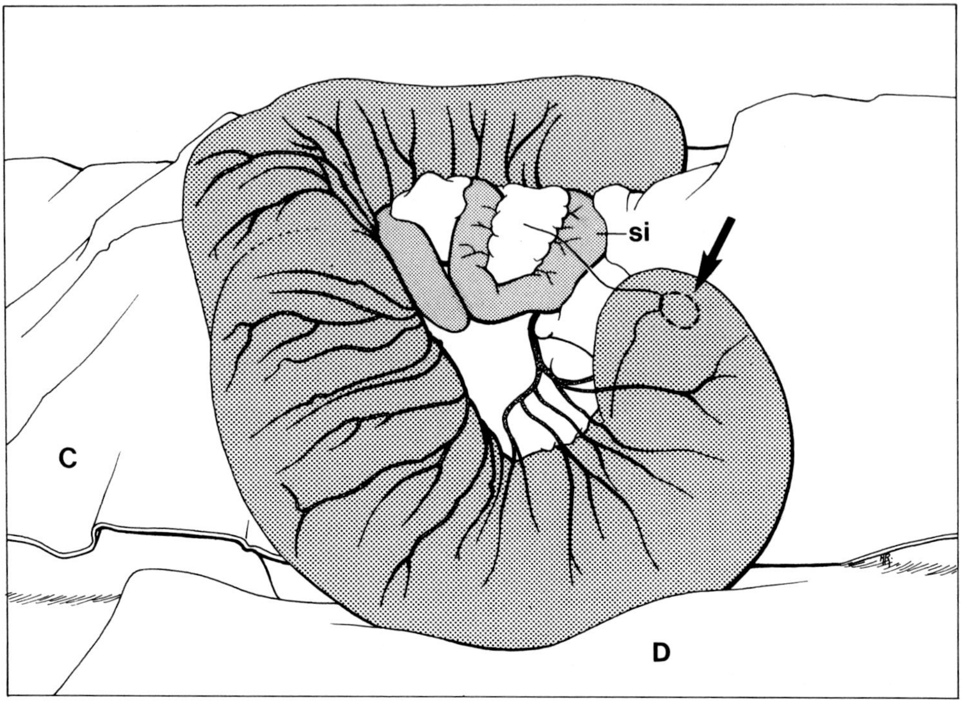

Figure 16.2.2. Placing the purse-string suture (II).
The purse-string suture has been placed in the wall of the uterus (arrow).
C and D. Moistened gauzes.
si Small intestine.

→

Figure 16.2.3. Cutting the wall.
Using jewellers forceps and iridectomy scissors, an aperture is cut inside the suture exposing the fetal membranes. These membranes are cut in exactly the same way.
E. Purse-string suture.
F. Fetal membranes.
G. Straight jewellers forceps.
H. Iridectomy scissors.

Figure 16.2.4. Exteriorization of the fetal foreleg.
The left foreleg of the fetus is exteriorized using two cotton-wool sticks applying slight pressure in the directions indicated by the arrows.

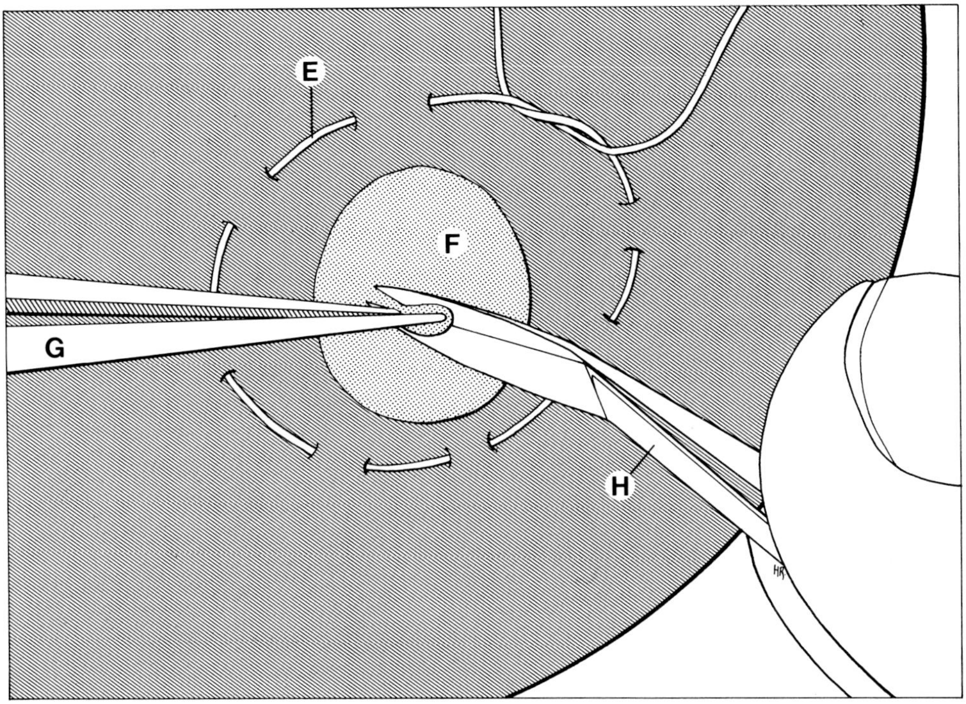

Fig. 16.2.3.

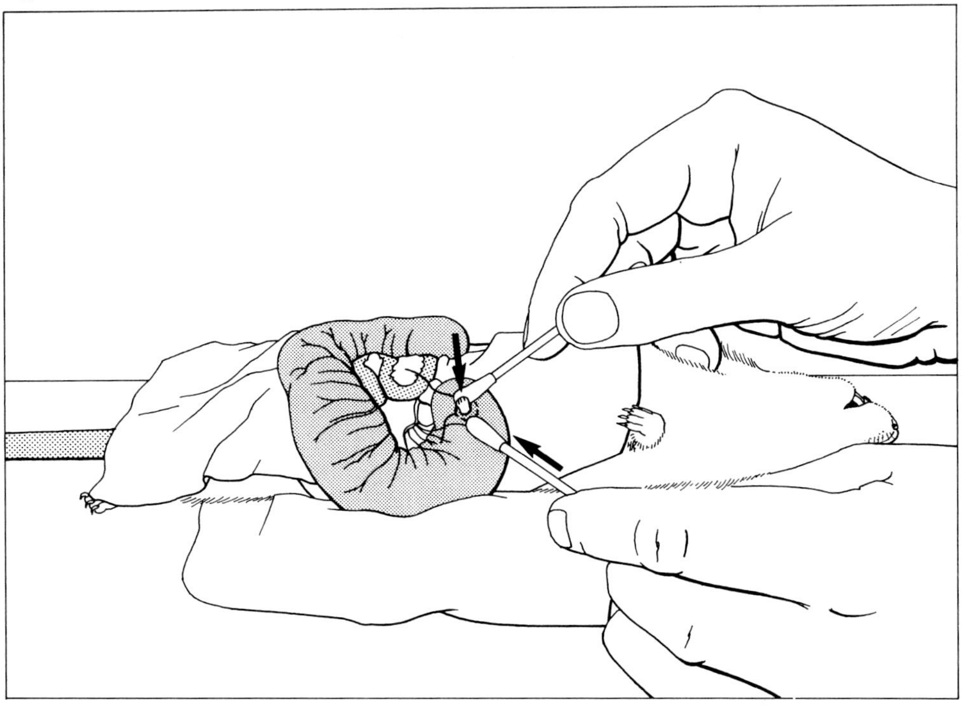

Fig. 16.2.4.

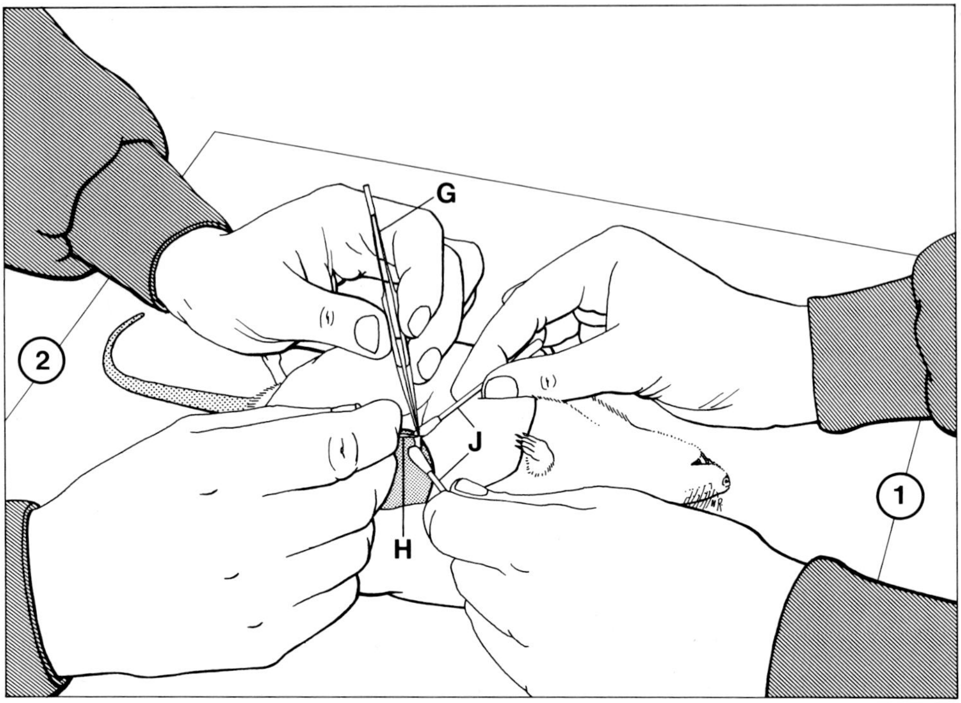

Figure 16.2.5. Incision in the fetal foreleg (I).
A small incision is made in the extensor side of the wrist by surgeon 2, using straight jewellers forceps and iridectomy scissors. Surgeon 1 keeps the wrist of the fetus in flexion with two cotton-wool sticks.

G. Straight jewellers forceps.
H. Iridectomy scissors.
J. Cotton wool sticks.

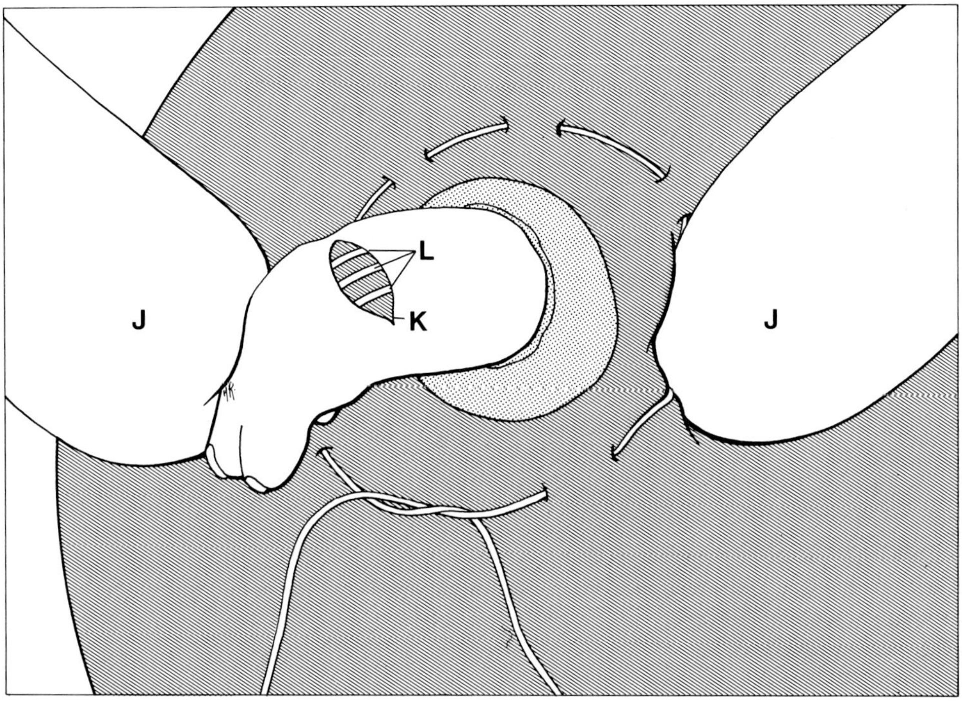

Figure 16.2.6. Incision in the fetal foreleg (II).
The skin incision at the extensor side of the wrist has been made.
J. Cotton-wool sticks of surgeon 2.
K. Incision.
L. Tendons of the extensor muscles.

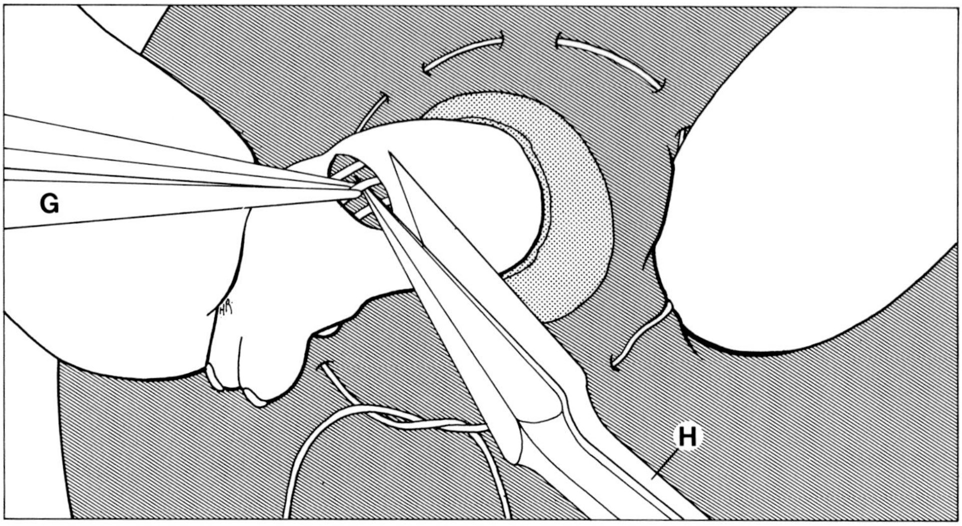

Figure 16.2.7. Cutting the tendon (I).
The proximal side of the tendon is cut using straight jewellers forceps and iridectomy scissors.
G. Straight jewellers forceps.
H. Iridectomy scissors.

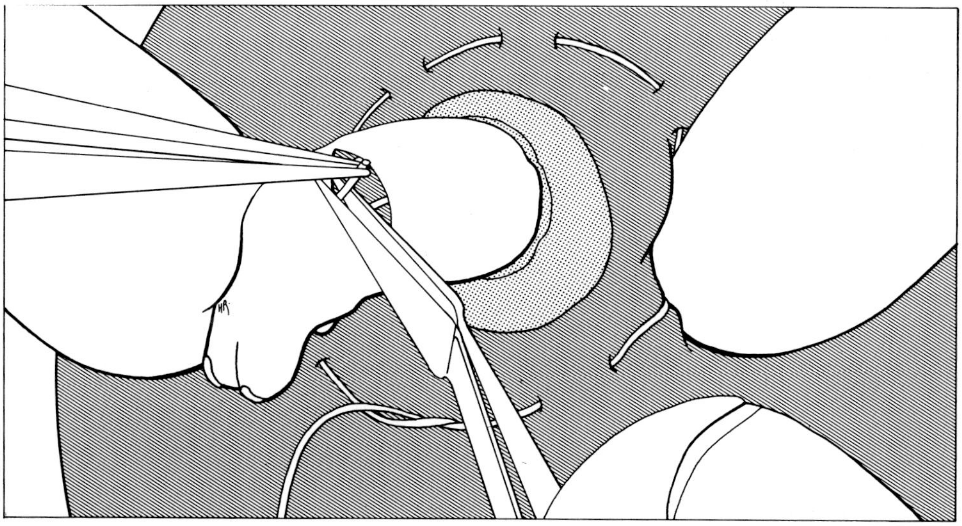

Figure 16.2.8. Cutting the tendon (II).
The cut end of the tendon is slightly reversed and cut distally, removing as much tendon as possible.

Manual of Microsurgery on the Laboratory Rat, Part I
Van Dongen, Remie, Rensema and Van Wunnik (eds)
© 1990 Elsevier Science Publishers B.V. (Biomedical Division)

Miscellaneous

1. Selected normative data

Respiration rate (breaths/min)		70–150
Heart rate (beats/min)		300–500
Body temperature (° C)		37.5–38.0
Body weight at birth (g)		4.5–6
Body weight at weaning (g)		50
Body weight of adult male rats, 3–6 months (g)		300–400
Body weight of adult male rats, 2–4 years (g)		400–600
Body weight of adult female rats, 3–6 months (g)		250–300
Body weight of adult female rats, 2–4 years (g)		300–500
Chromosome number (diploid)		42
Life span under conventional conditions (years)		2
Life span under laboratory conditions (years)		2–4
Gestation period (days)		21–23
Postpartum gestation period (days)		24–28
Age at weaning (days)		21
Age at puberty (weeks)		6–8
Age at mating (months)		3–4
Duration of the partus (hours)		1–3
No. of pups/litter (depending on the strain)		4–12
Length of pseudopregnancy (days)		10–12
Polyoestrus: Stage I.	dioestrus (h)	6
Stage II.	pro oestrus, early (h)	55–60
Stage III.	pro oestrus, late (h)	12
Stage IV.	oestrus (h)	12–20
Stage V.	metoestrus (h)	8

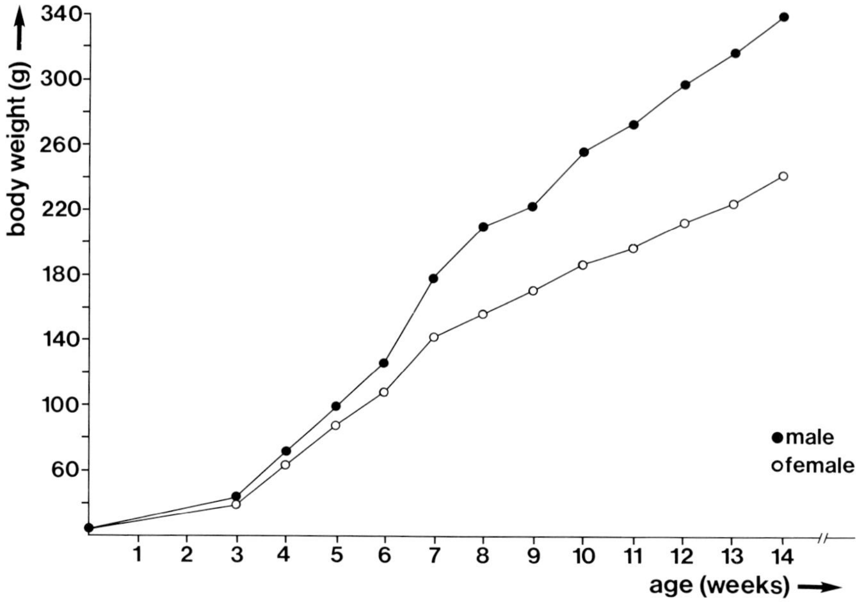

Figure I. The growth curves for a male and a female rat.

Cardiac output (ml/min)	15–80
Systolic blood pressure (mm Hg)	90–180
Diastolic blood pressure (mm Hg)	60–150
Daily food intake (g/100 g B.W.)	5
Daily water intake (ml/100 g B.W.)	10
Defaecation (g/24 h)	9–13
Urine production (ml/24 h)	10–15
Bile production (ml/h)	1–1.5
Pancreatic juice production (ml/h)	0.5–1

2. Housing conditions

Temperature, stock unit (° C)	20–24
Temperature, at recovery (° C)	28
Relative humidity (%)	60–70
Ventilation (changes/h)	15–40
Light (h/day)	12–14
Floor area solitary rat (cm^2)	350
Floor area rat with litter (cm^2)	800
Floor area in group (cm^2)	250/rat
Minimum height of cage (cm)	14

3. Blood values

Blood volume (ml/100 g B.W.)	5.5–6.5
Plasma volume (ml/100 g B.W.)	3.5–4.5
Erythrocyte sedimentation rate in male (mm/hr)	1.6
Erythrocyte sedimentation rate in female (mm/hr)	0.7
Red blood cells (no/ml blood)	$7.3–9.5 \times 10^9$
White blood cells (no/ml blood)	1.4×10^7
Neutrophils (no/1.4×10^7 wbc/ml blood)	3.5×10^6
Lymphocytes (no/1.4×10^7 wbc/ml blood)	1×10^7
Eosiniphils (no/1.4×10^7 wbc/ml blood)	1.5×10^5
Basophils (no/1.4×10^7 wbc/ml blood)	6.5×10^4
Platelets (no/ml blood)	5.3×10^8
pCO_2 (mm Hg)	33–41
pO_2 (mm Hg)	91–94
pH (whole blood)	7.40–7.44
Coagulation time (min)	2.5
Packed cell volume	46–50
Haemoglobin (g/100 ml)	15.7

Index